MEDICAL
PROFESSIONALS
and the
ORGANIZATION
of KNOWLEDGE

MEDICAL PROFESSIONALS
and the
ORGANIZATION
of KNOWLEDGE

Eliot Freidson
Judith Lorber
editors

ALDINETRANSACTION
A Division of Transaction Publishers
New Brunswick (U.S.A.) and London (U.K.)

Second paperback printing 2009

Copyright © 1972 by Transaction Publishers, New Brunswick, NJ

All rights reserved under International and Pan-American Copyright Conventions. No part of this book may be reproduced or transmitted in any form or by any means, electronic or mechanical, including photocopy, recording, or any information storage and retrieval system, without prior permission in writing from the publisher. All inquiries should be addressed to AldineTransaction, A Division of Transaction Publishers, Rutgers—The State University, 35 Berrue Circle, Piscataway, New Jersey 08854-8042. www.transactionpub.com

This book is printed on acid-free paper that meets the American National Standard for Permanence of Paper for Printed Library Materials.

Library of Congress Catalog Number: 2008005498
ISBN: 978-0-202-36208-3
Printed in the United States of America

Library of Congress Cataloging-in-Publication Data

Medical professionals and the organization of knowledge / [edited by] Eliot
    Freidson and Judith Lorber.
        p. cm.
    Originally published: Chicago : Aldine-Atherton, 1972 under the title:
    Medical men and their work.
    Includes bibliographical references and index.
    ISBN 978-0-202-36208-3 (alk. paper)
    1. Social medicine. I. Freidson, Rliot, 1923-2005. II. Lorber, Judith.
III. Freidson, Eliot, 1923-2005. Medical men and their work.
    [DNLM: 1. Professional Practice—Collected Works. 2. Attitude of
Health Personnel—Collected Works. 3. Health Knowledge, Attitudes, Prac-
tice—Collected Works. 4. Professional Role—Collected Works. 5. Sick
Role—Collected Works. W 21 M4893 2008]

RA418.F73   2008
362.1—dc22   2008005498

For Our Parents—

Grace,
Sophie,
and
Henry

Foreword

This collection of papers is intended to convey, in as systematic a fashion as possible, an approach to the field of medical sociology which stresses the way in which men shape and organize the knowledge, perception, and experience of illness, and much of the substance of illness behavior, its management and treatment. While man is a biological organism, he responds to himself and others in terms of the social meanings he assigns to his experience with the physical and biological world. It is now well established in such medical fields as psychosomatic medicine and psychopharmacology that the unique symbolic equipment of the human animal is intimately connected with the functioning of the body. This being so, it stands to reason that proper understanding of specifically human rather than generally "animal" illness requires careful and systematic study of the social meanings surrounding illness.

The content of the social meanings surrounding ascribed physical states (and indeed what *is* to be considered a physical state) varies from culture to culture, and from one historical period to another. At least as important as the content of those social meanings, however, is the organization of those groups of men who serve as their carriers and, sometimes, creators. In the case of illness, a critical difference exists between those considered to be competent to diagnose and treat the sick and those excluded from this special privilege—a separation as old and as ubiquitous as the shaman or medicine-man. This difference becomes solidified when the expert healer becomes a member of an organized, full-time occupation, sustained in a monopoly over the work of diagnosis and treatment by the force of the state, and invested with the authority to make *official* designation of the social meanings to be ascribed to physical states. When this stage of social organization occurs, only the expert healers are permitted to say what is and what is not legitimate illness, and who is and who is not legitimately ill.

The medical profession is today in that position in the United States and in other advanced nations. Its organization and its knowledge set many of the conditions for being recognizably and legitimately ill, and it controls many of the circumstances of treatment. It thus plays a central role in shaping the experience of being ill. It is with this fact of modern life in mind that we emphasize in this collection papers on the character of experts or professionals in general, and of medicine as a profession in particular. Similarly, we sample the literature on other occupations working with medicine in shaping the experience of being ill. Only after presenting materials that lay out the occupational and institutional boundaries set by health workers and their institutions do we present papers exploring the social identity of the sick person who, in interaction with health workers, also participates in the creation of the experience of being ill. This interactional process surrounding the invocation and negotiation of the social meanings of illness is, it must be remembered, precisely the process that makes illness among humans a phenomenon different from that to be found among other animals. It is the process about which medical science has virtually no systematic knowledge and about which it is the task of sociology to learn.

In sum, by our selection of papers we have tried to emphasize the role of medicine as a profession, and of other health occupations and health institutions in creating and maintaining some of the more powerful social meanings and consequences of illness. We have, furthermore, emphasized that health or health care is a form of work organized into special institutionalized practices. Given the limited space available to us, we have had to leave out a whole universe of literature devoted to specific administrative details of the various modes of financing and organizing health care. Such literature, which is growing rapidly at present because of the concern with developing a better and more equitable system of national medical care, is certainly useful and important. We are convinced, however, that attention to generic sociological analyses of healing as a form of work, of health workers in interaction with patients, and of the social meanings of health and illness, the well and the sick, the healer, the healed and the unhealed, are likely to be more useful in the long run for the solution of practical problems of medical care than a preoccupation with comparatively mechanical administrative and financial issues. We believe that the papers in this volume can suggest the source of organization of the behavior of the people involved in the health care system, and so some of the strategies required for improving the operation of that system.

Contents

II. MEDICAL WORK

I

Medical Men

Medical Men as Professionals

It is regarded as self-evident that medicine is a profession, but the nature of professions is by no means self-evident. While there is some rough agreement among sociologists that a profession is a distinct form of occupation characterized by both a comparatively long period of training in some abstract subject matter and commitment to the service of humanity, these criteria are extremely difficult to establish empirically and precisely in such a way as to discriminate an occupation called a profession from other kinds of occupations. Because of the vagueness of the concept, we are not provided with an adequate guide for discriminating what is distinctively professional about the occupation of medicine. It seems possible to gain more insight by making systematic comparisons between medicine and other professions and would-be professions. It is by this comparative, contrastive method that medicine is examined in this section.

Rueschemeyer provides us with an excellent statement of the "functionalist" theory of professions, which stresses, first, systematic theory, and second, the application of such theories to the problems surrounding the central values of society. The "functionalist" theory emphasizes the need for control of the behavior of the professional, control based fundamentally on the individual himself; "grounded in a long socialization process" and supplemented by colleague control. Society protects the profession against interference from other people such as clients and employers.

However, as Rueschemeyer points out, the concept of profession is based largely on the model of medicine. Law, which is considered by most analysts to be a profession, has characteristics quite different from medicine. Law differs from medicine in the nature of its technical competence and in the social values toward which its work is oriented. Rueschemeyer shows in detail how these differences make problematic the conception that the professional possesses special knowledge which the layman does not. The "gap in competence" between layman and professional does not hold

1

firmly in the case of law. On the basis of his analysis, he suggests modifying the usual model of profession so as to deemphasize scientific knowledge and rationality and readiness to change and to emphasize instead more "normative and evaluative elements in the knowledge base of all professions." He emphasizes the divergent and possibly conflicting value orientations to be found within a profession and in its relationship to society, and in the course of doing so he deemphasizes the gap in competence between practitioner and client. He also deemphasizes the significance of the profession's own conception that it is concerned with sustaining and advancing the central values of society (or, as Parsonian sociologists would put it, collectivity-orientation). More than special knowledge and ethics, the position of the profession in a system of social stratification is emphasized. By comparing medicine with law, then, Rueschemeyer refines the usual concept of profession and suggests that insofar as medicine is a member of that general class, its special knowledge and ethicality should be emphasized less than is common.

Consonant with Rueschemeyer's analysis, we may note that an essential element in successful professionalization involves the capacity on the part of an occupation to attain a position of some autonomy, a position which is usually sustained by some special form of occupational organization. Occupational organization is often intimately related to the state and its political support, for it is the state which grants both legal recognition and protection of the profession's status. The critical roles of the state and of such substantive characteristics of the occupation as its work and its prestige in the public mind become quite clear in Joseph Ben-David's article on unions in Israel, where he analyzes the conditions surrounding the maintenance of professional autonomy. Ben-David shows how, even in the face of extensive power on the part of both the state and an unusually powerful quasi-public labor organization, the traditional professions succeed in maintaining a considerable amount of autonomy while other occupations which call themselves professions nonetheless go through a process of "deprofessionalization." Indeed, Ben-David's paper implies that no matter what the aspirations of an occupation, the characteristics of its work within a given historical setting seem to limit the possibilities for professionalization.

The question of professionalization is pursued further in an entirely different context by Charles Leslie. Following a summary discussion of a classic work on the professions in England, Leslie sketches the relation of an ancient tradition of medicine in India to Western medicine. This tradition has led to the spurious, or at least thus far unsuccessful, professionalization of the traditional Indian practitioners. Critical to the problem of developing a secure profession out of traditional medicine seems to be the nature of the technical knowledge available to it in comparison to other occupations, the prestige (even if not the sentiment) attached to the Western rather than Indian tradition, and the lack of a self-sustaining, formal organization which joins practitioners together in such a way as to be able to assure the public of basic standards and essential processes of self-regulation.

In the next paper, Denzin deals with a fairly old occupation by Western standards and, using the notion of incomplete professionalization, describes the circumstances surrounding the failure of pharmacy to achieve a position of professional autonomy in the medical division of labor of the contemporary United States.

The usual conception of professions is that they are self-regulating occupational groups, "free" to define the nature of their work and to work as they see fit. Patently, however, the state is sovereign, and this "freedom" rests upon the mandate and license provided by the state to the profession. In the United States the medical profession is inclined to feel that the state should provide it with protection from the incursion of other occupations, and should help it drive other competitors considered "quacks" out of business. Beyond this, the state should leave the practitioner free to do what he will. The official spokesmen for the medical profession in the United States have long prophesied that when the state "socializes" medicine, a "third party" will come between the professional and his client and that the quality of service will suffer. However, what evidence there is seems to indicate that even when medicine is socialized, it remains quite free in a number of areas of its work and seems to continue as a "free profession" with working autonomy which is markedly different from that of other kinds of occupations.

Stimulated by the initiation of Medicare, the Health Insurance for the Aged Act of 1965, William Glaser attempts in his paper to evaluate how state schemes for paying the costs of medical care and organizing medical care have influenced the autonomy of the profession. At the same time, on the basis of the experience of other countries, he attempts to predict what some of the future problems of Medicare will be in the United States. His conclusion is that by virtue both of the special technical knowledge of medicine itself, and of the power of physicians as a political interest group, the socialization of payment for medical care will not lead to any significant diminution in the autonomy of the profession. Indeed, it seems that a true profession may be characterized more accurately and precisely by its autonomy than by anything else.

BIBLIOGRAPHIC SUGGESTIONS

The reader wishing to explore the problem of conceptualizing professions in general and the profession of medicine in particular would do well to begin by examining the historically outdated but nonetheless conceptually useful analysis of professions in England to be found in E. M. Carr-Saunders and P. A. Wilson, *The Professions* (Oxford; Oxford University Press, 1933). A general work which is rich in ideas about professions is Everett C. Hughes, *Men and Their Work* (New York: The Free Press, 1958). A recent study of the frequently neglected problem of the relations between professions and the state is Corinne Lathrop Gilb, *Hidden Hierarchies: The Professions and Government* (New York: Harper & Row, 1966). And finally, for a collection of many important articles on professions, there is Howard M. Vollmer and Donald L. Mills, eds., *Professionalization* (Englewood Cliffs, N.J.: Prentice-Hall, 1966).

Turning to medicine in particular, the classic sociological analysis is Talcott Parsons, *The Social System* (New York: The Free Press, 1951), Chapter 10. A recent full-length sociological analysis is Eliot Freidson, *Profession of Medicine: A Study of the Sociology of Applied Knowledge* (New York: Dodd, Mead, 1970), and, focusing particularly on medical care, Eliot Freidson, *Professional Dominance: The Social Structure of Medical Care* (New York: Atherton Press, 1970). A somewhat dated but still important legal and political analysis of the American Medical Association is David R. Hyde, et al., "The American Medical Association: Power, Purpose and Politics in Organized Medicine," *Yale Law Journal, 63* (May, 1954), 938-1022. A recent analysis of organized medicine's economic policies, with fairly up-to-date references, is Elton Rayack, *Professional Power and American Medicine: The Economics of the American Medical Association* (Cleveland: World Publishing, 1967). For another economic analysis, see Seymour E. Harris, *The Economics of American Medicine* (New York: Macmillan, 1964). And for a cross-national comparative analysis of the influence of methods of paying the physician, see William A. Glaser, *Paying the Doctor: Systems of Remuneration and Their Effects* (Baltimore: The Johns Hopkins Press, 1970).

1

DIETRICH RUESCHEMEYER

Doctors and Lawyers: A Comment on the Theory of the Professions

I

The current, predominantly functionalist, theory of the professions stresses two characteristics as strategic for the explanation of their position and functioning in society.[1] The professions are conceived of as service occupations that (1) apply a systematic body of knowledge to problems which (2) are highly relevant to central values of the society. Their high degree of learned competence creates special problems of social control: laymen cannot judge the professional performance; in many cases they cannot even set the concrete goals for the professional's work. This means that the two most common forms of social control of work in industrial societies, bureaucratic supervision by virtue of a formal position and judgment by the customer, are of only limited applicability. The need for social control is, on the other hand, especially urgent because of the values and interests that are at stake.

Reprinted from *The Canadian Review of Sociology and Anthropology* 1 (1964), 17-30, by permission of the author and the publisher.

1. The most complete development of this theory will be found in William J. Goode, Robert K. Merton and Mary Jean Huntington, *The Professions in American Society*, unpublished manuscript. Several articles by Goode treat various aspects of the theory: "Community within a Community: The Professions," *American Sociological Review*, 22 (April, 1957), 194-200; "Encroachment, Charlatanism, and the Emergent Profession: Psychology, Medicine, and Sociology," *American Sociological Review*, 25 (December, 1960), 902-914; "The Librarian: From Occupation to Profession?" P. E. Ennis and H. W. Winger, eds., *Seven Questions about the Profession of Librarianship* (Chicago, 1962), pp. 8-22. Cf. also Robert K. Merton, George G. Reader, and Patricia L. Kendall, eds., *The Student-Physician: Introductory Studies in the Sociology of Medical Education* (Cambridge, Mass., 1957). This approach is in many ways an outgrowth of older analyses such as those of A. M. Carr-Saunders and P. A. Wilson, E. C. Hughes, T. Parsons, and T. H. Marshall.

The following presentation of the theoretical model differs slightly from the one given by its authors in treating the "service" or "collectivity" orientation of the professions as a dependent variable, rather than counting it among the two basic independent variables. It is suggested, however, that this is only a difference in explicit formulation.

5

The dilemma is solved by a strong emphasis on individual self-control, which is grounded in a long socialization process designed to build up the required technical competence and to establish a firm commitment to the values and norms central to the tasks of the professional.[2] The values and norms are, furthermore, institutionalized in the structure and culture of the profession. Individual self-control is therefore supplemented by the formal and informal control of the community of colleagues. Accepting the pledge to a self-controlled "collectivity orientation" as trustworthy, society grants in return privileges and advantages, such as high income and prestige, and protects the profession's autonomy against lay control and interference. Nonprofessional competitors, customers, mass media, and especially government agencies exert control too, but the autonomy of the profession is sheltered against them by such means as laws against "quacks," professional referral patterns and norms which restrict certain forms of competition, insistence on exclusive professional competence in judging performance, and professional personnel in and professional advice to government agencies.

This structure of social control specific to the professions, at least in its extreme forms, is the focus for a series of interrelated hypotheses explaining other features of these occupations. One example may be sufficient. All professions have norms restricting or prohibiting advertising. This seemingly trivial fact is in various ways related to the outlined focal problem. (1) The restriction of advertising serves to emphasize symbolically the subcultural distinction between the professions and the business world, where, supposedly, monetary success is important in itself and as the main basis for esteem

---

2. This socialization is by no means confined to the professional schools. The required value commitments especially are developed largely in earlier socialization experiences. Professional school and early practice articulate these orientations with the specific traditions and practices of the profession. This becomes quite clear in Howard S. Becker, Blanche Geer, Everett C. Hughes, and Anselm L. Strauss, *Boys in White: Student Culture in Medical School* (Chicago, 1961). Discussing the alleged cynicism of medical students that is induced by medical school, the authors argue: "We believe that medical students enter medical school openly idealistic about the practice of medicine and the medical profession" (422). "They come in with a complement of ideas about healing the sick and rendering service to mankind" (*ibid.*). During school "they do not lose this idealistic long-range perspective but realistically develop a 'cynical' concern with the day-to-day details of getting through medical school" (*ibid.*). At the end of his training in medical school "the medical student is...idealistic with a difference. . . .His idealism is more specific and more professional than it was when he entered" (425).

I would suggest that the "collectivity orientation" of the professional is in part based on some latent functions of very long school attendance: over a prolonged period of time the students are relatively sheltered from the survival problems of adult life and exposed to the idealized version of culture presented by school and college teachers who, in turn, are professionals and sheltered from many personal and social problems prevalent in other segments of society. The relationship between the idealistic elements in certain forms of youth culture and the moral subculture of academically trained people deserves further exploration.

from significant others and for self-respect.[3] (2) Advertising would presuppose that the customer can legitimately make up his mind about the qualities of the various members of the profession. It would give the customer a controlling influence incompatible with the maintenance of high technical standards.[4] (3) Advertising would increase competition among the professionals who under pressure might give in to temptations to deviate from professional norms. (4) The restriction of advertising serves to make the members of the profession concerned with the performance of their "brethren," since it limits the possibilities to excel individually. It thus reinforces other mechanisms that make for indentification with the professional community and strengthens collective social control.

The study of the medical profession has dominated this field of sociology and has strongly influenced the development and elaboration of the theoretical model. In this article I shall make some comparisons between the legal and medical professions and attempt to point out modifications of the theoretical model that they suggest.

II

The legal and medical professions differ significantly in the two respects that form the core of the theoretical model under discussion: the nature of their specific competence and the social values toward which the professional work is oriented.

Apart from borderline cases there exists a near-universal *consensus about the central value* toward which the medical profession is oriented. Physician and patient, the doctor's colleague group and the patient's family, his friends, and his role partners in other contexts, as well as the larger community and its various agencies, agree essentially on the substantive definition of health and on its importance compared with other values.

The situation is far more complex for the legal profession. Justice, like health, ranks high in the societal value hierachy. In the substantive definition of justice, however, there are considerable ambiguities and wide discrepancies, as well as areas that are clearly understood and largely agreed upon. Certainly, enacted laws and established legal rulings carry the presumption of being accepted as "just," but the notion of unjust law is by no means uncommon.

These different conceptions of justice are not identical with divergent interests. Interests which stand against a given conception of justice may or may not lay claim to a different conception of justice, and the prevalent ambiguity allows for different shadings between. Divergent interests make for a second difference between the legal and the medical profession that is

---

3. Cf. Talcott Parsons' discussion of components of "success" and the multiple significance of monetary income in this respect in "The Motivation of Economic Activities," *Essays in Sociological Theory*, rev. ed. (Glencoe, Ill., 1954), pp. 50-68.
4. Cf. Goode, "Community within a Community."

relevant here. While the interests of the attorney's client may be at odds with what the lawyer considers just, it is rare that the patient's interests stand against the attainment of health.[5]

Divergent interests and the different more or less articulate conceptions of justice are not randomly distributed in the social structure. They are associated with various subgroups, particularly different socioeconomic strata and ethnic and religious groups. A relatively low degree of overall consensus may contrast with a relatively high degree of consensus within these subgroups. This constellation of societal value dissensus and subgroup value consensus also confronts the religious professional, the minister, priest, or rabbi. However, the diversity of religious commitments is, at least in liberal Western societies, established as legitimate, while the diversity of conceptions of justice finds only an indirect legitimate expression in the realm of politics. Moreover, the clergyman's work centers in the context of his subgroup, while the lawyer's activity often cuts across the boundaries of subgroups[6] and his primary loyalty is expected to be to an overarching system of value orientations that represents, beyond a clear-cut core, an ambiguous compromise among several influential conceptions of justice.

It may be argued that people act and think only to a very limited extent with respect to ultimate social values. The norms and values that actually guide men are those incorporated in the more immediate institutional arrangements and role expectations. Therefore, conflicting notions of justice, especially if they are vaguely or ambiguously defined and rarely formulated explicitly, and if they are not anchored in specific institutions and organizations, are of little consequence for the structure and functioning of the legal profession.

It would seem, however, that the argument refers chiefly to those ultimate values that are not fully compatible with the requirements of institutionalized social life and for those that function as integrating mechanisms for concretely divergent notions precisely because they are left vague. It should be noted that the value of health falls into neither of these categories, while the generalized notion of justice in an important sense fits the second. But even ultimate values of this kind are not completely without consequence for behavior. Furthermore, the conflicting conceptions of justice are to some degree associated with interests and anchored in specific groups, organizations, and institutions.

In spite of partial dissensus on the substantive definition of justice, the institutions of the medical and legal professions are similar in a related

5. The importance of conflicting interests for the situation of the legal profession is emphasized by Parsons in "A Sociologist Looks at the Legal Profession," *Essays in Sociological Theory*, pp. 370-385. Parsons' analysis neglects, however, the problem of value dissensus. It is thus implicitly treated as a simple by-product of conflicting interests with no significant consequences of its own.

6. I deliberately neglect differentiations inside the legal or medical profession. The most obvious exception to the proposition above would be the corporation counsel

dimension, and this makes the value dissensus even more consequential. The public exhibits a high degree of concern about the implementation of the central values of both professions. Open neglect or violation of the values of health and of justice, however understood, elicits considerable moral indignation from disinterested third parties.

In this context the emphasis on procedural law that is characteristic of a developed legal profession may be interpreted as a defense against an open clash of emotionally charged conceptions of justice and not solely a safeguard against the emotions, biases, and the political violence that grow out of a conflict of interests. However, a strongly procedural conception of justice creates at the same time a new source of alienation between the value orientation of the profession and the substantively defined orientations of the different "publics" of the profession.

The *technical competence* of the physician rests on a body of systematic scientific theory. In the actual application of this knowledge other elements that are less rationalized and may be called the "art of medicine" play an important role, for instance, the art of diagnosing on the basis of vague and insufficient clues, certain manual skills, and the use of interpersonal relations in the healing process. All these are, however, intimately connected with the main area of the physician's competence, medical knowledge.

If we compare the technical competence of physician and lawyer, three important differences emerge.

First, the lawyer's knowledge is not scientific. It is concerned not with the prediction and explanation of events on the basis of natural laws, but rather with a body of social norms and with rules for their application. These norms and rules can be systematized for the convenience of teaching or for avoiding inconsistencies and contradictions. But the resulting body of knowledge remains a description of a single normative system, designed for aiding its application and preparing its further development.

This development again requires comment. Legal norms are, in contrast to natural laws, subject to human decisions. Changes in the body of medical knowledge are due to new discoveries; changes in the body of legal knowledge are due to decisions of legislatures and of courts, decisions significantly influenced by members of the legal profession acting as legislators, judges, counsels, legal writers, and law professors. The value orientation of the legal profession, which is subject to patterned social conflict, thus plays a role in the substantive development of the law, while the content of medical knowledge is largely independent of the value orientation of the medical profession.

Second, a good deal of the lawyer's competence is connected with his legal knowledge only indirectly or not at all. Since the law is a generalized

---

who does little or no litigation. But although he maintains a considerable loyalty to the dominant conception of justice, he is by some legal quarters looked down upon as a "captive lawyer."

mechanism of social control, its application covers a great variety of
social situations. Different applications require a grasp of these social contexts as well as of the law. From the good lawyer we may therefore expect
a generalized capacity for defining situations and a great variety of "world-
ly knowledge." On the basis of this nonlegal knowledge and ability lawyers act often outside their specialty, giving economic advice or providing
their clients with organizational "know-how." The basic propositions of
the theoretical model under discussion do not apply fully to these activities:
they are not based on systematic theory, the customer may be in a position
to judge them for himself, and society does not imbue them with the same
moral significance as strictly legal activities.

Finally, it may be suggested that nonrationalized interpersonal skills
play, at least manifestly, a greater role in the lawyer's work than the
physician's. His relationship to the client shows significant similarities to the
doctor-patient relationship[7] but, in addition, interpersonal skills are of
extreme importance in litigation and negotiation, major fields of his professional work.

We have seen, then, that in comparison with the medical profession the
lawyer's special technical competence, his legal knowledge, covers less of
his work, while generalized intellectual skills, various areas of knowledge
outside his specialty, and skills in handling interpersonal relations play a
more important role. In these nonlegal activities the gap in competence
between professional and laymen may be considerably reduced. The part
of the cultural tradition that is the basis of his learned competence is not a
body of scientific knowledge, but a system of legal principles and norms,
the application and development of which are substantively influenced by
the value orientation of the profession. This value orientation is far from
clear-cut and, in addition, is subject to societal value dissensus and to the
impact of conflicting interests that may be at odds with any given conception
of justice. At the same time, the public's concern with the implementation of
these variously conceived values is quite intense.

III

Up to this point we have compared the legal and medical professions in
those characteristics that are the basic independent variables of the theoretical model, technical competence and the social values toward which the professional work is oriented. We should expect corresponding differences
between the two professions in those characteristics that are treated as de-

---

7. Cf. Parsons, "A Sociologist Looks at the Legal Profession," pp. 381 ff., and
The Social System, chaps. VII and X, where the lawyer-client relationship and the
physician-patient relationship are each analyzed in terms of a paradigm of social control that was originally developed from an analysis of the interaction between psychotherapist and patient.

pendent variables, such as their self-control. Several such differences may be found.

Ultimate values are important for the legitimation of more specific and concrete normative patterns. To the degree that within a society there is dissensus and ambiguity about the concrete meaning of the ultimate values underlying the specific norms and orientations of a profession, we should expect these values to be seen by the practitioner as less immediately binding and the specific norms to be more often taken as conventional rules the breach of which is of little consequence if "one can get away with it."

Societal dissensus and ambiguity about the central "reference values" of a profession should also strongly influence how the profession is perceived and evaluated by various more or less distant groups. The public image of the legal profession seems indeed to be characterized by suspicions and ambivalences. These are reinforced if the legal profession is seen as linked to certain social classes or religious and ethnic groups and if the most visible work of the profession is concerned with conflict situations and the defense of morally suspect or already condemned persons. Deprecatory elements in the public image of a profession will probably reduce the identification with the profession and its solidarity as a group, unless it is united by very strong common value orientations and interests.

With reference to the norms and values that are incorporated in institutional patterns and role expectations of immediate concern to lawyers, a full analysis would have to investigate the total role set and the reference groups for the various segments of the legal profession. In assessing the balance of social control in these relationships, the relative level of competence of lawyers and their role partners would require special consideration. Such analysis will have to await the accumulation of more empirical evidence.[8] It seems possible, however, to indicate some of the consequences for the profession as a group that grow out of the relationship between lawyers and their clientele.

Professional services are extremely costly. Therefore, although nearly every profession holds up the ideal of serving all segments of the population, the middle and upper classes are more strongly represented in the clientele of self-employed professions than the lower classes, unless tax or charity funds supply the professional fees. Compared with the medical profession, this tendency is reinforced in the legal profession by three factors: first, the incidence of problems defined as legal tends to be higher in the middle and upper classes; second, the elasticity of demand for legal services is greater than for medical services; third, tax and charity funds tend to be more generously supplied for medical than for legal problems. This situation structurally shields the legal profession against the full impact of the

---

8. The research of Jerome E. Carlin on New York lawyers will contribute significantly to such an analysis; cf. his *Lawyers' Ethics* (New York, 1966).

dissensus about relevant values while associating it more closely with the middle and upper classes.[9]

The clientele of a profession is distributed differentially among its practitioners. In addition to technical specialization, and often connected with it, we find a tendency toward specialization in clients and patients of a particular ethnic and class background.[10] Although the general class range of the legal clientele is narrower than the class range of medical patients, certain factors seem to strengthen the trend toward specialization in terms of client background for the legal profession and to lend special significance to such a differentiation of the clientele. There is, first, a rough connection between the position of clients and the legal character and difficulty of their problems. Furthermore, not all lawyers are trusted with problems the adequate solution of which, in the eyes of the client, not only require legal competence but a certain set of attitudes and value orientations. Finally, the nonlegal competence of the lawyer, especially his interpersonal skills, is highly class specific: for example, skill in negotiating with executives is quite different from competence in handling minor officials in local administration.

Association with clients of a particular social class or ethnic background not only seems to be more characteristic of the legal than of the medical profession; it also has more significant consequences for the lawyer than for the physician. Among the factors that give special significance to this differential association are divergent interests and conflicting conceptions of justice and the fact that, compared with scientific knowledge, "secular law is considerably looser in its points of reference" which could provide a stable orientation when facing pressures from clients.[11] Furthermore, clients will probably attempt to exert such pressures more often than patients, and they are often in a better position to do so: their health is not impaired; their education, to a high degree associated with class position, is better than average; their own occupational competence is often related to the issues at hand, and if the lawyer does not confine himself completely to strictly legal matters the gap in competence between client and lawyer may disappear completely.

9. In 1938, nearly three-quarters of all families in the United States had annual incomes between $500 and $2500, with an average of $1500. These families paid on the average $60 for health and less than $1 for legal services. "Plainly, lawyers were getting their paying clients largely from the highest-income groups, including only about 13 percent of the families in the United States. The mass of the people had practically no contact with the lawyer in a client relationship." James Willard Hurst, *The Growth of American Law*, (Boston, 1950), p. 255. This book is of considerable value for general information about the legal profession in the United States; cf. also Albert P. Blaustein and Charles O. Porter, *The American Lawyer: A Summary of the Survey of the Legal Profession* (Chicago, 1954). Some of the recent sociological studies on the legal profession are cited in note 14.

10. Examples outside the legal profession would be the role of the specialist in internal medicine as the general practitioner of the upper middle and upper classes, and the clienteles of psychotherapist and psychiatric social worker which are similar in problems, but clearly differentiated in social class.

11. Parsons, "A Sociologist Looks at the Legal Profession," p. 376.

One last difference between the medical and the legal profession may be mentioned in this context. The doctor's patients are, with some modifications, individual persons, while the lawyer's clients are very often formal organizations. Organizations provide more recurrent business than the average individual client or patient and they can often, especially if they have their own legal staff, check on the lawyer's performance. They are, in addition, in multiple and complex ways linked to other organizations with similar legal problems. Organizational clients exert, therefore, a more powerful social control over the practitioner than individual clients or patients do. Their large share in the lawyer's business further reduces the importance of the gap in competence between professional and client.[12]

These factors lead to an internal stratification of the bar in terms of income and professional esteem; this is found in other professions too, although probably to a lesser extent. They also expose the various segments of the bar to powerful influences from different client groups with their characteristic interests and value orientations, thus creating pressures to deviate from the traditional orientation of the profession or to emphasize and depreciate selectively some elements of the professional ethos.

A differentiation of the bar in terms of different client milieux that partially determine the attitudes and value orientations of lawyers will place considerable strain on professional solidarity. It will reduce identification with the profession as a group[13] and severely limit the possibilities of the social control, informal as well as formal, that the profession is supposed to exercise. It also will impede the moral commitment of the profession to values that transcend the lawyer-client relationship and its attendant virtues.

These tendencies could be counterbalanced by a strong internalization of common value orientations in the process of socialization toward the professional role. In the United States the socialization of lawyers shows considerable variation, and this heterogeneity is tied with the societal class structure on the one hand and the internal stratification of the bar on the other. Ethnic origin and class background are varied and show a high

---

12. That the lawyer's clients often are organizations has many other implications which cannot be discussed in this article. One point, brought out in a discussion with Arnold Feldman, modifies the propositions above. The work of important segments of the legal profession is associated with managerial foci of power. To the extent that a definition of the managerial role as the role of a relatively independent fiduciary for the interests of shareholders, employees, consumers, and the larger community gains in importance, these segments of the profession would be under less one-sided pressure and in a better position to assert their own professional orientation.

Together with a stronger backing by a more established legal system and a possibly better bargaining position of large law firms resulting from differential growth rates of law firms and client firms, this tendency could explain why the corporation lawyer in the United States is a professionally better respected figure than he was around the turn of the century.

13. A factor that may limit this tendency is the ignorance which stems from a near-complete segregation of several segments within the profession. It seems that lawyers in the upper brackets of the stratification system often are only dimly aware of the existence and the condition of the lowest strata.

correlation with length and quality of prelaw schooling, type and quality
of legal education, the incidence of nonlegal jobs as part of the work career, and, finally, the type and status of legal practice.[14] The structure of
recruitment and socialization is not simply a consequence of the special
features of the legal profession which have been discussed. It is largely
due to the general structure of higher education in the United States and
to the specific time at which formal legal education was institutionalized
in the United States.[15] It is, on the other hand, not unrelated to a professional tradition that is ambiguous to begin with and is subject to divergent
influences from clients and other reference groups and to a professional
competence that includes a good many nontechnical elements which are
largely subcultural and class-specific. Once developed, the heterogeneity of
professional socialization is reinforced by the heterogeneity of the profession
itself.[16]

1. Societies differ in the incidence and intensity of conflicting interests and
in subcultural differentiation. To the degree that a society shows less patterned conflict and value dissensus the hypotheses derived from dissensus
about justice should apply less.

Although this analysis has been developed on the basis of American
materials, the distinctive characteristics of the legal profession presented
here are not confined to the United States and its legal, economic, and
political system. Their incidence and their implications vary considerably,
however, according to different societal conditions.

14. Cf. Dan C. Lortie, *The Striving Young Lawyer: A Study of Early Career Dif-
ferentiation in the Chicago Bar*, unpubl. Ph.D. diss. (University of Chicago, 1958);
Dan C. Lortie, "Laymen to Lawmen: Law Schools, Careers, and Professional So-
cialization," *Harvard Educational Review*, 29 (Autumn, 1959); Erwin O. Smigel,
"The Impact of Recruitment on the Organization of the Large Law Firm," *American
Sociological Review*, 25 (February, 1960); Jerome E. Carlin, *Lawyers on Their Own:
A Study of Individual Practitioners in Chicago*, (New Brunswick, N.J., 1962); Jack
Ladinsky, "Careers of Lawyers, Law Practice, and Legal Institutions," *American
Sociological Review*, 28 (February, 1963), 47-54; Seymour Warkow, "Allocation to
American Law Schools," paper presented at the annual meeting of the American So-
ciological Association, Los Angeles, August, 1963. For a comparison of the American
and the German legal professions in this respect, see Dietrich Rueschemeyer, "Re-
krutierung, Ausbildung und Berufsstruktur: Zur Soziologie der Anwaltschaft in den
Vereinigten Staaten und in Deutschland," *Sonderheft* 5 der *Koelner Zeitschrift
für Soziologie und Sozialpsychologie*, 1961, 122-144.
15. This institutionalization dates back only to the turn of the century. Rapid urbanization and a large influx of immigrants increased the heterogeneity of the potential recruits of the bar. The proportion of night school students rose from 10 percent to nearly 50 per cent in 25 years, while for other reasons large law firms began
to develop which recruited their lawyers increasingly from the best schools in the
country. Cf. Hurst, *The Growth of American Law*, and Carlin, *Lawyers on Their
Own*, for a convenient summary of the relevant sources.
16. Attempts to raise the level of legal education met with much stronger resistance
than similar efforts in medical education. One frequent argument pointed directly
toward value dissensus: the quasi-political character of the profession makes a relatively open access to it desirable, and this consideration outweighs the disadvantages of
night schools and similar low-cost institutions. Cf. Albert J. Harno, *Legal Education
in the United States* (San Francisco, 1953).

2. Radical social change upsets legitimate arrangements and requires complex innovations in the legal system. The area of substantive consensus is reduced and the system of legal norms is probably more subject to the impact of contending notions of justice and of conflicting interests than an established legal order of long standing that meets more or less standardized legal problems. The profession or significant parts of it are more subject to divergent pressures, while the cultural reference points are at the same time most fluid and ambiguous.[17]

3. Cultural and political traditions differ in dealing with social conflict and value dissensus. If, for instance, we compare schematically the dominant cultural definitions in nineteen-century Prussia and nineteenth-century America, we see on the one side a conception of justice and the common good as determined by *a priori* solutions to be found and formulated by experts and a rather low level of tolerance of conflict and dissensus, and on the other a conception of justice and the common good as determined by ordered dispute and compromise and a rather high level of tolerance of conflict and dissensus. These different cultural and political traditions rest, of course, on structural conditions, contemporary and antecedent, among which are the position and structure of the legal profession, as Max Weber has shown. At any given time, however, they are relatively independent of the legal profession and determine the sociocultural situation in which the legal profession has to operate. These differences pervade the whole legal system: the system of legal norms, the administration of justice, the political and legal position of government bureaucracy, the role of law professors as quasi-legislators and quasi-judges, as well as the dominant attitudes in major client groups and in major sources of public opinion.

To the degree that the dominant cultural definitions and social institutions shelter the legal profession from the impact of conflict and value dissensus, and create the fiction of law as being derived by scholars, the hypotheses about the consequences of value dissensus and the nonscientific character of legal knowledge would have to be modified considerably.

17. It would be instructive to analyze from this perspective certain features in the historical development of the legal profession in the United States. The hypothesis may explain partially the increased independence from client pressures that now seems to prevail in large law firms dealing with big business clients, compared with their situation around the turn of the century. The relatively stabilized legal situation of big business in the post-New Deal period has interacted, according to the hypothesis, with the development of a better bargaining position of large law firms on the market for highly competent legal services and the embryonic emergence of a fiduciary definition of the business executive's role to result in fewer conflicts of orientation in the lawyer-client interaction and better possibilities for resistance on the part of the law firm (cf. note 12). For material on the position of the large law firm in various periods, see Joseph Katz, *The Legal Profession, 1890-1915: The Lawyer's Role in Society: A Study of Attitudes*, unpubl. M.A. thesis, Columbia University, 1953; Robert T. Swaine, *The Cravath Firm*, 3 vols. (New York, 1946-48); R. T. Swaine, "Impact of Big Business on the Profession: An Answer to the Critics of the Modern Bar," American Bar Association Journal, 35 (1949); Erwin O. Smigel, *The Wall Street Lawyer* (New York, 1964).

4. The gap of competence between layman and lawman depends on the relative legal competence of lawyers and their various role partners as well as on the importance of nonlegal skills in the lawyers' role performance and the relative skill in these respects of lawyers and their role partners. All the factors involved, such as complexity of the system of legal norms, most prevalent types of client, their legal and nonlegal competence, and extension of the lawyer's role performance into nonlegal areas, are subject to conditions that vary greatly from society to society; important variations occur even between industrial societies which show considerable similarity in their economic and occupational structure.

IV

What are the implications of these comparisons of the legal and the medical profession for the model underlying much of current sociological thinking about the professions?

With respect to those variables the model treats as independent, three distinctive aspects of the legal profession have been emphasized. (1) The body of systematic knowledge does not have scientific character. (2) The values to which the profession is committed are subject to societal dissensus and patterned conflict of interests. (3) Various factors tend to reduce the gap in competence between the lawyer and his role partners.

The first two points are not taken into account by the original model, although what is currently known and surmised about the legal profession suggests that they do have significant implications for the models' dependent variables. The third point places the legal profession relatively low in one of the essential dimensions of professionalism. The model states more or less clearly certain consequences for this case. To the degree that they are not fully borne out, the question arises whether other factors have to be considered as functional equivalents for the independent variables of the model.

Neither these specific initial points nor their implications can be confined in any sense to the legal profession. To a greater or lesser degree they are relevant for other professions, including medicine. Several suggestions for a revision of the model may be stated as "general orientation" theses rather than as specific hypotheses.

1. The model under discussion does not differentiate enough between different types of knowledge; it overemphasizes the role of scientific knowledge and its attendant consequences, such as a rationality and readiness for change.[18] Among the classical professions, the emphasis fits neither the legal

18. In "Encroachment, Charlatanism, and the Emergent Profession," William J. Goode develops some interesting hypotheses about different types of knowledge in several professions and concomitant differences in their social structure. Consider, however, the following generalization of Ernest Greenwood as one exmple for the tendency noted above: "The importance of theory precipitates a form of activity normally not encountered in the nonprofessional occupation, viz., theory construction via systematic research. . . Continued employment of the scientific method is nurtured by and in turn

profession nor the ministry, and the military profession only to a limited extent. It does fit many of the new professions which grew up during industrialization; but their growth did not provide substitutes for the professions without a scientific base nor did it transform them into a similar pattern.[19] The professions of law and religion deal with parts of the cultural tradition the core of which does not consist of scientific propositions.

If we, in turn, focus our attention on normative and evaluative elements in the "knowledge" base of all professions and semiprofessions, we discover that knowledge about norms, evaluative definitions of situations, and metaphysical assertions play a more or less important role in many of these occupations. Thus, what constitutes health and how it may be achieved seem to depend much more on nonscientific assumptions in psychiatry than in medicine, although the line between the two is becoming more and more blurred.

2. Much has been said about a neglect of dissensus and conflict by "functionalist" theory; often, the criticisms are oversimplified and the proposed alternatives show even more neglect for other dimensions of social reality. The model of the theory of the profession, built as it is on the paradigm of medicine, assumes a high degree of societal and intraprofessional value consensus.[20] In the legal profession such a societal consensus is combined with dissensus about the substantive definition of important

reinforces the element of *rationality*. As an orientation, rationality is the antithesis to traditionalism. . .It implies a perpetual readiness to discard any portion [of the theoretical system], no matter how time honored it may be, with a formulation demonstrated to be more valid." "Attributes of a Profession," in S. Nosow and W. H. Form, eds., *Man, Work, and Society* (New York, 1962), p. 209, first published in *Social Work*, 2 (July, 1957), 45-55.

Lawyers often refer to the conservatism of their profession and explain it by pointing to the element of tradition inherent in any system of legal norms and especially in those of the Common Law type. It seems doubtful, though, whether such an hypothesis of the lawyer's "immanent conservatism" is correct. Attorneys played an important role in liberal revolutions and bourgeois modernization and reform movements and in the attendant legal changes. It may be suggested that progressive or conservative attitudes in the legal profession are largely an outgrowth of the attitudes of clientele rather than an outgrowth of commitment to a body of knowledge and its furtherance. For a suggestive example from a non-Western society that fits this interpretation, see Richard William Rabinowitz, *The Japanese Lawyer: A Study in the Sociology of the Legal Profession*, unpubl. Ph.D. diss., Harvard University, 1955.

19. The cultural predominance of the sciences did result in legal and theological movements that interpreted themselves as scientific. These were, however, based on misunderstandings of what science is or they developed into auxiliary disciplines such as the sociology of law and religion.

20. Rue Bucher and Anselm L. Strauss emphasize in "Professions in Process," *American Journal of Sociology*, 66 (1960-61), 325-334, diversity and conflict of interests within a profession against the model of functional theory. They conceive of profession as congeries of "segments" with distinctive identities and divergent interests which tend to take on the character of social movements within the larger profession. This conception is illustrated with suggestive examples from the American medical profession.

The relationship between such internal conflict and dissensus about the orientation toward a profession's central values in other segments of the larger society is pre-

aspects of what is required by justice. In addition, we find strong conflicting interests that may be at odds with any of these conceptions of justice.

It is suggested that focusing explicit attention on divergent and possibly conflicting value orientations and interests would be profitable for the study of all professions, including medicine. The analysis could be more differentiated and go beyond the general concepts used above, like the values of "health," "justice," or "order." The character of relevant value orientations, that is, the substantive definition and relative ranking, the intensity of moral sentiment and the concern for implementation, the relationship to interests, ambivalent elements, has to be identified for various groups and subcultures that are important for the profession as recruitment fields, socialization environments, actual and potential clientele, sources of public opinion, and supervisory and control agencies. The impact of these various orientations and interests on the profession can be analyzed largely in terms of existing middle-range theories about role, role set and role strain, reference groups, and deviant behavior.

3. The third characteristic more clearly seen in the legal profession seems easiest to deal with in terms of the theoretical model. If the gap in competence between the lawyer and his role partners is in various ways and degrees reduced, then members of the legal profession simply score low on one primary characteristic of the ideal-type of a profession. The situation seems to be similar to that of librarians,[21] social workers, and other semi-professionals. One would expect this to result in their being granted less autonomy as well as lower rewards in income, prestige, and respect. The expectation seems to be borne out for some segments of the bar, especially the metropolitan solo practitioner in the United States; it is clearly not confirmed for the higher strata of the legal profession. It may be suggested that these last groups of lawyers score high in the dependent variables of the model in part because of their affiliation with the highest segments of the societal stratification system, that is, for reasons that lie outside the model of professionalism.

This point may be generalized. The core of the theoretical model is identical with the assertions used by the professions to legitimize their claims for maintaining old and acquiring new privileges. It seems likely that the structure of legitimation is only a part of the causal matrix underlying the pattern of professionalism. The advantages of a recognized professional position seem attractive enough to mobilize all means of power, prestige, and ideology for the acquisition or maintenance of that position, whether legitimate or not. The differential access to these means, however, is strongly influenced by factors other than specialized expertise and impor-

---

sumably quite complex. As one hypothesis it may be suggested that the incidence of organized intraprofessional segmental movements is inversely related to the degree of dissensus in the various publics relevant to the profession. In an "embattled group" internal factionalism is less likely to emerge openly and to be tolerated.

21. Cf. Goode, "The Librarian: From Occupation to Profession?"

tance for core values of a society. One should avoid being misled by the collectivity-oriented self-definition of the professions into separating their analysis from the analysis of social stratification. Many features that are considered specific characteristics of the professions seem to be in fact aspects of upper-class and upper-middle-class life and subculture. Thus, autonomy at work and many facets of professional ethics seem buttressed not only by professional norms and granted claims, but also by the class status of the practitioner, his social origin, and the class positions of his clients and his other role partners.

2

JOSEPH BEN-DAVID

Professionals and Unions in Israel

There is little agreement on the sociological implications of professional-ism.[1] There is no generally accepted definition of what professionals are, other than that they require higher education and possess researchable technologies.[2] Some sociologists predict that eventually a broad range of occupations will model themselves on medicine and the law (in that they will seek status and self-regulation in return for observing ethical standards and performing altruistic service). Others disagree. Some think that wide-spread professionalism is desirable because it leads to technical efficiency and a better integration of society. Others regard professionalism as a socially harmful, monopoly-oriented fossil of a bygone corporate society.[3] Under the circumstances, the best way to deal with these questions is to strive for a more systematic and complete description of the relevant phenomena. This in turn will help us to assess the extent of the tendency to professionalize and the conditions under which different aspects of the typical structure appear or are absent.

Israel as a Special Case

Israel provides an unusually interesting locale for such a study. Profes-sionals and kindred groups constituted 11 to 12 percent of the labor force of the Jewish community in Palestine from 1918 to 1948 and the same

Reprinted from *Industrial Relations*, 5 (1965), pp. 48-66, by permission of the author and the publisher.

1. I am indebted for assistance to Harold L. Wilensky, Randall Collins, and the Institute of International Studies, University of California, Berkeley.

2. See J. Ben-David, "Professions in the Class System of Present-Day Societies," *Current Sociology*, 12 (1963-1964), chap. 1, and Harold L. Wilensky, "The Profes-sionalization of Everyone?" *American Journal of Sociology*, 70 (September, 1964), 137-158.

3. For a survey of these views, see Ben-David, *loc. cit.*

percentage of the total labor force of Israel after 1948.[4] This was the world's highest level of professionalization until the figures were matched by the United States in 1960. And, for a country whose economy is relatively undeveloped, Israel has an exceptionally high proportion of college graduates.[5] But, to the extent that bargaining power is determined by supply and demand, the position of professionals in Israel and preindependence Palestine is and has been worse than anywhere else in the world.

Other factors have contributed to making the Israeli case exceptional. An overwhelmingly socialized economy has led to most professionals being employed by large public bureaucracies, a condition much like that in communist countries. At the same time, unlike the situation in communist countries, professional organizations have complete freedom to express membership views. Furthermore, the behavior of professionals can be studied against a background of rapid and dramatic change: Zionist immigration started in 1881; Palestine was a Turkish province until the end of World War I; then it came under British rule and existed as a plural colonial society until 1948, when Israel gained its independence.

The Status of Professional Work

BEFORE INDEPENDENCE

Owing to the peculiar nature of immigration patterns, professionals were denied a secure middle-class status until about 1947. Although over 11 percent of immigrants (from 1919 to 1947) were professionals, many did not continue to work in their respective fields. Teachers were unable to find employment in teaching because of language difficulties; many lawyers failed local bar exams which were based to a considerable extent on British and Turkish law. A perhaps more important source of downward mobility was the number of young people from middle-class families who went to Israel as students or had joined Zionist youth movements and had trained themselves in agriculture in order to join pioneering collective settlements. The extent of deprofessionalization and downward mobility is indicated by a 1937 survey of wage and salaried workers.[6] Of those who had been teachers abroad, 16.7 percent became farmers in Israel and an additional

4. A. Nitzan, "Miyne Koah Haadam Bammeshek Hayyisr'eli" ("The Structure of the Labor Force in the Israel Economy"), *Riv'on L'kalkala*, · No. 9-10, 1955: for 1916-1918, 11.4 percent; 1931, 12.8 percent; 1939, 10.9 percent; 1948, 11 percent (of the Jewish labor force only); and *Statistical Abstracts of Israel*, No. 14, p. 510, for 1962; 11 percent of total 1962 labor force (including Jews and Arabs). The composition of the professional and kindred component has changed little over time. See Joseph Ben-David and H. Muhsam, "Miktzooth Hofshiyyim," in the volume *Eretz Yisrael* of the *Hebrew Encyclopedia*.

5. In 1954, 6.1 percent of Jewish males 25 years and older in Israel were college graduates. The comparable figure in the United States was 7.3 percent for 1950. *Basic Facts and Figures* (Paris: UNESCO, 1959), pp. 15-23, Table 3.

6. Excluding managers, but including salaried professionals. Havvaad Happoel shel

10 to 15 percent became manual workers of other kinds. Of former students, 29.2 percent became farmers and an additional 35 percent manual workers.

Why did professionals and students continue to go to Palestine despite the prospects of downward occupational mobility? Leaving one's studies or profession to become a worker was regarded not as a sign of failure but as an act of heroism and selfless devotion to cause, somewhat like volunteering for a difficult mission in wartime or joining the United States Peace Corps today. As a consequence, the word "worker" acquired an ambiguous meaning which it still possesses to some degree in Israel. On the one hand, it refers to a person who earns his living through physical effort and is therefore at the bottom of the occupational prestige ladder; on the other hand, it refers to a selfless pioneer who has claim to moral leadership. The Marxist ideal of a society in which status inequalities would disappear came to be tied up with the new nation's special need for individual sacrifice. These ideas had a particularly strong appeal to the young and to intellectuals as they were more able to perceive the hopelessness of their future in Europe and at the same time possessed the time perspective and imagination to envisage the rise of a new society. The paradoxical result was that an extremely anti-intellectual and antiprofessional ideology selectively attracted intellectuals. Even though in terms of economic opportunity they were likely to lose more than other groups, they still tended to go to Palestine in relatively great numbers.

It should be noted that there have been other instances in history of intellectuals (mainly students and professionals) being attracted to equalitarian movements which were striving to eliminate the privileged status of professionals, e.g., the French and Russian revolutions.[7] But the difference is that in the latter cases the attempt to create an equalitarian state took place in rigidly stratified societies and involved, owing to economic scarcity, the compulsion of terror. By contrast, in Palestine a high percentage of the working class came from middle-class backgrounds and the ideological claim for equality had in consequence a more realistic social basis. In addition, the economic cost of the experiment in Palestine was greatly alleviated by foreign aid and by the provision of certain services by the colonial administration and other foreign agencies. Among Palestinian Jews there was a greater degree of economic equality than existed in any other country and this equality was generally acceptable to all classes of the population.

SINCE INDEPENDENCE

Conditions have changed since Israel gained its independence in 1948. In the first place, the proportion of immigrants of African and Middle Eastern

Hahisthadruth Hakklalith shel Haovdim, *Pinkes Hahisthadruth Hakklalith shel Haorvdim (Bulletin of the General Federation of Labor)*, No. 8 (1938), p. 36.

7. Robert Michels, *Political Parties* (Glencoe, Ill.: The Free Press, 1958), pp. 332-

origin increased from 10.5 percent during the period 1918 to 1948 to some 40 percent during the years 1948 to 1962.[8] Owing to a higher birth rate in this group, they now constitute probably more than 40 percent of the total population. While it would be grossly misleading to describe these immigrants, mostly petty traders and artisans, as working class, they are certainly accustomed to lower standards of living and education than immigrants from Europe and they have mainly become manual and clerical workers.

As the economy developed, occupational differences became increasingly important. The implications of these differences in terms of education, responsibility, authority, and social contact have become more obvious. The ideology of pioneering and equality still has great meaning to the oldtimers, but for youth and the newcomers it is but a legend from bygone days. Fewer immigrants plan to be pioneers and immigrant professionals and students are no longer prepared to do manual work.

Finally, the market situation of professionals has improved. The supply of professionals has remained stable (the relatively greater scarcity of professionals among new immigrants has been balanced by the rapid growth of higher education), but the growth of the economy has definitely increased the demand for such workers. International developments have also improved the professionals' bargaining power. Between the two world wars there was little unmet demand for professionals anywhere in the world and there was unemployment among professionals in many countries. This situation has changed since World War II, so that professional people, dissatisfied with their lot in Israel, can relatively easily look for employment elsewhere.

To sum up, conditions prior to 1948 were unique and temporary. There was a trend towards occupational and social de-differentiation which led at times to a situation where unskilled manual work actually received higher prestige than specialized intellectual work. This reflected both ideology and conditions of supply and demand for different kinds of workers.[9]

Conditions became more normal after 1948. From the professional point of view the state of supply and demand is still probably among the least favorable in the world. This is correctly reflected in low income differentials between professional work and clerical or manual work.[10] But there has

---

346; Daniel Bell, "The Background and Development of Marxist Socialism in the U.S.," in D. D. Egbert and S. Persons, eds., *Socialism in American Life* (Princeton, N.J.: Princeton University Press, 1952), 294-296.

8. *Statistical Abstracts of Israel*. No. 14 (1963), p. 110.

9. It has to be emphasized that this de-differentiation and reversal of the scale was characteristic only of the Jewish population of Palestine. The country as a whole, which was a British mandated territory, was "normal" in both respects.

10. Occupational prestige scales were administered in Israel by M. Lissak to a sample of young people and by the present author to a sample of teachers.

been a definite trend toward differentiation, and the professions are on top of the prestige scale, as elsewhere.

Histradruth and the Foreign Agencies

The role of professionals in Israel has been made even more unique by the preeminent influence of the Histadruth or General Federation of Labor and by the existence before 1948 of institutions which employed professionals but which were controlled by foreigners or the mandatory government.

THE HISTRADRUTH

The Histadruth, founded after World War I, functions both as a union and an employer. Its founders looked on it as the core of a totally organized socialist society. It was to include unions of all "workers" and aimed at complete equality of income among all ranks. The separate existence of professional unions was therefore seen as a potentially disruptive factor.[11] In addition, the Histadruth owns many industries and services. Its Sick Fund today insures 70 percent of the population; it operated a special network of schools until they were absorbed by the state; and it is an increasingly important employer of architects and engineers in its various construction and manufacturing operations. Thus, both as an employer and an organization which regarded itself as the nucleus of a socialist equalitarian society, it was interested in bringing the professional unions within its authority and exerted considerable pressure on all except the lawyers to join.

FOREIGN AGENCIES

Before independence many professional services and positions were almost monopolized by foreigners and conditions of work, pay, and social prestige met European standards in these cases. Schools run by foreign philanthropic bodies, such as the Alliance Israélite Universelle, the Hilfsverein für Deutsche Juden, and the Anglo-Jewish Association, were set up before World War I. Later, there was the American-run Hadassa Medical Organization and some other organizations controlled to a large extent from abroad, e.g., the Hebrew University and the Jewish Agency. In addition, there were the few, but conspicuous professional positions of the Mandatory Government (especially in the judiciary and legal services).

Thus the growing number of professional immigrants, while encouraged by the prevailing political atmosphere and actual conditions in the

---

11. For similar opposition to the existence of separate professional associations, see H. E. Sigerist, *Socialized Medicine in the Soviet Union* (New York: Norton, 1937), pp. 147-152.

Jewish community to abandon their occupations and become workers, or at least put up with an entirely new bureaucratic and socialist pattern of professional work, were on the other hand frustrated by the fact that although high quality and high cost professional services existed, these did not provide opportunities for employment. The principal aim of these professional immigrants was to obtain employment for themselves, particularly in the elite positions, and one of the main functions of professional organizations was to create, or induce others to create, suitable employment opportunities.

Professions Before Independence

TEACHING

The teacher's union was founded in 1904.[12] Even in its early years there existed workers' parties which denied the justification for separate professional organizations and insisted there should be an overall, politically active organization for all workers, led by those in manual work and agriculture. Nevertheless, optimal conditions existed for teachers to realize professional objectives before World War I. Considerable sympathy existed for the replacement of foreign language schools, which spread a spirit alien to the population, with Hebrew language schools. The fight for an opportunity for the Hebrew teacher was, therefore, a fight for a widely accepted community aim. The end result was that the teachers' union was charged to run schools financed by the Zionist organization.

After World War I, when the self-governing organizations of the Jewish community were developed, they took over the school system. The teachers' union, which had established the core of a Department of Education, maintained its hold on the department's professional staff, however. It willingly abandoned the responsibility for finances, but it did not trust either the various political parties or the mandatory government with the making of educational policy.

Until the early twenties, the teachers' union was the prototype of a professional association. It concerned itself primarily with educational policy and safeguarded the right of the profession to determine its own practices. It strove to raise standards and controlled appointments and promotions. No academic senate has ever been more self-governing than this union of teachers. It enjoyed widespread membership support and its leadership included the elite of the profession. There seems to have existed ideal conditions for professionalism since the educational system was established by the teachers themselves. What is considered as the goal of the teaching profession in many countries, namely the official recognition of the profes-

12. The following account, where not otherwise indicated, is based on a study of teachers, doctors, and lawyers in Israel by the author: *Hammivne Hahevrathi shel Hammiktzooth Hahofshiyyim B'Yisrael (The Social Structure of the Professions in*

sional status of the teachers and the granting of most far-reaching control over all matters of teaching and educational policy to the organized profession, was here attained at the very outset.

Notwithstanding its authority, the attempts of the union to raise the standards of the profession were only moderately successful. It was, and has been, unable to prevent the inflow of poorly qualified people. To defend the interests of this significant minority, the union had to adopt the same goals as traditional unions, namely, job security, seniority rights, and across-the-board benefits. By the early thirties the union's interest in educational policy had become clearly subordinated to its economic interests. Its means became those employed by tough labor unions, including strikes. Nevertheless, the union was passively supported by its members as the most desirable alternative to domination by the mandatory administration or the Histadruth with its avowedly deprofessionalizing tendencies. Support was given with some reservation, however, as was evidenced by the withdrawal of the elite of the profession—secondary school teachers—from leadership. Indeed the leaders were increasingly regarded as bureaucrats or strong-men.[13]

MEDICINE

The Medical Association originally followed the path of the teachers by attempting to foster a public health committee which would be charged with the organization of national health services. According to its plan, the organization was to have as decisive an influence as the Teacher's Union had in education. However, none of the enterprises launched by the organization, such as a sickness insurance scheme, have become important. Unlike the teachers, who started their organization before there was an educational system acceptable to the population, the medical organization started its activities after the establishment of services and enterprises by others

---

Israel) (unpublished Ph.D. thesis, Hebrew University, Jerusalem, 1955). Some of the material is also included in my "Professions and Social Structure in Israel," *Scripta Hierosolymitana*, Vol. III (Jerusalem, 1956), and "The Professional Role of the Physician in Israel," *Human Relations*, 11 (August, 1958), 255-274.

13. A parallel case of deprofessionalization in spite of early success and a distinctly professionalistic ideology occurred in nursing. The profession was introduced to Israel from the United States in the early twenties and was intended to play a decisive and highly professional role in the health services planned by the United States social security expert Dr. Rubinov and Henrietta Szold, a U.S. philanthropist who had settled in Israel. Neither was a medical doctor, and both thought that the place of the M.D. in preventive medical services should be rather limited. They also considered the doctors too conservative and status-conscious a group to be useful in the creation of a complete public health service based on new ideas. On the other hand, they were convinced of the usefulness of graduate nurses. Under the circumstances, nursing became a respected profession which attracted highly educated and very able young women. Gradually a decline set in, however, and the profession is today engaged in the same struggle for status as it is elsewhere. See J. Shuval, "Perceived Role Components of Nursing in Israel," *American Sociological Review*, 28 (February, 1963), 37-46;

(the same is true in the case of engineers).[14] They had to face an unfavorable market situation without a reasonable chance to alleviate it by some original enterprise of their own. Medical services were monopolized by the American-sponsored Hadassa Organization and later the Histadruth Sick Fund. This left only some private ambulatory practice and two or three old-fashioned hospitals founded by local practitioners.

The Medical Association has never abandoned its claim both to represent the profession as a whole and to combine furthering the economic interests of its members with raising the standards of the profession, enforcing a code of ethics, and serving as the guardian of the public interest in matters of health. For twenty years its effort had seemed rather quixotic. In trying to protect the economic interests of its members, which in practice meant those in need of protection, it precluded the possibility of living up to its other aims. It tried to uphold the ideals of the old-time private practitioner and organize the profession in the manner of the European medical profession (i.e., lucrative individual practices, no competition between members, high ethical standards, much free aid to the needy, and voluntary public service) in a situation where the best hospitals were part of a foreign-controlled network which employed senior members from abroad and where an increasing proportion of patients was being drawn away from private practice by the Sick Fund.

The shrinkage of private practice created vicious competition among the doctors and considerable bitterness about the policy of the leading medical organizations (Hadassa, and later the Sick Fund). The large numbers of chronically underemployed private practitioners coveted the modest security of their salaried colleagues, while the few well-to-do practitioners resented their exclusion from hospital practice as well as the threat to their incomes represented by the cheap services of public and insurance medicine.

Since at the same time the Histadruth was interested in organizing the salaried doctors, and, in fact, compelled those employed in the Sick Fund to join a Histadruth-sponsored separate union, one would have expected the Medical Association to succumb to the pressure. Such a development often seemed imminent. There were times in the thirties when the Sick Fund doctors refused to cooperate, and the heads of hospital departments usually showed little interest in the association. Nevertheless, a formal split has never occurred, and as soon as the unemployment situation eased somewhat (during World War II when many doctors enlisted in the army and immigration came to a virtual standstill), the association managed to close its ranks.

---

and for the earlier period, Ben-David, *Hammivne....*

14. "L'ahar Arbaim Shana" ("After Forty Years"), interview with Engineer R. G. Pasovsky, *Handasa V'Adrikhaluth (Journal of the Association of Engineers and Architects in Israel)*, 20 (September-October, 1962), 311.

ENGINEERING

The engineering field was not monopolised by as few employers as was
medicine. Nevertheless, engineers suffered too from the meagerness of the
private market due to the channeling of most investments through public
bodies dominated by Histadruth or by the parties attached to Histadruth.

The engineers and architects reacted somewhat differently They established
two separate bodies, an association for the entire profession and a union
for the salaried part. At first the two bodies competed with each other, but
in 1948 the union surrendered its educational and training functions to the
association. Salaried engineers usually belong to both the union and the
association.

THE LAW

The development of the Bar Association was basically different and particularly interesting. The lawyers' problems were also less serious. Licensing
was conditional on the passing of a government-supervised law examination which, in addition to requiring knowledge of the rather complex
Palestinian law (an unorganic compound of Turkish and English law and
original Palestinian statutes), demanded good knowledge of English and of
either Arabic or Hebrew. This examination, the severity of which was con-
veniently manipulated, kept the numbers of licensed lawyers down to a
point where serious overcrowding was prevented. Furthermore, the colonial
government safeguarded the status of the lawyers, since it considered all
matters relating to law as part of its responsibility. This in itself made the
legal profession more a part of the external colonial society and rather
marginal to the Jewish community.

An additional reason for marginality was that while medicine, teaching,
or engineering were all considered essential services by the pioneering labor
movement (in spite of antiprofessional bias), legal services were not. The
Histadruth, like other unions, has an internal system of lay jurisdiction
and the tendency to such informal justice has been, and still is, quite
widespread in Israel. For the first few years after World War I there was
even an attempt to institute a network of lay courts which would act on the
basis of an undefined sense of popular justice and to exclude the official
courts and formal legal procedure. The fact that these so-called "courts
of peace" were not a success could be attributed partly to the fact that the
Jewish community was not sovereign.

In any case, the lack of any serious attempt to incorporate the legal
profession in the Histadruth has to be attributed to the lack of interest and
lack of appreciation of the service by the labor movement. In Palestine,
as elsewhere, there was no room for formal law in the socialist utopia.[15]

15. For a parallel see H. J. Berman, *Justice in Soviet Russia*, rev. ed. (Cambridge,
Mass.: Harvard University Press, 1963).

The unrealistic nature of this assumption went unnoticed there longer than elsewhere, owing to the fact that the practical need for formal law, like other "imperfections," could be attributed to the plural colonial aspects of Palestinian society.

All this made it possible for the Bar Association to emerge as the only professional organization whose structure and policies were strictly according to the ideal. National leadership consisted of the elite of the practicing profession, and local leadership was given to lawyers prominent in local affairs. The organization managed to keep its affairs separate from its members' personal political interests. In addition to the representation of Jewish national interests, the association's main activities were directed to improving legislation and legal administration. Its contribution was uncontroversial and was usually considered helpful.

The Impact of Independence

The establishment of the state of Israel in 1948 had several effects. The colonial society with its extraterritorial elites was abolished. The professional elites represented by the leadership of the Hadassa Medical Organization, the Hebrew University of Jerusalem, the Anglo-Palestinian judiciary and government legal service, etc., all became part and parcel of the local professional community. Professionals are now recruited locally and pay and conditions depend on the local economy and local politics.

The first result of these changed opportunities was a determined attempt by the Histadruth to take over all the professional organizations. The conditions justifying their autonomous existence in a plural colonial society disappeared. Important elements of the ruling socialist parties envisaged the imminent creation of a completely socialized economy, and the absorption of professional organizations was part of this general scheme.

The pressure exerted varied according to the extent to which the services involved were publicly organized. The teachers were under the greatest, the lawyers under the least pressure. Pressure came partly from within the organizations from the invariably large, but in no case decisive, proportion of members who accepted the idea of a socialist state and saw no danger to their professional interests in Histadruth affiliation, and partly from the government which, having become the direct employer of the teachers and of the second largest group of salaried doctors (in the government hospitals), made known its preference for Histadruth-affiliated unions.

TEACHING

The teachers' union succumbed immediately. Its differences with the Histadruth had nothing to do with educational policy, or even professional autonomy. By becoming part of the Histadruth it changed neither its structure, as it had been ruled over by a professional union oligarchy which fitted

into the Histadruth bureaucracy perfectly, nor its functions, i.e., defending
the security and seniority rights of the teachers by collective bargaining.
By the thirties it had practically become an industrial union representing
all "educational workers." Conceivably educational and bargaining functions could have been separated in 1948, as happened with engineers and
architects, but this step would probably have reduced the funds available
for each activity. There is no sign that joining the Histadruth has affected
either quality or quantity of such activities. The only important change
has been the rejection of the union's authority by the secondary school
teachers. Although their alienation from the union goes back to the thirties
(as noted above), they only began to bargain separately during the last
few years and they remain members of the union.

MEDICINE

A sharp, and for the development of the professional organizations in
Israel, crucial battle took place between the Medical Association on the
one hand and the combined forces of the Histadruth and the government
on the other. When the latter refused to negotiate with the Medical Association on the contract of government doctors and asked them to join the
Histadruth-sponsored government workers' union, the Association organized a strike which compelled the government to give in (1950-1951). In
this conflict, the Association obtained the support of the whole medical
profession, including that of the Sick Fund doctors. Since then the influence
of the Medical Association as the representative of salaried doctors has been
on the increase. There have been several disputes and strikes concerning
the salaries of doctors since 1951, and in no case has the authority of
the Association been seriously challenged. It has enjoyed the loyalty of its
members and has been relatively successful in gaining the support of public
opinion even for strikes.

THE LAW

Since the establishment of the state of Israel, the number of salaried lawyers has increased considerably. British government attorneys and legal
advisers to government departments have been replaced by local people
and all the services have expanded, introducing problems of collective
salary fixing. The suggestion of a separate union of salaried lawyers was
rejected in favor of government legal employees being represented through
a Histadruth-affiliated general union of government employees. By taking
exactly the opposite step, the lawyers have, however, achieved the same
result as the doctors. They are members of a single association which
represents the profession in all matters concerning legal practice. They
then have the added advantage that the profession appears to remain
above union types of conflict, since government lawyers also belong to a
general union which performs this "dirty" work for them. This more ad-

vantageous course was open to them because, unlike the doctors, most of the lawyers are not employed by public organizations. The main activities of the Association have continued to center around matters of legislation, the administration of the law, judicial practices, and professional ethics.

Other postindependence developments have been (1) the introduction of formal qualifications for, and protection of, medical specialties, and (2) legislation concerning the establishment of public medical and legal councils, which give considerable autonomy and rights of self-policing to these professions. While the interest of the respective professions in these matters does not need explanation, it is surprising that the legislation was passed by governments based principally on the support of socialist parties closely tied to the Histadruth, which has been in unceasing conflict with the professionals since 1950. It seems that these parties have dissociated this legislation, which indirectly strengthens the authority of the professional associations, from the conflict concerning union representation in salary negotiations. This may be taken as an indication of some public, non-political interest in preserving a kind of corporate identity and autonomy in these two professions.

The Emergence of Militance

Governmental attempts to create a unified wages and salaries policy, with all workers to be represented by the Histadruth, led to the 1951 doctors' strike and the combined resistance of all professional workers. Although a unified salary system may make sense in a socialized economy where the bulk of the labor force works for governmental or public bodies, professional people fear that Histadruth representation of their interests might result in a whittling away of the slight income differential which separates them from the bulk of white-collar workers.

Since the government's policy affects all professionals, all have united against it. They have adopted the methods of relatively militant unions. An informal coordinating committee was created in 1950-1951 for the purpose of combating the abolition of separate civil service professional grades. By now this committee is a more or less permanent affair. It organizes common resistance protests, memoranda, and usually strikes. In fact strikes have become as much part of the routine of collective bargaining of the professionals in Israel as of auto workers in America. The committee has managed to obtain the active support of all the university-trained professions, irrespective of whether their unions or associations are officially affiliated to the Histadruth. The organizations participating in this committee are: the Union of Engineers (affiliated with the Histadruth); the Medical Association (not affiliated); secondary school teachers (officially part of the Histadruth, affiliated with general teachers' union); government lawyers (officially part of the general Government Workers' Union); Association of Graduates in the Humanities and Social Sciences (affiliated); the Organization of University Professors and Lecturers (not affiliated); the Organization of University Instructors and Assistants (affiliated), and other small groups of salaried, university-trained professionals, such as social workers, dentists, veterinarians, and meteorologists (most of whom belong to general Histadruth-affiliated unions).

The committee is a very small-scale organization, dependent on the Medical Association for rudimentary office services. It has never attempted to replace, unify, or even serve as a central body for its constituent professional unions and associations, which jealously preserve their freedoms. Certainly any attempts at standardization would be against the committee's raison d'être, opposition to uniformity. Nevertheless, the committee's activities may lead to unintentional uniformity. The mere fact that negotiations are conducted through a committee representing the various associations reinforces a tendency to determine salaries of different types of professionals according to formal criteria, such as years of training or seniority—and these formal criteria tend to introduce uniformity.[16]

The committee's policies, on the other hand, recognize formal status differences within the various professions according to the level of training and specialization. The committee has made it possible for secondary school teachers and degree-holding social workers to rebel against the equalitarian general teachers' and social workers' unions, to seek greater emphasis on professional standards, such as reduction in class size and case loads, and to oppose their unions' policies of giving greatest weight to seniority, as opposed to formal specialized training. Furthermore, during this period the various specialties within medicine received formal recognition.

The final outcome of the conflict with the Histadruth cannot yet be predicted. The strained relationship has to be attributed partly to the emotional involvement of the current Histadruth leadership. Many of them are pioneers who abandoned studies out of real or feigned idealism and have a revulsion against any claim reminiscent of the superiority of the intellectual to the manual worker, even if this superiority is formulated in terms of returns on investment in education. This particular factor is bound to disappear as university-trained people become Histadruth leaders.[17]

There are real difficulties, of course, in attempting to represent manual and clerical workers (whose skills are relatively undifferentiated) and, at the

16. On the acceptance of a measure of standardization and further characteristics of this movement, see J. Ben-David, "The Rise of a Salaried Professional Class in Israel," *Transactions of the Third World Congress of Sociology* (London, 1956), pp. 302-310.

17. A somewhat similar takeover by career-oriented professionals from mission-oriented ones has been recorded in the United States by Harold L. Wilensky, *Intellectuals in Labor Unions* (Glencoe, Ill.: The Free Press, 1956), pp. 111-159.

same time, people with specialized training. Unlike the former group, the professional finds his best interests lie in emphasizing "product differentiation," rather than strength of organization.

The difficulty here is not ideological, but organizational: whatever social values people choose to adopt—barring the return to a state where specialized skill is not needed—the objective differences between professional and routine work cannot be eliminated. Attempts at single organization are bound to create tension and continued attempts to subordinate the interests of one category to another. Israel's professionals seem to be convinced today that, since in a single organization they are bound to be minority, it is their interests rather than those of manual workers which would suffer. This is why they almost unanimously support the autonomous policies of their respective unions and the Coordinating Committee, even though many are socialists in political conviction.[18] Under nondemocratic socialism or nondemocratic labor organizations, the inevitable takeover of leadership by professionals may, of course, tilt the balance in favor of the professional minority.

Types of Professional Organization

The large majority of Israel's professionals are salaried employees and practically all of these belong to organizations which are unions in the sense that they bargain collectively and use strikes to advance their economic interests.[19] Except in the cases of engineers, lawyers, and university professors, the unions also act as professional organizations. They publish journals and arrange meetings, conferences, and lectures designed to advance professional knowledge and public education; they represent the point of view of the profession on legislative and other matters.

Within this general framework three different types of organization have evolved.

1. Teachers, nurses, and social workers have organizations which are full-fledged unions in everything but name. They are run by career union organizers as part of the Histadruth. Union goals are determined in large part by the salary and wages policy worked out between the Histadruth and the government for publicly owned or publicly controlled industries[20] As a result, individual salary policies resemble those of clerical or manual

18. This is shown clearly in a forthcoming attitude study of Israeli engineers by Lester Seligman, as well as in the virtually complete observance of strikes by all the professional employees.

19 The only significant nonunion salaried groups are judges and professional employees of private law and chartered accountant firms—usually young people who are trainees and/or prospective partners.

20. For estimates of the overwhelming share of the socialized sector, see Haim Barkay, *The Public, Histadruth, and Private Sectors in the Israeli Economy,* Falk Project for Economic Research in Israel, Sixth Report (1961-1963), pp. 1-87.

workers' unions in their stress on relative equality, seniority, job security, and collective benefits. These unions emphasize the special "missions" and high moral and intellectual standing of these particular professions. However, it has not been possible—nor have the unions tried very hard—to resist dilution of professional standards.

2. In contrast, the organizations of university-trained professionals jealously safeguard the independence of their actions and policies from the Histadruth (whether they formally belong to it or not), insist on representation by professionally active colleagues, and are willing to cooperate only with other professionals in the loose and semiformal framework of the "Coordinating Committee." Their main aim is to maintain and, where possible, increase the income differential between professionals and other workers. One of the means typically employed is obtaining recognition for different grades of qualification and levels of specialization, thus adding higher salary grades to the existing scales of professional salaries.

3. In addition to following the same policies regarding independent action, doctors and lawyers have gained official recognition of the corporate status of their professions. This allows them important powers of internal legislation and jurisdiction in matters of professional practice ("professional ethics"). This recognition was gained in spite of ideologically based opposition to special privileges for professional workers. Other professional groups—except perhaps certain categories of social workers and clinical psychologists—have been much less persistent in their efforts to obtain such privileges, and none has had the success of the lawyers and the doctors.

Why These Differences

Differences in organization and policy can be explained by the existence of two unconnected components in professionalism which are of central importance in Israel as well as elsewhere.

SKILL

The first component is a high level of scientific, scholarly, or artistic training and skill, usually—but not necessarily—connected with university studies. Even though many engineers and doctors perform a fairly routine job, they are expected not only to master certain techniques and command a certain amount of existing knowledge but also to show initiative, inventiveness, and originality. Consequently, their roles are defined more flexibly than those of other workers and their careers usually have a wider span. In addition, they develop fewer institutional loyalties than other workers, probably because the character of their training creates a relatively greater feeling of community among them. As a result, they often have more commitment to profession than to place of work. Everywhere, in a variety of ways, professionals have resisted the traditional kind of bureaucratization which tends to treat human work as composed of interchangeable units. Those whose work can be done singlehandedly, such as doctors and lawyers, have, in countries where they could, resisted salaried employment. Others—university professors, researchers, and engineers—who cannot work privately, have adopted other means of loosening organizational restraints, such as faculty self-government or joining management.

These occupational patterns seem to be inconsistent with trade unionism, since the professional seeks to maximize professional potential—and presumably earning power—in a flexible way. Where, however, income and basic working conditions are determined by political considerations, rather than by relatively free economic forces, professionals apparently feel the need for some sort of union. A good example of this sort of union is the American Association of University Professors in the United States, which exists in one of the highest level professions which is exposed to political pressure. The Israeli brand of professional unionism is a similar attempt —much nearer to complete unionization—to secure for salaried professionals more autonomy in the determination of pay and conditions than is enjoyed by other salaried employees. These unions arose in a centrally controlled socialist economy where income distribution is an openly declared political process. Such independent unionism has been successful only in the higher professions, however. Those lower on the scale of education and skill, such as teachers and nurses—in Israel both professions still consist predominantly of persons not possessing university education—did not manage to maintain independence for their organizations and followed Histadruth policies.

CORPORATE AUTONOMY

A second component of professionalism, important only in the professions dealing with human affairs, is public recognition of the right to self-regulation on a nationwide basis. As pointed out by Parsons concerning law and medicine, personal trust is a major tool of these professions and their peculiar organization is designed to safeguard it.[21] They have to solicit the active cooperation of autonomous clients and accept responsibilities with potential legal consequences. The relative lack of success of teachers, nurses, and social workers in obtaining public recognition of their corporate standing is probably due to the fact that their work is not regarded as sophisticated enough to be given much autonomy.

THE SENSE OF MISSION

Another characteristic which is often connected with professionalism is that the work involves performance of an important public mission. This, however, turns out to be of secondary importance. The idea has helped

21. See T. Parsons, *The Social System* (Glencoe, Ill.: The Free Press, 1951), chap. X, and his "A Sociologist Looks at the Legal Profession," in *Essays In Sociological Theory*, rev. ed. (Glencoe, Ill.: The Free Press, 1954), pp. 370-385.

occupations such as teaching, nursing, and social work establish honorable images and claims for professional recognition. But, as long as the orientation is not accompanied by a sophisticated technology, the missionary ideology more often than not tends to hurt rather than help attempts at professionalization.[22] Elementary school teachers and nurses, for example, have both succeeded in convincing the public of the importance and necessity of their services. Rightly or wrongly, however, people assume that beyond a certain point (which can be attained relatively cheaply), further improvement in the quality of service is not needed or not possible. Attempts at improvement are resisted as immoral efforts to raise the price of an essential service and turn what ought to be a mission into a business. The only way the quality of manpower or, indeed, the supply of manpower, can be maintained, given such a set of circumstances, is by using cheap female labor and appealing to a certain kind of idealism to which women, badly handicapped in occupational careers, are sensitive.

When idealism fails to supply the manpower, recourse may be taken to bureaucratic measures. Governments create relatively cheap training institutions, "recruit" into them as many candidates as possible, and try to mass produce teachers. As their qualifications are poor, they have to be directed and supervised by inspectors and central offices. Education becomes a centrally directed operation, where the teacher is not considered as a person using his own knowledge and imagination, but as one who carries out orders under a uniform plan conceived for the nation as a whole. The ideology of mission has, in these cases, the same effect as in the army. It is a factor of deprofessionalization and hierarchic bureaucratization.

Where, on the other hand, the need for technological specialization is recognized, mission does not seriously interfere with professional autonomy. Doctors in bureaucratic settings, or specialists needed by the military, have not had much difficulty maintaining professional status.[23] Social work also seems to be an exception. In spite of its missionary ideology and, with few exceptions, not very advanced technology, it has had more success in getting professional recognition than teachers or nurses. The reasons may be that (1) social workers have been less successful in convincing the public of the importance of their mission, so that people care less that raising professional standards may reduce the general availability of the service, and (2) the element of trust is more important—social workers have to solicit the active cooperation of adults who can walk out on them.

Explanations Disproved

The above explanations of professionalism are plausible, since the changes which have occurred through time have disproved alternative

22. See Wilensky, "The Professionalization of Everyone?"
23. In fact professionalism is increasing in the military as a result of the need for

explanations. Had the corporate autonomy of certain professions been a survival of once-acquired privileges, then in Israel the teachers, nurses, and lawyers alone would possess such autonomy. Instead, however, the doctors managed to acquire it under most adverse circumstances, while teachers and nurses lost it. Teachers failed even before they surrendered the autonomy of their organization to the Histadruth. The theoretically significant thing about this development is that teachers and nurses ended up with a status similar to their counterparts elsewhere, in spite of the fact that they started out with practically complete professional recognition. This shows that professional status is not the function of history, but of factors inherent in the nature of the service, or at least of the public view of the service.

If the different arrangements in Israel were a function of purely economic interests, then doctors, like engineers, would have split openly into two competing organizations before 1948. Instead, the only separatist organization of doctors was the union of those employed by the Histadruth-owned Sick Fund, a company union for all intents and purposes, and even the members of this union never completely severed their allegiance to the Medical Association. Similarly, on purely economic grounds the salaried lawyers should have formed a separate union in 1948, as did the engineers. Instead, they insisted on the unity of the Bar Association.

This is not to say that economic conditions had no effect. The reverse is true. There was very great tension in the Medical Association between salaried and private doctors in the thirties, and there were suggestions to create a separate union of salaried lawyers in 1950. But other factors determined the final outcome.

Conclusion

The Israeli case provides independent evidence on the limits and conditions of professionalization. Some believe that all occupations will eventually become professional. It seems to me that the pattern is characteristic only of occupations with a high level of education and skill, roughly of university or equivalent standard. My data also indicate that corporate autonomy of a professional group (as opposed to an individual's autonomy in his work) is an important characteristic only of the professions which deal with matters of great personal trust and presumably involve legal responsibility. Finally, the situation in Israel indicates that some features of unionism (virtually compulsory membership and strikes) will be accepted by professionals when they feel their interests can be defended only by political pressure. In many Western countries the hesitation to adopt such measures is probably due to a tradition which makes working-class patterns of action

---

greater technological expertise. See Morris Janowitz, *The Professional Soldier* (Glencoe, Ill.: The Free Press, 1960).

not respectable and, therefore, politically inefficient.[24] Where these traditions are weakening, militant unionism is becoming a legitimate means for professionals.

24. This in my view explains the difference between the fortunes of engineering unionism in Israel as compared with the United States. As we have seen, engineers have reacted in Israel with complete rationality to the changing market and political situation. In the United States too, they seem to constitute a rationally acting group; it has not paid them to unionize, except for a very brief period in the late forties. See George Strauss, "Professional or Employee-Oriented: Dilemma for Engineering Unions," *Industrial and Labor Relations Review*, 17 (July, 1964), 519-533.

3

CHARLES LESLIE

The Professionalization of Ayurvedic and Unani Medicine

We come to most human affairs assuming that we know, in general, the direction of history. Our assumptions in this regard provide the context for our understanding of and curiosity about events. For example, if I discovered that one of my colleagues believed in astrology, that person would appear to me to be eccentric, and my curiosity would be aroused by the anachronistic character of his belief. In India I would be less inclined to perceive the believer in astrology as an eccentric, but his belief would seem no less anachronistic. Two principles are at work in these responses. In the first place there is the principle of cultural relativity by which I recognize differences between academic subcultures in America and India. Astrology has social and religious uses throughout Indian society that it lacks in the United States. The second principle limits cultural relativity by assuming that knowledge is cumulative, that it manifests elements of self-correction, and that it changes the conditions of life for the whole species. Thus, belief in astrology in New York or Calcutta would appear anachronistic.

Henry Adams expressed the direction of history by contrasting the Virgin and the Dynamo, collective representations of medieval and modern societies, which like the positive and negative poles of a magnet drew men's lives, like iron filings, along the lines of historical forces that traced their fields of power. Nowadays, social scientists analyze similar historical forces, though usually with less irony and less poetry than Adams. Mankind, in our view, is being shaped by processes of secularization, urbanization, industrialization, commercialization, modernization, rationalization, and so

Reprinted from *Transactions of the New York Academy of Sciences*, 30, No. 4 (1968), pp. 559-572, © The New York Academy of Sciences; 1968, by permission of the author and publisher.

The research upon which the paper is based has been sponsored by grants from the Center for Medical Research and Training of Johns Hopkins University, School of Hygiene and Public Health. W. T. Jones read the manuscript and helped clarify its language and ideas.

on. Our job is to analyze these processes, asking how they vary in degree, how they are causally related, and what consequences they have for the quality of life in various times and places.

The professionalization of occupations, knowledge, and the arts is one of the pervasive, long-term processes that orient the evolution of modern society. A generation ago A. M. Carr-Saunders and P. A. Wilson published the first comprehensive study of professionalization processes in English society. To them a primary criterion of professionalism was "the application of an intellectual technique to the ordinary business of life, acquired as the result of prolonged and specialized training."[1] In medicine, law, engineering, and various other professions, they traced the development of institutional structures that were designed to improve technical knowledge, educate novices, regulate standards of practice, exclude the unqualified and improve the status of qualified practitioners. Above all, these activities were initiated by professional associations.

Carr-Saunders and Wilson wrote,

> a technique may exist and men may practice it, and yet there may be no profession. Just as a number of families in primitive society do not form a State, so a number of men, though they perform similar functions, do not make a profession if they remain in isolation. A profession can only be said to exist when there are bonds between the practitioners, and these bonds can take but one shape—that of formal association.[2]

Accordingly, the evolution of contemporary professions has been largely the elaboration of institutional structures, some of which go back to the 11th century "when a great movement toward association began to sweep like a wave over the cities of Europe, "giving rise to medieval guilds and to the first universities.[3] Out of these institutions the traditional professions slowly began to assume new forms.

As a result of the rise in modern science in the sixteenth century, fields of knowledge began to develop which new professions cultivated and drew upon. But, according to Carr-Saunders and Wilson, "for some 200 years the scientific movement made so few additions to the arts that it exerted little influence upon the existing professions and brought no new professions into being."[4] They saw the Industrial Revolution as the great watershed in the growth of professionalism. As they put it, "Then the flood-gates opened. New vocations arose and filled the ears of the public with demands for places alongside the ancient professions."[5] Large-scale industrial organization, with the accompanying increase in the scale of other economic, political, and educational structures, radically changed

1. *The Professions* (Oxford: Clarendon Press, 1933), p. 491).
2. *Ibid.*, p. 298.
3. *Ibid.*, p. 289.
4. *Ibid.*, p. 296.
5. *Ibid.*, p. 295.

the division of labor and the dependence of society upon new, progressively specialized skills.

In the conclusion of their study, Carr-Saunders and Wilson predicted that

under a system of large-scale commercial and industrial organization, all those who occupy the important positions will gradually come within professional association, or at least under professional influences. . . . science advances and techniques multiply. In the long run technical advance implies an increase in the number of those doing more or less specialized intellectual work relative to the number of those who are engaged in manual labour or in unspecialized intellectual routine. It may be that, while the extension of professionalism upwards and outwards will be fairly rapid, its extension downwards, though gradual and almost imperceptible, will be continuous. Thus, taking the long view, the extension of professionalism over the whole field seems in the end not impossible.[6]

In their view, with the weakening of old forms of association based upon religion and locality, professional associations would progressively assume greater importance in the total organization of society. It is in this context that they suggested the way professionalism could contribute to the quality of life. They remarked how size, complex organization, and concentration of power of modern communities provoke feelings of helplessness, oppression, and alienation in many individuals. Professional associations might compensate for these deficiencies by giving individuals a sense of autonomy and responsibility.

If men found in vocational associations their permanent anchorage and shelter, they could set out from those secure positions to shape organizations into instruments for the fulfillment of their purposes. That which is important is that organizations should be regarded as instruments to be created and remodeled where necessary by those who, by these means, render specialized services: schools by teachers, newspapers by journalists, and so on.[7]

Men with special knowledge and skills, joined with other men devoted to similar vocations, would have something of the status of free-lance workers, in contrast to workers dependent on particular organizations.

The man who belongs to a profession which has won for itself prestige and a position of dignity, may pass from the service of one organization to that of another. Though he remains salaried all his life, he takes his stand upon his proved competence and experience; he serves one client after another much as does a free-lance worker. He is attached primarily to his profession whence he goes out, as occasion may offer, to render his services in some cooperative organization, and whither he returns.[8]

Thus, when Carr-Saunders and Wilson published their monumental study in 1933 they looked forward to the professionalization of everyone,

6. *Ibid.*, pp. 493-494.
7. *Ibid.*, p. 501.
8. *Ibid.*, p. 502.

or at least of everyone who was anyone. Recently, Harold Wilensky has challenged this notion. Though he admits "a general tendency for occupations to seek professional status," he asserts that only thirty or forty occupations have in fact become fully professionalized. Some occupations such as social work and city planning are still in process. Others, like nursing and optometry, are borderline professions. But many occupations assert claims to professional status without success.[9]

Although students of occupations describe events among realtors, barbers, and taxi drivers as if the whole labor force is becoming professionalized, to Wilensky "the idea that all occupations move toward professional authority—this notion of the professionalization of everyone—is a bit of sociological romance."[10]

The concept of professionalization is subject to controversy of this kind because it is a polytypical concept.[11] That is, it includes several parameters, and application of the concept to a particular case requires judgmental determination of the relationships and relative significance of these parameters. This does not mean that the concept should be abandoned for narrowly defined terms, but that like other concepts close to ordinary language usage, it must be used with the mental flexibility called common sense.

Harold Wilensky's skepticism about the professionalization of everyone has the value of focusing attention on the barriers to professionalism, and on the mixture of professional organizations and role orientations with other organizational structures and role orientations. Wilensky's ideas are, on the whole, compatible with those of Carr-Saunders and Wilson, and will help us consider the professionalization of Ayurvedic and Unani medicine in India. Our procedure will be first, to indicate the nature of these traditional systems, and secondly, to outline the history of the effort to improve their professional status. Finally, with reference to Wilensky's analysis, we will consider several barriers to their professionalization.

While Hindu scholars claim that all medical knowledge originated in India, Western scholars have assumed that Greek science diffused throughout the ancient world to become the basis for all subsequent development. A leading French Sanskritist, Jean Filliozat, has sought to correct both of these ideas by arguing that elements of Indian medicine said to have been borrowed from Hellenic science are based on widespread cosmological notions of preclassical antiquity that were independently elaborated in India. What in fact happened was that "the two medical traditions, Indian and Greek alike, developed in a parallel fashion."[12] Similarly, the diffusion

9. Harold L. Wilensky, "The Professionalization of Everyone?" *American Journal of Sociology* 70 (1964), 141.

10. *Ibid.*, p. 156.

11. Morton Beckner, *The Biological Way of Thought* (New York: Columbia University Press, 1960).

12. Jean Filliozat, *La doctrine classique de la médecine indienne* (Paris: Imprimerie Nationale, 1949), p. 6.

of classical Indian medicine throughout South and Southeast Asia, into Central Asia, and its influence through the spread of Buddhism on the medicine of China and Japan, are historical phenomena parallel to the diffusion of Greek medicine through the Western and the Near Eastern world.

The great tradition of Ayurvedic practice refers to three primary Sanskrit collections: the Caraka Samhitā, which in its present form goes back to the first century of this era; the Suśruta Saṁhitā, about the fourth century; and the texts of Vāgbhaṭa, about the eighth century. These works are the foundation of aṣṭāṅga ayurvēda, the eight-limbed science of longevity, including surgery (śalya), internal medicine (kāya cikitsā), eye-ear-nose-and-throat (śalakya), pediatrics (kaumāra bhṛtya), treatment for poisons (agada), illness inflicted by demons (bhūta vidyā), the maintenance of health (rasāyana), aphrodisiacs and the restoration of youth (vājīkarana). The Caraka Saṁhitā is supposed to excel in kāya cikitsā or internal medicine, Susruta in surgery, and Vāgbhaṭa, who claimed to synthesize the best work of the earlier authorities, is said to excel in the principles of medicine (sūtra).

Other works are important, particularly Māhava's Nidāna, a thesis on the diagnosis of illness composed in the twelfth century. In Tamilnad, vernacular texts emphasizing alchemy provide the authority for a variant of Ayurveda called Siddha. Although the three primary collections by Caraka, Suśruta, and Vāgbhaṭa prescribe detailed examination of patients, the idea that a patient's condition is expressed by his pulse apparently gained popularity in medieval times, and pulse reading came to symbolize the art and authority of the Ayurvedic physician. For example, Kaviraj Gangadhär Roy, a nineteenth century Bengali physician, is said to have known the entire course of a patient's affliction from his pulse.[13]

The argument we are developing about the professionalization of Ayurveda requires further description of the traditional system.

Ayurvedic theories as they are taught by learned practitioners in relation to the classic texts are based on Nyāya, Vaiśeṣika, and Sāṅkhya philosophies. They conceive of man as a conglomerate (samūdaya) of the panchabhūtas, or five elements: earth, water, fire, air, and ether. There are subtle and material forms of the elements, each element possessing five subtle and five material forms. The physiological expression of these elements are the dhātus: chyle, blood, flesh, fat, bone, marrow, and semen. Semen (ojas) stored in the heart and diffused through the body sustains its vital tone. In addition, the tridosas, or three humors, in their role as supporters of the body are called dhātus. The aggregation of elements in the human body is a microcosmic version of the universe in which an equilibrium of the humors, wind (vāyu), bile (pitta), and mucus (kapha

---

13. Prabhakar Chatterjee, "Kaviraj Gangadhar Roy Kaviratna: Who Inundated British India with Ayurvedic Waters Brought from Heaven," *Nagarjun* (Calcutta) 2 (February, 1959), pp. 400-401.

or śleṣman) is necessary to health. The nature and severity of illnesses are diagnosed according to the dominant humor and the number of humors involved. Filliozat writes,

> Therapeutics is dominated by the ideas conceived about calming or stimulating action of drugs, aliments, diet, and habitat upon wind, bile, and mucus. . . .Once the role played by such and such a doṣa has been determined, the Indian doctor must prescribe a medication whose effects are antagonistic to those of the doṣa in question. . . . . The theory was supple and vague enough to accommodate itself to the data of pure experience, appearing to dominate them. In effect, the action of the remedies was known through usage, and if a given drug calmed a given morbid manifestation reputedly due to the wind, this drug would be classified among the antagonists of the wind, even if they had to invent an explanation of this fact. It was thus quite definitely experience which directed the choice of medications and the general theory was only an effort to explain after the fact the mechanism of the normal functioning of the body, pathological accidents, and the action of treatment. The Ayurvedic system is, therefore, a dogmatism interpreting experience.[14]

Ayurvedic practitioners would, of course, dispute our description of their science. They claim that the Sanskritic vocabulary cannot be translated as I have done, using the word "humor" for dosa, "wind" for vāyu, and so on. Since the theories of Ayurveda are for them eternal truths, they cannot be translated into demonstratably obsolete or false propositions. They reject, also, the imputation that their therapies are grounded in empiricism. They claim thousands of years of accumulated empirical knowledge, but they hold that this knowledge has accumulated only because it has been guided by theories of the panchabhūta, tridosa, etc.

Whatever one thinks about these claims, it is a fact that the vast majority of Indians still resort to Ayurvedic treatment, along with other forms of therapy. Even Indian doctors trained in modern medicine occasionally use medications, ideas of diet, and other elements from Ayurveda. Some of them refer patients to Ayurvedic physicians and accept patients referred to them by Ayurvedic physicians. Also, it should be said that European residents in India sometimes resort to Ayurvedic treatment, usually on the advice of Indian friends, and, in the cases one hears about, with satisfactory results.

The point is that various people, some of them with considerable training and experience, testify that there are useful Ayurvedic therapies.

However, contrary to Filliozat, it is probably not true that experience primarily guided the creation and selection of Ayurvedic therapies. Putting aside the placebo effect and the achievement of a certain level of efficacious knowledge, the classical Hindu medicine, like Greek and Chinese medicine, was often guided by its theories rather than by experience. To the outside observer its fancifulness indicates this quite clearly. For example,

14. Filliozat, *op. cit.*, p. 24.

one of the earliest known Ayurvedic manuscripts recommends a preparation as follows:

> The two truth-seeking Asvins, the divine physicians, honored by the Devas, have declared the following oil which promotes plumpness, relieves all diseases, is fit for a king, and is as good as ambrosia. . . . At the time of Pushya, after having said prayers, performed purificatory rites, and asked the Brahman's blessing in a few words, take out liquorice-roots grown in a favorable place. Of the fresh juice of these roots let a clever physician take four patra, and add four pala each of the following drugs. . . .[15]

The list that follows is quite elaborate and though we do not know to what plants many of the Sanskrit names refer, an abbreviated account will give the idea. To the juice of licorice roots one should add Tinospora cordifolia; knots of rootstalks of lotus; asparagus racemosus; emblic myrobalan; the bark of five trees with a milky sap; roots of Kusa, Sara, and Virana; dates; coconut; plumbago-root and, the author added, "other astringent, sweet, or cooling drugs, as many as may be obtainable." All this was to be boiled in water until it was reduced to one-eighth the original quality. Then pastes made from powders of numerous substances were to be added, including Bala, Nagabala, mercury, cardamons, cinnamon, blue lotus, saffron, red and white sandal, coral, conch-shell, moonstone, sapphire, silver, gold, pearls, and so on and on. Oil, milk, and rice vinegar should be added and the whole mixture boiled gently, allowed to cool, and boiled again a "hundred or even a thousand times." It is ready for use when exposure to the sun stiffens the oil. Then, after purificatory rites, it can be taken orally, used as a liniment, or administered through the nose, anus, and urethra.[16]

In the classic tradition, members of all twice-born castes could receive Ayurvedic training from a master physician, but only Brahmins should be taught the sacred knowledge required to grasp completely the metaphysical principles of the science. In the traditional society of the 18th and early 19th centuries, Ayurvedic physicians belonged to various castes, even where, as in Bengal and Kerala, there were castes for whom medicine was a traditional occupation. A few practitioners were learned scholars of the ancient texts, others possessed limited and, not infrequently, garbled knowledge, while the majority were folk practitioners. Practitioners were often known for special therapies which supposedly descended through many generations as closely guarded family secrets. Secret nostrums continue to be a part of Ayurvedic lore. As I write this paper, I notice a report in the *New York Times*[17] that credits Dr. Chandrasekhar, who heads the family planning program for the government of India, with having solicited the aid of

15. A. F. Rudolf Hoernle, *The Bower Manuscript* (Calcutta: Archeological Survey of India, New Imperial Series XII, 1893-1912), p. 106.

16. *Ibid.*, pp. 106-107.

17. Kasturi Rangan, *New York Times*, January 19, 1968, p. 67.

Ayurvedic physicians. It notes that "government laboratories are processing several of the 'secret' formulas offered by these men for contraception."

Traditional medical education followed the pattern, so admired in India,
in which the student entered into a deep spiritual relationship with his guru,
symbolized by an initiation rite. He joined the household of his teacher and
was supported by him through years of apprenticeship. During this time he
observed the master diagnose illnesses and acted as a compounder in preparing medications suited to each case. In theory, at least, each individual's illness was unique, varying according to the humoral character of
the patient, astrological conditions, climate, and other circumstances.
The large number of variables emphasized the tacit knowledge of the master
in grasping and evaluating their relationships, and tacit knowledge was
learned by example rather than by exposition. More teachable were the
medical texts, which the student memorized and the guru explicated. By
the eighteenth and nineteenth centuries, a major portion of the textural
material was no longer practiced. For example, the surgery and dissection
described in the texts had been entirely abandoned, though the Sanskritic
verses describing them were still memorized and speculated about. Similarly, much botanical lore had become unintelligible, but the verses were
memorized for their own sake and subjected to undisciplined interpretation.

I have taken a good deal of space to define the subject of professionalization and to describe the traditional system of Ayurveda with the hope that
by laying this foundation we will be able to move with greater understanding and rapidity through the modern history of Ayurvedic and Unani
medicine, focusing on the effort to professionalize the status of learned Vaids
and Hakims.

I have waited until now to mention the Unani system because, with
notable exceptions, Vaids, or Ayurvedic physicians, rather than Hakims
have been the more persistent and active proponents of professionalization.
The word Unani means Greek, and Unani Tibbia is based upon Aristo-
telian science elaborated in Islamic centers of learning, and brought to
India by the spread of Islamic civilization. In practice, Ayurvedic and
Unani medicine have greatly influenced each other. In the rest of this paper
I will often refer to them together as indigenous medicine in contrast to
allopathic, or modern, medicine. Modern medicine is called allopathy because the nineteenth-century system of homeopathy is extensively used by
urbanized Indians.

With the exception of surgery there was little to choose between European
and indigenous medicine until the nineteenth century. A sixteenth-century
visitor to Goa remarked that "the Portuguese, from the Viceroy and Arch-
bishop down to the monks and friars, put more trust in the 'heathen
physicians' than in their own doctors."[18] During the seventeenth and eigh-

18. L. S. S. O'Malley, *Modern India and the West* (London: Oxford University Press,
1941), p. 635.

teenth centuries various European surgeons were employed at the courts of ruling princes,[19] and in 1839 Sir William Sleeman observed that "The educated classes sought the aid of European surgeons wherever they could obtain it, surgery being an art in which they felt that they were helpless; but they had no confidence in the prescriptions of European physicians and preferred the services of their countrymen."[20]

Indigenous physicians were employed by the British as early as 1690, and by 1762 the East India Company's Bengal army employed nineteen native doctors. In the Madras Presidency, too, Vaids and Hakims found employment with the Company, and from the middle of the eighteenth century were titled Sub-Assistant Surgeons.[21]

By the beginning of the nineteenth century there were proposals to use indigenous physicians on the cruisers of the Bombay Marine and to train Compounders for similar service. In Calcutta approval was given to a plan to train Indians "as compounders and dressers, and ultimately as Apothecaries and Sub-Assistant Surgeons," and in Madras an institution referred to as the "medical pupil establishment" was enlarged from thirty to forty boys, to be trained as Apothecaries.[22]

The most notable of these developments—because it was at the center of a policy struggle within the British administration between the Orientalists, who wanted to protect traditional institutions, and the Anglicists, who wanted to introduce European knowledge by means of English language schools— was the Native Medical Institution in Calcutta. Dr. John Tytler, who became Superintendent of the school shortly after it was established in 1822, was an active member of the Orientalist faction. The purpose of the school was to combine indigenous medicine with training in modern anatomy and medical skills. Instruction in modern subjects was in Urdu and students were educated in Ayurveda at the Sanskrit College or in Unani Tibbia at the Calcutta Madrassa. In 1835, the Anglicists secured the patronage of the company for a system of English-language education. The Native Medical Institution was abolished and a new medical college was founded. Pandit Madhusudan Gupta, who had taught medical courses at the Sanskrit College, joined the new college and became the first Indian in modern times to dissect a human body.[23] During the decade of its existence, the Native Medical Institution trained 166 "native doctors" in the combined system of indigenous and European medicine. In 1839, the Company employed 305 "native doctors" in Bengal Presidency, of which 124 had been trained by the short-lived Native Medical Institution.[24]

19. D. G. Crawford, *A History of the Indian Medical Service, 1600-1913* (London: W. Thacker, 1914), vol. 1, pp. 7-16.
20. L. S. S. O'Malley, *op. cit.*, p. 636.
21. D. G. Crawford, *op. cit.*, vol. 2, pp. 101-109
22. *Ibid.*
23. *Ibid.*, vol. 2, p. 438.
24. K. C. Sarbadhikari, "Western Medical Education in India During the Early Days of British Occupation," *Indian Journal of Medical Education* (New Delhi) 1:1 (1961), 32.

The point of this abbreviated history is that by the first quarter of the nineteenth century there had arisen a series of new bureaucratic statuses which were occupied by practitioners of indigenous medicine who also drew upon knowledge of European medicine with various degrees of eclecticism we cannot now reconstruct. Some had been trained in apprenticeship relations to European practitioners, while others had received more formal training in institutions especially created for that purpose. Not all of these individuals spent their whole careers in the employ of the company, and there had grown up in the centers of British administration a class of private practitioners of indigenous medicine with some knowledge of European techniques. These Vaids and Hakims served the local Indian population and, by virtue of their acquaintance with European medicine, claimed superior status to other indigenous practitioners. In Bengal, caste Vaidyas came into conflict with Brahmins, who by tradition were supposed to practice Ayurveda as a philanthropic avocation but who increasingly adopted medicine as an occupation. The earliest record of an association of indigenous practitioners is of the Native Medical Society, founded in Calcutta in 1832 "with the object of confining medical practice to members of the Vaidya caste."[25]

We have seen, in addition, that the new native medical institutions had their advocates as well as their critics. The Orientalists found virtues in Ayurveda and Unani Tibbia and were more tolerant of their foibles than were the Anglicists. Quackery, obsolete theories, the legitimate course of training for various kinds of practice, state patronage for educational institutions, and positions in the medical services of governmental bureaucracies—all these perennial issues in the professionalization of occupations were contested with reference to Ayurvedic and Unani medicine in the early nineteenth century, and continue to be contested to the present day.

Another thread of this story of the professionalization of indigenous medicine is illustrated by the career of a renowned practitioner, Kaviraj Gangadhār Roy. Kaviraj, prince of poetry, is the common title of Bengali Vaidyas. Gangadhar was born in 1798 and was trained by a guru in the traditional manner before moving, when he was twenty-one years old, to Calcutta. A member of the Vaidya caste, he established a successful practice and remained in Calcutta for sixteen years. We mentioned earlier his fame for knowledge of the pulse, but legend has it that his insight was so great that he did not even have to read a patient's pulse; by a glance he could penetrate the nature of the most obscure maladies. He opposed the Hindu social reformers of the period, debating the Principal of the Sanskrit College on the textural authority for sacred injunctions against widow remarriage. He did not learn English, and he is said to have abandoned Calcutta in 1835 because the first dissection of a human cadaver by Kaviraj

25. D. G. Crawford, *op. cit.*, vol. 2, p. 453.

Gupta was honored by a 50-gun salute. He was, in short, a traditionalist, and refused to accept Brahmins or other non-Vaidya caste students (chela) in the traditional establishment for Sanskritic instruction, or tol, that he founded on the eastern bank of the Ganges after leaving Calcutta. But—and this is the point—he initiated another important step in the professionalization of Ayurveda by purchasing a printing press and publishing his commentaries on the Caraka Samhitä. He moved the press to his tol and continued to edit, write, and publish Ayurvedic and other Sanskritic works until his death in 1885, by which time his disciples were spread throughout Bengal and he was known to Sanskritic scholars in other parts of South Asia. A guru with a printing press was something new to Ayurvedic tradition.

Gangadhär's students and the students of his students constitute many of the late nineteenth- and twentieth-century innovators who gave Bengal the reputation in other parts of India for leading a movement to professionalize or, as they began to say, to revive the glories of Ayurveda. Some of these innovations would have given Gangadhär the shakes, for later generations have been modernizers even while claiming the mantle of traditionalism. They have reinterpreted the ancient texts to discover in them the modern theory of the circulation of the blood, the germ theory of disease, contemporary anatomy, the vitamin conception of diet, and so on. They have founded colleges, open to the public, and companies that manufacture Ayurvedic preparations for commercial distribution in modern packagings and in such modern forms as pills, capsules, and hypodermic injections. And, where possible, they have sent their sons to get university educations in the English language, frequently in allopathic medicine or in one of the natural sciences.

The professionalization of Ayurvedic and Unani medicine became a self-conscious revival movement after the setback of the decision to found English language medical colleges. It received the patronage of rulers of native states, the Arya Samaj movement, and the emerging class of bourgeois entrepreneurs and Western-educated Indians. In the last decades of the nineteenth century it gained momentum. One pattern was for a practitioner to have his son educated in allopathic medicine, and for father and son to engage in the combined practice of indigenous and modern medicine. They would found a company to manufacture indigenous medicines, a school to give training in both systems, and a journal or other publication to advertise their enterprise.

For example, the Adi-Ayurvedic Aushadhalaya was founded in 1870 by Kaviraj Binod Lal Sen, whose son continued the business. In 1897, in a journal advertising its products, he published this typical complaint:

> Remembering the ancient glories of his caste, the Editor. . .views with sorrow the present backward condition of his caste-men. In the sciences which it was

their special privilege to learn . . . they have been far outstripped by Western nations. When the Editor, after he had studied the ancient medical works under proper preceptors and passed out as a Kabiraj or physician according to the Hindu Sastras, entered the Medical College of Calcutta, he was simply astounded to find the progress which the Western nations have achieved. . . .[26]

He went on to contrast the standardized nomenclature in modern botany to the confusion of Ayurvedic texts and practices, calling on Indians to regain their ancient lead in scientific excellence and warning that, if they did not, other nations would look down on them. The English, he said, called Indians "natives," and "have classed us among the Sioux of America, the Hottentots of Africa, and the Maoris of Polynesia."[27]

We will leap, now, to the conclusions toward which this paper is headed, at the same time commenting on the movement in the twentieth century to establish state-supported and state-regulated institutions that would provide full professional status for qualified Vaids and Hakims.

Both Carr-Saunders and Wilensky emphasized that professions are based on technical skills founded in systematic knowledge requiring long, prescribed training. Professionalization processes tend to center upon the development and regulation of educational institutions. In this century, the characteristic skills and knowledge of Vaids and Hakims have been exposed as a barrier to the professionalization of Ayurveda and Unani Tibbia by the creation and expansion of modern colleges of indigenous medicine. To understand what happened, we need to distinguish technical knowledge from tacit knowledge.

Technical knowledge is highly teachable. It can be explicated in textbooks and manuals and organized into courses or other units of study arranged in sequences of increasing complexity and inclusiveness. Thus, it can be standardized, and it can be externalized in the manipulation of tools, machines, laboratory equipment, and abstract figures such as graphs, charts, and equations. Tacit knowledge cannot be explicated with the effectiveness of technical knowledge; it must be learned by imitating the example of a master. This is one source of the moral bond between teacher and student, and the legitimate foundation for the ritualization of professional training. Because a profession is an art as well as a skill, the best instructors are practitioners as well as teachers. And because they communicate the tacit knowledge of the profession by example, they have need of ceremony. Tacit knowledge lends mystery to a profession and enhances its authority.

We have already observed that Ayurvedic and Unani traditions emphasize the tacit knowledge of Vaids and Hakims. From hundreds of subtle variations in the pulse, and other signs imperceptible to ordinary cogni-

26. Ashutosh Sen, "Notes by the Editor," *The Wealth of India: Monthly Journal of Indian Industries, Products, and Trade* (Calcutta) 1:1 (1897), 6.
27. *Ibid.*, p.8.

tion, they claim to foresee the entire course of a patient's affliction. Their technical knowledge, on the other hand, is limited to Sanskrit grammar, drill in philosophical argumentation, the memorization of medical verses, and cookbook instructions for the preparation of medicines. Their theories, rather than being submitted to tests of reality, are, in Filliozat's fine phrase, "a dogmatism interpreting experience," or even, as we suggested, a dogmatism that creates experience.

The new schools of indigenous medicine, such as the Tibbia College founded in Hyderabad in 1890, the Aryan Medical School founded in Bombay in 1896, and the Government Ayurvedic College founded in Mysore in 1905, were for a time simply elaborations in urban settings of Gangadhār's tol-with-a-printing-press. They were dominated by a master physician, lacked access to hospital wards for clinical instruction, were without laboratories or libraries beyond the personal library of the teacher, and were unsupervised by outside authorities. On the other hand, they purchased modern anatomical charts and models, published brochures and medical tracts in the vernacular and English languages, and introduced students to the stethoscope along with a few other devices. The spirit of these colleges may be judged from the statement in 1905 of the Mysore government:

> The Government observed that the Ayurvedic system of medicine has fallen into much neglect. . . . The fact that Hindu medicine is sometimes practiced by quacks and charlatans is . . . reason why it should be rescued . . . and proper provisions made for combining Ayurvedic teaching with sound European methods. A strong desire to revive the ancient method of Hindu medicine is spreading to the country and any steps . . . to revive . . . Hindu learning while providing also for the students thereof being trained so far as possible in . . . modern medicine are sure to be welcomed by the people of the State.[28]

Gradually some of these schools enlarged their plants, and additional schools were built so that by the time of Independence there were 51 hospitals and 57 urban Ayurvedic and Unani schools with an enrollment of over 3,000 students. Some of these schools were equipped with modern classrooms, laboratories, dissection halls, libraries, hospitals, outpatient clinics, pharmacies, and student dormitories—though in all these facilities they were vastly inferior to the allopathic colleges. The setting was enough, however, to expose the scandal of the inadequate technical foundations of the ancient medical systems.

My interviews with physicians educated in these institutions, many of them leaders in the movement to revive indigenous medicine, reveal their unfavorable impression of the technical knowledge of indigenous medicine compared to allopathic medicine. Before Independence, however, the

28. Reprinted in *Mysore* (Magazine of the Government College of Indian Medicine) (May, 1958), p. 87.

missionary spirit of a newly awakened nationalism overcame the disappointment they felt when they made such comparisons. One physician, recalling the atmosphere of the government-sponsored college at Madras, wrote:

> The big and inspiring banyan trees, the palm leaf thatched sheds, the white-robed saint, the old boys who tasted life already, sanctified the school of Indian Medicine when I entered it in 1927. It presented an appearance and piety of the historic universities, read in books viz., Nalanda, Taxila, Amaravati, etc., etc. To us the Principal was the teacher, philosopher, guide, guardian, and a father. . . . That the students might not get depressed, comparing this school with the palatial mansions of the sister schools and colleges, they used to be encouraged by sermons that they are the torch-bearers of new light—progressive Indian Medicine—and that the great universities of historic times flourished under similar circumstances and environments. . . . The students consisted of all elderly men and none almost fresh from any school or college. Most of the men were sufferers as N.C.O.s (noncooperation), some went to jails in C.D. (civil disobedience) movements, some lost employment in railway strikes, etc., and some who were dissatisfied with the previous concerns in life and wanted a new mission to carry.[29]

Missionaries of professionalized Ayurveda and Unani Tibbia, they resolved to create the technical knowledge that would revive indigenous medicine. But they could not create from whole cloth. As Marx said, "Men make their own history, but they do not make it just as they please; they do not make it under circumstances chosen by themselves, but under circumstances directly found, given and transmitted from the past."[30] The progress of modern science left them no choice but to draw upon its theories and instruments, and to do this while maintaining the appearance of loyalty to the categories of ancient thought and a humoral pathology. The effort required monumental acts of self-deception.

It is necessary, I believe, to distinguish spurious from genuine professionalization processes. The pretense of discovering modern knowledge in ancient texts was widely practiced by individual medical revivalists, even by those who ridiculed the practice in others. And, whatever the theoretical claims, the technical skills associated with this knowledge remained firmly associated with allopathic medicine and modern science. It is just the disassociation of theoretical claims and demonstrable skills that made Ayurvedic teachers appear to be spurious professionals to their students in modern colleges. The chronic problem for these colleges has been to recruit students. When they have recruited students the problem has been to overcome the negative impression of instruction in indigenous compared to modern knowledge.

29. V. S. Rao, "Our Struggles," *Silver Jubilee Souvenir Magazine* (College of Indian Medicine, Madras, 1950), 61.

30. Karl Marx, *Selected Works in Two Volumes*, prepared by Marx-Engels-Lenin Institute, V. Adoratsky, ed. (New York: International Publishers, no date), p. 315.

Since Independence the symbolic opposition between Indian and Western medicine has lost much of its resonance. The popular culture of the nation simplifies the elaborate forms of traditional culture, adapting Indian music, dance, and costume to the media of mass entertainment, mass education, and mass production. Commercially manufactured Ayurvedic and Unani medicines now have a place in Indian society beside aspirin and other patent medicines. They are popular and cheap home remedies that anyone can prescribe for himself and purchase at the neighborhood store. Thus, the tacit knowledge of Vaids and Hakims has become less precious.

There is another sense in which spurious elements subvert modern Ayurvedic institutions: the organizations created to raise the professional status of practitioners have not developed what Wilensky calls "colleague control." That is, they have been opportunistic organizations subject to the manipulation of individuals, and so without the power to set standards of training and practice or to set up bureaucratic frameworks for stable, professional careers. Instead, in this century, the Ayurvedic and Unani colleges, the State Boards of indigenous medicine, the regional and national associations of practitioners, and the various committees of state and central government have been helplessly exposed to factionalism and the schemes of individuals. In short, though organizational instruments to professionalize indigenous medicine were created, they have failed to achieve the substance of professionalism. That substance inheres in professional norms: respect for colleagues, commitment to objective standards for judging competence, deference to the more qualified, and so on.

There is another barrier to the professionalization of indigenous medicine that I cannot refrain from mentioning in conclusion. Paradoxically, this is the very popularity of Ayurvedic and Unani medicine in Indian society. Commenting on Everett Hughes' suggestion that "The quack is the man who continues through time to please his customers but not his colleagues," Wilensky wrote,

> In any work context where the professional lacks strong colleague constraints, the customer's complaints, real or imaginary, are likely to receive prompt and costly attention; his real problems, if they require professional skill, may be overlooked. In the extreme case, the client-oriented practitioner makes a point of maligning the techniques and motives of his professional competitors and, like the proverbial ambulance chaser, solicits work where no work needs doing.[31]

Throughout urban India, the Vaids and Hakims whom I have interviewed malign their colleagues. When asked about their own practices, they complain that their patients want antibiotics and other quick-acting medications; so, although they personally believe in the more gentle and life-sustaining indigenous preparations, they are forced to bend to their clients' corrupting desires. Still, they point out, many complaints do not yield to modern

31. H. L. Wilensky, *op. cit.*, p. 154.

drugs, and laymen as well as practitioners testify to the wonderful qualities of Ayurveda and Unani Tibbia.

Had it been possible for the professionalization of indigenous medicine to proceed directly from the stage achieved by the first quarter of the nineteenth century, it might have matured in union with allopathic medicine. But with the intervening development of the modern medical curricula, the systematic recording of case histories, experimental medicine, the germ theory of disease, and all of the other advances in medical institutions and knowledge during the nineteenth and twentieth centuries, historical forces aligned men and institutions in patterned relationships that made the professionalization of Ayurvedic and Unani medicine progressively anachronistic, rather than a magnetic pole of Indian culture—a force in itself, like the dynamo in Adams' vision of modern history.

4

NORMAN K. DENZIN

Incomplete Professionalization: The Case of Pharmacy

While sociologists have successfully defined and described the characteristics which differentiate an occupation from a profession, they have yet to deal systematically with those occupations which attempted to become professions, perhaps achieved some modicum of success, and then failed to maintain this prestigious title.[1] The present paper proposes to discuss just these sorts of problems by giving specific attention to the case of pharmacy and the recent and historical developments which have moved this ancient occupation into a present-day position commonly labeled as a marginal occupation or a quasi-profession.[2]

Characteristics of Professions

Before we turn to the special case of the pharmacist, it is necessary first to discuss just what characteristics are commonly employed to define a profession.[3] Following Carr-Saunders we define a profession as an

. . . occupation which is based upon specialized intellectual study and training,

Reprinted from *Social Forces*, 46 (1968), pp. 375-382, by permission of the author and publisher. With the assistance of Curtis J. Mettlin.

1. Walter I. Wardwell, "Limited Marginal and Quasi-Practitioners," in Howard E. Freeman, Sol Levine, and Leo G. Reeder, *Handbook of Medical Sociology* (Englewood Cliffs, N.J.: Prentice-Hall, 1963), pp. 213-240, discusses a number of occupations which attempted to transform themselves into professions but failed. Wardwell's discussion is one of the few treatments of this problem.

2. *Ibid.*, pp. 215-219, treats pharmacy as a "special case" of his limited, marginal and quasi-practitioner model. Just exactly why he does so is never made clear, and in the present case each of Wardwell's types are considered special cases of occupations which achieved what we call "incomplete professionalization." That is, each has attempted to become professional, but has failed to attain all the necessary characteristics to be so labeled. See also Thelma Herman McCormack, "The Druggist's Dilemma: Problems of a Marginal Occupation," *American Journal of Sociology*, 61 (January, 1956), 308-315, where pharmacy is called a "marginal occupation" because its structure and functions as an occupation are unclear, and because it has incorporated the conflicting goals of business and profession into its organization. We shall return to these points in greater detail.

the purpose of which is to supply skilled service or advice to others for a definite fee or salary.[4]

Specialized training and a skilled service are not, however, the only characteristics of professions, for a number of occupations also possess these elements.[5] Carr-Saunders goes on to note that occupations transforming themselves into professional groupings develop special codes of ethics, engage in formalized recruitment patterns, establish formal institutions to transmit the knowledge of the occupation, develop social organizations to insure the perpetuation of the profession through time, and finally, take on the characteristics of self-governing, autonomous institutions; in short they claim what Hughes calls a *license* to carry out certain actions and a *mandate* to define what is proper conduct of others toward their work.[6]

Another element of a profession, not mentioned by Carr-Saunders, or other recent observers, is the fact that with the license, professions set up formal mechanisms which insure their continued control over the social object around which they organize their services and activities. Law, for example, has insured its long-lasting control over the social object of the law—no other occupation or profession can legitimately attempt to carve out activities and services around this social object.

It is important to note that contrary to current functionalist arguments, professions are not homogeneous, static institutions or groupings of persons sharing the same title.[7] They are, rather, moving, shifting, growing, splitting, assimilating bodies of persons held together at one point in time by a common name or label.[8] Viewed from this perspective, professions are like social movements. They recruit only certain types of persons, they develop highly elaborate ideologies and supra-individual values, they have their own mechanisms of socialization, and they often attempt to proselytize and bring new persons into the fold.[9]

Incomplete Professionalization: The Case of Pharmacy

We turn now to the case of pharmacy—an occupation which has achieved what we will call *incomplete professionalization*.[10] That is, they have taken

3. A. M. Carr-Saunders and P. A. Wilson, *The Professions* (Oxford: Clarendon Press, 1933), pp. 3-31. See also Howard M. Vollmer and Donald L. Mills, eds., *Professionalization* (Englewood Cliffs, N.J.: Prentice-Hall, 1966), for the most recent treatment and definition of professions.

4. Carr-Saunders and Wilson, *op. cit.*

5. *Ibid.*

6. *Ibid.*; also Everett C. Hughes, *Men and Their Work* (Glencoe, Ill.: The Free Press, 1953), pp. 78-87.

7. Rue Bucher, "Pathology: A Study of Social Movements Within a Profession," in this volume; Rue Bucher and Anselm Strauss, "Professions in Process," *American Journal of Sociology*, 66 (January, 1961), 325-334.

8. *Ibid.*

9. *Ibid.*

on a number of the characteristics of a profession, but they failed to escape the marginality associated with professions which still contain within themselves elements of an occupation. Specifically, pharmacy has failed to abide by the requirement of a profession that "you do not advertise." Similarly, they have failed to recruit into their instituitions of learning truly committed persons who would go out and commit their lives to the altruistic goals and values of the profession.[11] They have likewise failed to engaged in long-term activities which insure their control over the social object around which their activities are organized—e.g., the drug.[12] Furthermore, they have failed to accumulate a systematic body of scientific knowledge which can only be learned by socialization in their own institutions, and which is needed for the enactment of their professional role.[13] Due to the proliferation of subspecialties

10. Professionalization in this context refers to the process whereby occupations attempt to transform themselves into professions. Incomplete professionalization is then the failure to achieve the final condition of professionalization which accords the occupation the title of a "profession." See Vollmer and Mills, *op. cit.*, pp. v-ix. We do not mean to imply that we are studying what Hughes called the false question "Is this occupation a profession?" This is largely irrelevant. Rather we ask: What processes have prevented the members of this particular occupation from calling themselves professionals?

The following quotation from the *American Druggist* (March 5, 1962), highlights this particular problem with respect to pharmacy: "In America, the professional profile is hazy and soft" (p. 18). Or as a recent comment from the same journal (September 14, 1966) notes: "The pharmacist has the possibility of regaining his professional stature which has been steadily corroded of late." (p. 30).

11. Edward Harvey, "Some Implications of Value Differentiation in Pharmacy," *Canadian Review of Anthropology and Sociology*, 3 (February, 1966), 23-37, indicates that a large proportion of pharmacists enter the work world with the hopes of advancing their own careers as opposed to committing themselves to the goals and objectives of the profession. These finding are similar to McCormack's *op. cit.*, which indicated that 85 percent of her respondents wanted to own their own retail outlet. See also Paul R. Dommermuth, "Retail Pharmacists: Professional Contingencies in Business Settings," paper presented at the annual meeting of the American Sociological Association, 1966.

A recent issue of the *Iowa Pharmacist* (June, 1966), 23, ran the following advertisement which is indicative of the pressure within the occupation to be nonprofessional: "Boost your store traffic, build sales...with this exclusive *professional pharmacist* advertising program!"

12. We have reference here to trends within the occupation which have taken the drug out of the hands of the pharmacist. These include "detail men" who sell drugs for the pharmaceutical houses, the tendency for retail outlets to sell nondrug items and the trend for industry to produce all the drugs formerly compounded and prepared by the pharmacist.

13. The recent trend for pharmacy schools to expand their education program from four to five years indicated a response to retail pressures to teach more business management matters in schools with less emphasis on the technical and chemical aspects of drugs themselves. Thus the educational institutions of pharmacy have themselves incorporated elements which stress the business as opposed to the professional aspects of the occupation into their curriculum. See, for example: Charles L. Braucher and Robert V. Evanson, "Academic Factors Related to Success in Community Pharmacy Management," *American Journal of Pharmacy Education* (Winter, 1963), 56-66; and T. S. Grosicki, "History of Pharmacy in the Five-Year Program," *American Journal of Hospital Pharmacy* (Spring, 1963), 237-241.

within the profession, pharmacy has failed to hold together a cohesive social organization which would exercise strict control over its members and which would ensure its perpetuation through time.[14]

Pharmacy has not failed on all counts, and it is for this reason that we call it a marginal or quasi-profession. It has developed a systematic code of ethics, it has established formal institutions for transmitting its body of knowledge, it has set up some types of recruitment policies, it does have a specialized skill to offer and this skill is offered for a definite fee or salary.[15] Most importantly, pharmacy is a moving, shifting conglomeration of persons sharing the common label of *pharmacist*. Also, pharmacy has established some legislative and self-controlling patterns by virtue of the fact that it and it alone has the power to determine who practices and who does not practice pharmacy.[16]

Thus at this point in time, *pharmacy as an occupation contains within itself elements which are both professional and nonprofessional.* Certain segments within the profession are clearly more professional—as for example the hospital pharmacist, who does not advertise, does recruit stringently but has also lost control over the drug.[17] Retail pharmacists clearly represent the most nonprofessional aspects of the profession. It is in the retail outlets that the rule of "no advertising" is seldom abided by.[18] It is in the retail outlet that the pharmacist subordinates professional goals to personal goals.[19] It is in the retail setting that the pharmacist takes little interest in the fact that he does not engage in professional activities—that he does sell nonprofessional items and objects seems not to bother him.[20]

WHY THE FAILURE NOT TO BE FULLY PROFESSIONAL?

If pharmacy as an occupation has taken on these formal characteristics of a profession, why has it failed to go all the way and become fully professional in the sense that medicine has, for example?

THE SOCIAL OBJECT

The major problem which prevents pharmacy from stepping across the line of marginality is its failure to gain control over the social object which

14. Dommermuth, *op. cit.*, noted, for example, three distinct types of retail pharmacists. The profession itself recognizes at least ten distinct specialties which range from hospital pharmacy, to pharmaceutical administration, to production planning in industry. See, for example, Richard A. Deno, Thomas D. Rowe, and Donald C. Brodie, *The Profession of Pharmacy* (Philadelphia: J. B. Lippincott, 1964).

15. Deno, Rowe, and Brodie, *op. cit.*

16. *Ibid.*

17. Troy C. Daniels, "The Hospital Pharmacist and the Pharmacy Profession," *American Journal of Hospital Pharmacy* 18 (December, 1961), 691-693; and Don E. Francke et al., *Mirror to Hospital Pharmacy* (Washington, D.C.: American Society of Hospital Pharmacists, 1964).

18. Dommermuth, *op. cit.*; Deno, Rowe, and Brodie, *op. cit.*, p. 14.

19. *Ibid.*

20. Hospital pharmacists frequently refer to their retail counterparts as "garden hose druggists" implying by the label that nonprofessional drug items are sold in the retail setting.

justified the existence of its professional qualities in the first place. Pharmacy has not developed an ideology to limit the manner in which its members will view the drug. Medicine has agreed that the illness and disease are the social objects which their services are to be directed toward. Physicians cure, control, and eliminate illness and disease. No other use is made of these objects. While illness and disease are sometimes used in teaching institutions as learning tools, this activity is still only a method of developing other practitioners to combat their existence. In the case of pharmacy no such agreement has been reached in regard to the drug. Some practitioners, particularly in the retail setting, view the drug as a product to be sold rather than as an object to direct a service toward.[21] Viewing the drug as a product, the pharmacist is forced to violate some of the basic rules of being a professional. The drug as a product necessitates advertising for a profit rather than a salary or fee.[22] As a further consequence of the product view of the social object the pharmacist becomes the agency through which the drug may be obtained rather than an individual who makes some service contribution.

A recent trend in pharmacy has been to alter this view of the drug as a product and shift the attention to the service of filling the prescription. A professional fee-pricing system has been developed.[23] In contrast to the price of the prescription being arrived at by adding a fairly standard percentage markup to the cost of the drug, the professional fee system adds a set service fee to the wholesale cost of the drug so that the income of the pharmacist is more directly related to the service provided rather than to the cost of the product. However, even this approach has problems for the retail pharmacist. The public sees very little service being provided, and objects to paying a fee to someone for counting out pills and typing a label. No longer is their service visible to the public which demands "specialized intellectual study and training" from professions.[24]

Other pharmacists feel that the service they provide concerns the supplying of information about the drug.[25] They claim that they are the best quali-

21. *Iowa Pharmacist, op. cit.*

22. Carr-Saunders, *op. cit.*, notes that one of the cardinal rules of a profession is that you do not advertise your services to the public.

23. Jon J. Tanja, "The Professional Fee," paper presented to the Iowa Pharmaceutical Association Convention, 1966.

24. A recent article in the *American Druggist* (March, 1962), entitled "Public Doesn't Know or Care if Pharmacists are Professionals," documents this point. The article goes on to note "the public recognizes that the phamacist has considered himself a merchant and they think....a prescription is a commodity, a product, so why not, they say, buy it at the discount house" (p. 18).

25. The *American Journal of Hospital Pharmacy* has published a series of articles on this newly expanding role of the pharmacist. See for example: Donald C. Brodie and Frederick H. Meyers, "Role of the Pharmacist as Drug Consultant," 18 (January, 1961), 11-13; Don E. Francke, "The Expanding Role of the Hospital Pharmacist in Drug Information Services," 22 (January, 1965), 33-37; and Phillip H. Greth, William W. Tester, and Harold J. Black, "Decentralized Pharmacy Operations Utilizing the Unit Dose Concept II: Drug Information Services in a Decentralized Pharmacy Substation," 22 (October, 1965), 558-563.

fied in interpreting and guiding the flow of drug information through medical institutions and to the lay public.[26] Pharmacy meets serious difficulty in attempting to explain to the medical profession that they are really "experts on drugs" when physicians, who control institutions and prescribe to and provide medical consultation for the patient, believe that they are the most qualified source of information on drugs.

In the hospital the pharmacist has failed to associate with the dispensing of drugs a set of skills which only he possesses. As a consequence drug distribution systems have evolved which allow lesser-trained individuals to engage in the dispensing of the drug while the pharmacist is relegated to providing outpatient services, supplying the nursing stations with bulk quantities, and manufacturing special preparations. Typically in the hospital the pharmacist has no contact with his client, the patient, and little communication of a professional nature with the other medical professions because of the drug distribution systems that have evolved.[27]

Some groups of pharmacists are currently forming a social movement to revolutionize the role of the pharmacist in the hospital.[28] They have attacked the nurses' competence in the handling of drugs by citing the high occurrence of medication errors in the hospital. Thus they are developing systems that demand that they alone dispense each dose of the medication, and only allow the nurse to "administer" the medication, claiming the dispensing operation as an exclusive operation of the pharmacist.

Although pharmacy has been able to limit the access of the public to their product through legislation, they have not been able to gain exclusive control over this social object. Some physicians engage in the dispensing and charging of drugs to the patient. Even more common is the practice on the part of the physician to provide their patients with manufacturers' samples. In this instance both the physician and the drug industry circumvent the pharmacist in the distribution of "his" social object. Even more threatening to the pharmacist is the growing number of physician-owned pharmacies.[29] Pharmacy has taken this problem, which endangers the autonomy of the pro-

26. *Ibid.*
27. *Ibid.*; Harold J. Black and William W. Tester, "Pharmacy Operation Utilizing Unit Dose Concept," *American Journal of Hospital Pharmacy*, 21 (August, 1964), 345-350, note, for example, that under the conventional system of drug distribution the nurse, the physician and the pharmacist are all performing roles for which they were ill-trained and which deny them the activities they are best equipped to handle.
28. This movement consists of several groups of pharmacists located in hospital pharmacies who are experimenting with a new method of drug distribution (the unit-dose concept) which entails movement of the pharmacist onto the hospital ward and into more direct contact with the physician, nurse and patient. See Norman K. Denzin and Curtis J. Mettlin, "A Sociological View of Hospital Pharmacy: The Case of the Unit Dose Concept," *American Journal of Hospital Pharmacy* (in press).
29. A recent article in *Life* magazine (June, 1966), 87-102, "Doctors and the Rx Scandal: How Some M.D.s Short-cut Ethics and Profit from Their Own Prescriptions," details the growing problem of physician-owned pharmacies and the threat this poses for the pharmacist.

fession, to the popular press in an attempt to gain support from the public.[30]

THE RECRUIT

Aside from the occupation's ambiguous view and control of their social object, pharmacy has recruited a larger number of students who subscribe to more of the unprofessional qualities of the occupation than to its professional elements. McCormack found that pharmacy students chose the profession of pharmacy because it suited a particular aptitude or promised economic security.[31] A comparatively small group of respondents claimed that they entered pharmacy school out of a desire to provide some humanitarian service to the public.[32]

Similarly, Harvey observed that pharmacy tends to recruit persons into the work world who are not committed to one dominant value-orientation.[33] Contrary to medicine, for example, which recruits persons who are committed to humanitarian and people-oriented endeavors, pharmacy recruits are not committed to a dominant value-orientation. Rather it attracts persons who have mixed interests which range from the humanitarian goal to intrinsic-self-rewarding activities to extrinsic-economically based ideals.[34]

This failure of the occupation to recruit persons who are truly committed to altruistic and supra-individual values and goals can be explained in part by the failure of pharmacy itself to decide just what its dominant values should be. As McCormack noted the occupation is caught between two dominant value-orientations, business versus profession.[35] Should it stress the remunerative rewards which accrue from its practice or should it stress the humanitarian rewards which come from serving the public in a professional manner? Pharmacy educators themselves are unclear as to which of these paths should be taken and in fact tend to encourage the merging of the two. As a recent textbook argues:

> In exclusive prescription and semiprofessional pharmacies, a major part of the time of the pharmacist is devoted to professional activities: compounding and dispensing prescriptions, advising patrons on health problems, and serving as consultant on drugs to physicians and other health workers.[36]

Setting up this professional image of the prescription shop the text goes on to argue:

> . . . however, the pharmacist operating a prescription pharmacy also has need for business "know-how." He must buy countless prescription items, pay rent,

30. *Ibid.*
31. McCormack, *op. cit.*
32. *Ibid.*
33. Harvey, *op. cit.*
34. *Ibid.*
35. McCormack, *op. cit.*
36. Deno, Rowe, and Brodie, *op. cit.*, p. 5.

calculate overhead expenses, and realize a fair profit at the end of the year if he is to remain in business.[37]

Informing the prospective pharmacist that even in the purest of retail outlets he must necessarily be a businessman the text concludes by noting that:

Even in the most exclusive presscription pharmacies, the pharmacist will uses a cash register. *In this respect—inherent combination of professional and busness activities—his work differs from that of his fellow professional workers both within and outside the health fields*[38] (italics inserted).

It is not surprising then that pharmacy has failed to send practitioners out into the field who could correct the deficient aspects of its professional image. "True" professions demand greater commitment from their students than does pharmacy—and similarly, "true" professions—like medicine, organize the activities of their members around consensually held supra-individual humanitarian goals and values. On both of these counts pharmacy has failed to achieve a stance which would accord it the status of a profession.

A SELF-GOVERNING ORGANIZATION

As has been previously stated, professions also maintain themselves through time by forming organizational structures which direct the efforts and activities of their members. Although pharmacy has its several national, state, and local societies, these organizations have been ineffective in representing and controlling the total profession.[39] Segments of the profession often move in opposite directions without strict censure from the pharmacy societies. An example of this is the current dual trend in the retail segment of the occupation to proliferate the small apothecary shop on the one hand and the large chain, discount drug store on the other. Clearly the small apothecary shop which avoids selling nondrug items fits more closely the professional model pharmacy is aspiring to.[40] However, there has been little attempt on the part of pharmacy societies to take a definite stance toward either movement and as a result these two segments prosper by derogating each other.[41]

MANDATE

As Hughes has cogently noted, those occupations which have license will:

. . . if they have any sense of self-consciousness and solidarity, also claim a

37. *Ibid.*
38. *Ibid.*
39. The major professional society is the American Pharmaceutical Association. In addition, there are segmental societies such as the American Society for Hospital Pharmacy and the National Association of Retail Druggists.
40. This is the implication made by McCormack, *op. cit.* As Deno, Rowe, and Brodie, *op. cit.*, point out, for the profession as a whole the emphasis on the professional aspects of the small apothecary shop implies that the large retail outlet is unethical. Thus the stance taken by the profession has been ambiguous and somewhat contradictory.
41. *Ibid.*

mandate to define what is proper conduct of others toward the matters concerned with their work.[42]

This mandate may go no further than an insistence that other people stand back and give the workers a bit of elbowroom while they do their work. Or it may, as Hughes notes:

> . . . in the case of the modern physician include a successful claim to supervise and determine the conditions of work of many kinds of people.[43]

The mandate forces upon the relevant others of the occupation a consistent self-image of the occupation and tells them how to act toward that occupation. The mandate that the pharmacist has attempted to develop and present to its relevant others revolves around its image of self which claims superior knowledge about drugs, their distribution, their chemical composition, and their therapeutic side effects. They have attempted to legislate this mandate in the modern hospital through a definite structuring of the drug distributional system. However, as was noted earlier, they have largely failed in this endeavor, and have of late become in the eyes of most nurses and physicians "the person who gets the drug up here when I want it." Their inability to maintain a mandate is further documented by the fact that when nurses, medical residents, interns, and students were recently asked where they would fit the pharmacist in the organizational structure of the hospital they ranged in their opinions from placing the pharmacist in the third highest echelon of the structure of the two lowest positions possible. Pharmacists, on the other hand, were quite clear as to where they fit—in the three highest structural positions. Pharmacy has then failed to achieve and maintain a mandate which guides and directs the behavior of its relevant others toward them.

Discussion

We have attempted in this paper to pose and answer a number of questions about the characteristics of an occupation which attempted to turn itself into a profession but failed to achieve the professional status so desired. Rather than asking "is pharmacy a profession?" we have focused on the circumstances which have prevented its members from calling themselves professionals.[44] Arguing that sociologists have quite adequately discussed and analyzed the characteristics of professions, we chose to focus on the special case of the occupation which strives to become professional but never quite succeeds.

This inability of pharmacy to maintain license and mandate, to recruit committed persons, to develop a professionally pure set of humanitarian values, to become completely self-governing and self-legislating, and to

42. Hughes, *op. cit.*, p. 78.
43. *Ibid.*
44. *Ibid.*

maintain control over its social object is also shared by such marginal occupations or quasi-professions as optometry, osteopathy, chiropractory, and librarianship.[45]

Goode has noted, for example, librarianship is an occupation that is moving toward a profession in that it has developed prolonged specialized training programs and does have a service-orientation with a somewhat clearly defined client.[46] However, as an occupational group it has not achieved professional status because the public will not allow it to become a purely self-controlling group. In short just as pharmacy has failed to achieve a clear license and mandate, so too has librarianship.

Similarly, optometry and chiropractory have failed to achieve professional status because they have not maintained full control over the object around which their occupation is organized and in the case of chiropractory the ideology and values behind the occupation were never accepted by the public-at-large or by the powers-that-be (eg., the profession of medicine).[47]

In conclusion, it is hoped that this analysis of the occupation of pharmacy has served to shed light on the process which we have labeled incomplete professionalization. It is hoped that future investigations will be able to examine in greater detail the more generic elements of those occupations which attempt to turn themselves from ordinary occupations into the prestigious groupings called professions.

45. Wardwell, *op. cit.*; William Goode, "Professions and Non-Professions," in Vollmer and Mills, *op. cit.*, pp. 33-43, discusses the case of librarianship.
46. *Ibid.*
47. Wardwell, *op. cit.*

5

WILLIAM A. GLASER

"Socialized Medicine" in Practice

Long resisted albeit ambiguously defined, "socialized" medicine seems finally to have come in America. To its proponents, the Health Insurance for the Aged Act of 1965 promises to alleviate the anxieties and satisfy the health needs of the aged; to its critics, it threatens to create a massive bureaucracy that will permit politically motivated laymen to dictate to doctors and hospitals. Who is right?

A close reading of the statute gives no clear answer. It reveals the Act to be a general framework rather than a specific plan. The Act provides that money shall be collected from taxes and paid for the medical care of the aged—but the precise administrative structure is left for future negotiation. Thus one cannot be certain whether the Medicare statute will achieve either the hopes that inspired it or the fears that it has provoked. One cannot even say, with precision, whether or not it truly establishes "socialized medicine" in America. At present, one can no more than make informed guesses, based on knowledge of American conditions and on facts from other countries with extensive public schemes of medical care.

This article will report how publicly sponsored systems of medical care actually operate abroad. From these generalizations about the workings of "socialized medicine" in practice, I will make inferences as to trends that might occur in American medicine, as a result of the Medicare program. I shall concentrate on the topics customarily emphasized in American discussions about the dangers and merits of "socialized medicine"— namely, the relationships between doctors and public agencies, and the effects of public programs on the performance of doctors. A fuller examination of "socialized medicine" would say considerably more about the effects on hospitals, private health insurance schemes, medical schools, and other medical institutions.

Reprinted from *The Public Interest*, 1 (1966), pp. 90-106, © National Affairs, Inc., by permission of the author and publisher.

The article is based on my research into the organization of medical care in Europe, the Soviet bloc, and the Middle East. This research, extending over a period of a year and a half, involved visits to sixteen countries and interviews with officials in Ministries of Health, officials in health insurance programs, secretaries of medical associations, members of hospital medical staffs, private practitioners, and others.

Kinds of Socialized Medicine

Extensive public systems for providing medical care are of two types: national health insurance and national health services. Most developed countries, particularly in Europe, have some type of national health insurance. Basically, this is simply a method of paying the doctor for care given subscribers, and the conditions of private office practice or of hospital inpatient care are changed very little. National health insurance usually evolves out of a long history of private health insurance sponsored by labor unions and cooperatives. It is based on employment; workers and their employers contribute to funds, and the funds pay for medical care for these workers, usually for their dependents, and also usually for retired workers. In order to ensure collections, to extend coverage, and to improve fiscal efficiency, these programs are almost invariably given a public character by statute, at some point in their history. Instead of relying on voluntary contributions by workers and employers, social security taxes are levied on both; and, further, instead of having to live within the limited income generated by social security taxes, insurance funds in many countries are given large grants by the Treasury from general tax revenues. Usually the insurance funds enjoy considerable administrative autonomy, within the limits of general policy laid down by legislatures. In many countries, the funds are supervised by the Ministry of Labor; elsewhere, they are governed by their own boards. It is common that the insurance system involves no newly created government agencies, but is simply composed of the pre-existing private funds, now strengthened with legal authority and public subsidies.

Because an insurance principle is based on employment, most national insurance schemes cover only employed persons, their dependents, and some recently retired workers. In the most developed countries, about three-quarters of the population is so covered; in some of the less affluent countries along the Mediterranean, a quarter or half of the population is covered. The groups who are not covered usually are the unemployed, the unemployable, the elderly with no continuous work experience, businessmen, and some of the wealthier classes. Only recently are the farmers being included. The sick fund will usually pay the doctor's fees directly to the doctor; in a few countries, it reimburses the patient after he has paid the doctor. The funds also pay the hospitalization costs of subscribers;

in most countries the funds pay the full hospital bill, including the cost of all drugs.

When most Americans speak of "socialized medicine," however, they usually visualize, not a system of national health insurance, but a national health service. This is a nationwide administrative structure that dispenses medical care and that may be used *as a matter of right* by all citizens, regardless of their status as workers or taxpayers. Such a system is very rare among developed countries, and is adopted only because national health insurance is incomplete or cannot be financed adequately through payroll taxes. Great Britain created such a national health service after several decades of experience with national health insurance; there was a desire to expand coverage of the population; more money was required to pay for hospitalization and physicians' fees than was available in the insurance funds; and the hospitals needed to be reorganized and improved. The English system does not "bureaucratize" the doctors, in the sense of arranging them in a chain of command. Instead, the National Health Service is a loosely arranged hierarchy of committees composed of laymen and medical representatives, functioning according to general directives from the Ministry of Health, and acting primarily as the dispensers of money. British doctors have contracts with these committees, but are not their employees or subordinates.

National health services are found more commonly in underdeveloped countries. Usually the colonial government maintained a small corps of salaried doctors to give care to the general public in polyclinics and hospitals. After independence, the new government confronts a society that has poor health, few doctors and facilities, and too little private purchasing power to support private practice. Therefore the new government expands its salaried medical corps, most of the country's doctors join it, and all but the rich use it. In many such systems, the doctors are arranged in a hierarchy of ranks and are employees of the Ministry of Health. The Soviet Union has the most extensive system of this type today. With various modification, the pattern will become standard in Asia, Africa, and Latin America.

American Medicare in World Perspective

The Health Insurance for the Aged Act creates, not a national health service, but a national health insurance program of limited scope. All employed and self-employed persons are taxed, but only two categories are covered—the aged who are eligible for social security benefits and other aged persons who become voluntary subscribers. The program is simply a way of coping with hospital and doctors' bills; it does not specifically reorganize the working conditions of doctors.

In every country, a comprehensive system of national health insurance usually evolves out of modest beginnings. By starting coverage with one group, the American program is typical. But by beginning with a special program for the aged, the U.S. is unique. In other countries, coverage is first sought for industrial workers, and the aged are included later or never. In most countries where national health insurance does cover the aged, these persons usually must have built up eligibility during prior years as subscribers and users of the sick funds; thus, care for the aged is simply an extension of care for the economically active. Italy is one of the few countries with a special fund for the aged, while Holland and Sweden are among the few countries where large numbers of aged are covered by the general health insurance program, regardless of whether these persons were eligible for treatment through the same sick funds during their economically active years. Because the aged are so expensive to treat, care can be financed only if hospitals and doctors agree to accept lower fees (as in Italy) or only if the government subsidizes the sick funds from general taxation (as in Holland and Sweden).

Demands for national health insurance, or for a national health service, arise in any country when medical care is unavailable or too expensive for large segments of the population. If the pressures for national health insurance occurred first on behalf of the aged in America, and first on behalf of industrial workers elsewhere in the world, the different priorities reflect the numerous unique characteristics of this country. America's wealth means that many people are capable of paying doctors and hospitals, albeit with the complaints that accompany medical expenditures everywhere. The strength of labor unions has resulted in well-financed private health insurance programs paid for, in large part, by employers; such extensive private coverage of large categories of workers has never been achieved in any other country, because of the weakness of private collective bargaining. In order to head off socialized medicine in America, the medical and hospital associations themselves have created extensive hospitalization and medical insurance; medical societies abroad rarely sponsor health insurance. In most countries, a program is either wholly public or wholly private, but America has a tradition of government grants to supplement inadequate private finances, and thus private hospitals, medical schools, and research centers have been able to survive and flourish with government help.

Thus the problems in America are selective gaps in coverage (rather than large deficits in care), high prices, and the control of undue hospitalization and drug costs. These problems have not been sufficiently acute and widespread to generate demands for a sweeping reorganization of American health insurance and medical care—unlike the critical situations that have led to general changes abroad. Inadequate insurance coverage and high medical costs for the aged have been one of the special and persistent problems in America, and consequently national health insurance in America has begun at a point where it started nowhere else. In other countries, coverage spread by subsequent amendments to the original legislation; but there is no assurance that America will follow the same evolution, unless a general breakdown in medical care unexpectedly occurs.

The Power of The Medical Profession

One might think that "socialized medicine" potentially could transfer power over medical services from the doctors to the laymen—especially the laymen in strategic government posts. But in practice abroad, national health insurance and national health services are dominated by doctors. It would be very surprising if the same were not true of the actual administration of Medicare in America.

A fundamental reason for domination by the doctors, of course, is lay deference to professional expertise. In practice, most medical work is technical and naturally gravitates into the hands of the persons with the special training to do it. In most of the world, laymen greatly respect medicine and doctors, and the lay administrators in socialized medical systems invariably treat the doctors with much deference. Consequently, in most administrative decisions made by mixed committees with lay and professional members, the doctors exercise weight beyond their numbers; and in decisions made by lay administrators in the health services, the laymen often act on professional advice.

The Health Insurance for the Aged Act creates many openings for such domination by the doctors. It establishes all-medical or mixed medical-lay advisory committees in several key areas of decision-making, such as the approval of participating hospitals, the definition of reasonable charges, and the review of utilization. The statute requires the Department of Health, Education, and Welfare to consult associations representing doctors and hospitals. In practice—just as occurs in other countries—the Department will probably make no decisions unacceptable to the doctors on these committees or to the professional associations. Other clauses offer even greater potential scope for professional authority in the administration of the act: the insurance of medical fees (as distinct from hospitalization fees) is supposed to be conducted wherever possible through existing carriers, and thus the Blue Shield Plans sponsored by medical societies might take over this portion of Medicare. Only in Holland did a large proportion of the officially recognized sick funds evolve out of private funds originally created by the doctors themselves, and the Dutch evolution ensured a dominant voice for the doctors in the administration of national health insurance. American Medicare may well develop similarly.

Usually socialized medical institutions are not created abroad unless they have been made acceptable to the medical profession. If the scheme is national health insurance or a national health service enacted by a democratic legislature, the conservative political parties are usually strong enough to delay passage until the medical association's principal objections are met. Whether the government is authoritarian or democratic, the co-operation of the doctors is necessary to make the system work success-fully, and therefore the officials modify the scheme to please them. Almost never is any new medical system adopted over the opposition of the doctors; in the rare cases when that happens—as in Belgium and Saskatche-wan during recent years—the government usually is forced to make changes in subsequent negotiations. The American Medicare statute bears much evidence of caution and a desire to avoid confrontations with the doctors.

There are several concessions that the medical association seeks and usually obtains abroad. It demands and usually succeeds in getting a stipulation that all licensed physicians shall have the right to treat patients under health insurance or to join the health service. Such language appears at the beginning of the American Medicare statute.

In some countries the doctors fear the adoption of payment systems that will restrict their income and freedom, and they usually successfully insist that a traditional form of payment will be used in the official system. For example, fears that their governments would make them salaried employees led the English general practitioners to insist on a fixed payment per patient each year ("capitation fees"), while Swedish doctors practicing under national health insurance preserved payment for each act ("fee-for-service"); fears that the government would control their fees by direct payments led the French doctors to press for a reimbursement system by which the patient pays the doctor and then is repaid by the sick fund. The American Medicare program attempts to avoid involvement in the explosive subject of doctors' pay: bills in earlier years covered only hospitalization and not payment for care by doctors; the bill in 1965 finally included the payment of doctors, but delegated the compensation formulas to private insurance carriers, which presumably will negotiate agreements acceptable to the doctors. So that doctors' incomes do not decline relative to the rest of the economy, the profession in foreign systems usually obtains some negotiating machinery that regularly reviews and increases fees and salaries.

Lest all medical care be given through the socialized medical system and lest all doctors' incomes be controlled by it, the medical society usually obtains guarantees that every doctor has the right not to join, and that every participant may conduct a part-time private practice. In many European countries, medical associations have induced sick funds to pledge that they will never create polyclinics but will always allow their subscribers to be treated in the doctors' private offices. Also in Europe, the medical associations have secured various formulas to give the doctors statuses different from the ordinary employees of the governments: in the British National Health Service and in most of the continental hospitals, the doctor has a contract to give time and services, and thus can still retain the aura of a free professional; the salaried district medical officers who care for the poor and rural inhabitants of Sweden are the only local government functionaries who are technically appointees of the King; hospital specialists in England are classified as "officers" of the Regional Hospital Boards, while all other hospital staff members are employees of local hospital committees; after many years of complaint about the power of the sick funds, the German medical profession obtained a new arrangement whereby the funds would deal only with a collective organization of the entire profession, and this organization alone would pay and discipline individual doctors.

The Crucial Link

Usually doctors occupy all the jobs where controls can be exerted over other doctors. In the bureaucratized national health services maintained by the Soviet Union and underdeveloped countries, usually all the administrative posts—often including the position of Minister of Health—are occupied by physicians. In national health insurance schemes, the sick funds employ physicians who conduct nearly all the contacts with the doctors treating insured persons. These physicians handle the particularly sensitive task of judging whether certain doctors are doing medically unjustified work in order to earn extra money from the funds, and they alone confer with such miscreants. Instead of identifying themselves with laymen in the government and trade unions, these doctors seem to feel a sense of professional solidarity with the practitioners; for example, during my interviews, the physicians in sick funds and Ministries of Health repeatedly referred to the rest of the medical profession as "we" and referred to their fellow officials as "they" or "the government."

The medical association becomes a crucial link between the medical profession and any "socialized" medical system, and it becomes an important element in the administration of the system. In the past, medical associations in most countries were mere pressure groups for the doctors, but they always grew in importance and power after creation of national health insurance or a national health service. Usually, regular consultative meetings are held with the sick funds and with the Ministry of Health. The medical association usually becomes the bargaining agent for the doctors in all questions of pay and working conditions. In England and in some other countries, the national health service establishes committees of doctors to discipline those who violate their contracts, and these committees in practice are branches of the medical association. Doubtless the several advisory committees created by the American Medicare statute will also be filled by representatives of the medical and hospital associations, and the legislative requirement that the Secretary of Health, Education, and Welfare regularly consult with the professional associations will further cement their interlocking relationship with the health insurance structure.

The requirement of responsible participation in a "socialized" medical system has usually transformed the leaderships of medical associations abroad; before such a change, the leaders are militant representatives of the private office practitioners; afterwards, they are replaced by new leaders who are favorable to the new system and who are skilled in negotiation and in administration rather than in the techniques of pressure group warfare. The decision of the American Medical Association convention in 1965 to negotiate with the Johnson Administration for a satisfactory administrative structure, rather than to boycott Medicare, foreshadows a similar taming of the medical association's mutinous impulses in America.

Because of the concessions obtained from the system, "socialized medicine" often works to the benefit of the doctors. Unpaid bills cease. The right of private practice enables many to earn a considerable income from high private fees, in addition to the fees and salaries earned under the official scheme. In most countries, doctors are eager to get this mixture of public and private practice, since their incomes and economic security surpass those of full-time private practitioners. In countries with many doctors and a low-income population, such as Italy and India, few doctors can survive financially without a part-time public appointment. In countries with few doctors and heavy demand, such as Sweden, the medical association can press successfully for high salaries, high fees, and therefore very high incomes. In most of the world, the greatest ambition of a doctor is to become a professor of medicine in a public medical school or chief of service in a public hospital; with this certificate of eminence, the physician enjoys high prestige and a large income from private practice. Although the professors and service chiefs are powerful and prosperous everywhere, "socialized medicine" does not always guarantee contentment for other doctors; in countries with many doctors and low national incomes, fees and salaries may be low and doctors are often angry—although they still may earn more money than if "socialized medicine" did not exist.

The Limits of Lay Domination

One of the great fears of American critics of "socialized medicine" is that the doctors will be controlled by laymen and that technical medical problems will be decided by political criteria. Laymen always play an important role in the establishment of national health insurance or of a national health service. Complaints about the distribution, maintenance, or costs of preexisting private medical services come primarily from the trade unions and from the political parties of the Left. "Socialized medicine" sometimes is enacted by democratic legislatures with the votes of these groups; or it sometimes is decreed by dictatorships either to please these groups or to swing public support from these groups to the dictatorship itself. Once national health insurance or a national health service is adopted, the trade unions and the political parties of the Left remain to criticize any general deficiencies in the services rendered, but the details of daily work almost always are turned over to the doctors and medical administrators. In some countries, the governing committees of health insurance or the health service contain representatives from the trade unions and political parties, but usually these committees meet only occasionally, they are concerned with general policies, and they leave specific matters to their staffs.

In practice, the medical services are insulated from politics because politicians, trade union leaders, and most other pressure group leaders have little interest in medicine and little knowledge of medical services. This is true whether the government is totalitarian, authoritarian, or democratic. A totalitarian government is supposed to try to mobilize all social institutions, but in practice its leaders are preoccupied with matters far removed from medicine, such as foreign policy, industrialization, and the military. Even unusually energetic dictators such as Josef Stalin take notice of the medical services only if there are drastic breakdowns or if too much money is requested during the annual preparation of the national budget.

If any of these programs are induced to make certain decisions on non-medical grounds, it involves the location of hospitals and clinics. Occasionally, influential members of parliaments and of governing committees secure facilities for their home communities in order to please their political constituents, when rational planning might locate them elsewhere. But instead of being peculiar to "socialized medicine," the wasteful distribution of facilities can occur in all systems. For example, the United States has many small hospitals that were established from community pride or from a voluntary association's desire to have its own facilities, when economy might have dictated fewer and larger installations arranged according to regional plans.

One might expect considerable political interference with the appointment of doctors to key posts, such as professorships in medical schools and the jobs of chiefs of service in hospitals. And one might expect such pressures to be greatest in totalitarian and authoritarian governments; totalitarian regimes are dedicated to transforming and mobilizing the society, while authoritarian governments distribute the spoils among the ruling cliques. Much less of this occurs than one thinks. Very few doctors belong to totalitarian parties, authoritarian parties, or democratic political machines, and thus few are available for such patronage. For example, the proportion of doctors belonging to the Nazi and Communist Parties was much lower than the membership rates of other occupations, and thus the Nazi and Soviet governments always had to fill the great majority of posts with doctors who cared little about politics. At the early stages of their existence, totalitarian and authoritarian governments often try to install some "more acceptable" doctors in place of professors and chiefs of service who were closely identified with the old regime, but after a few years, such political appointments cease. In most countries, the professors and chiefs of service are screened and selected by committees on which doctors hold most of the seats, and in practice the members resent outside interference from the politicians, from the Church, or from other laymen. (In practice, of course, the factional influences within the medical profession are thereby allowed to replace lay politics in determining selections.) Conforming to this tradition, the American Medicare statute explicitly guarantees that health insurance is a payment mechanism without leverage to affect appointments; in one of the law's several concessions to the doctors and hospital administrators, an introductory clause says that no "Federal officer or employee [shall] exercise any supervision or control . . . over the selection, tenure, or compensation of any officer or employee of any institution, agency, or person providing health services."

There is one type of lay government official who wields considerable authority over "socialized" medical services: he is not a power-hungry ideologue but the humdrum budget officer. Left to their own discretion, doctors would modernize all the hospitals and clinics, increase staff, order more drugs, charge higher fees, and cause spectacular increases in costs. Under privately organized medical care, they are inhibited by patients' inability to pay too much. In some wealthy countries, such as the United States, doctors and hospitals are able to give steadily more expensive care because of the population's wealth and because of the steadily increasing premiums that private health insurance schemes can collect from their subscribers. But under national health insurance, mounting costs would require an increase in social security payroll taxes and in Treasury subsidies. Under a national health service, higher medical costs would require higher income and excise taxes. Meanwhile, other government agencies are also seeking more funds. Thus, in the annual battle of the budget, the Treasury men tend to view the doctors as one of many special agencies that are trying to spend too much money on the basis of fancy claims. In order to maintain the fiscal integrity of the social security system, to prevent higher taxes, to prevent national deficits and the decline of the currency in international trade, and to give priority to other expenditures—such as national defense—the budget officers exercise considerable power over the functions of the medical services and over the pay of doctors.

Just as rapidly rising costs are troublesome in private American medical care, so rising costs will doubtless beset Medicare in the future. And just as conflicts between budget officers and the medical services wrack health schemes abroad, so they may torment American Medicare. The potential pressures on the sick funds are obvious: hospital costs are very high and rise steadily because of the lavish use of laboratory tests and drugs, heavy staffing, and numerous amenities for patients; doctors are accustomed to high incomes and freedom in setting their fees. The drafters of the Medicare statute appeared to anticipate trouble: the insurance funds are supposed to pay the "reasonable costs" of hospitalization and the "reasonable charges" for physicians' care; extensive research and negotiation are prescribed to fix the "reasonable costs" of hospitalization; the sensitive problem of deciding what medical fees are "reasonable charges" and can be paid from social security funds is handed over gingerly to the private health insurance carriers who will receive social security money and who will pay the doctors.

But the still vaguely defined system is full of potential conflicts that could be exacerbated by each group's single-minded preoccupation with its own ideas, although—as Holland's experience shows—wisdom and cooperation can avoid trouble. If the less commendable precedent of several other countries is followed, any of the following could occur: the budget officers of the sick funds and the hospitals could fight over payments, with the fiscal officers trying to keep within the resources of the social security taxes and with the hospitals trying to raise their services and salaries; the sick funds and hospitals could agree on "reasonable costs" exceeding the re-resources of the sick funds and could become involved in disputes with the Treasury over the need for supplementary grants from general tax funds; the public agency that pays the private medical insurance carriers for physicians' care might content that the carriers are not controlling fees sufficiently to keep within the budget, while the carriers and medical societies could claim that some of the ambiguous wording of the statute gives them exclusive power to make such judgments, regardless of the budgetary consequences; the Department of Health, Education, and Welfare might claim that it has the responsibility to protect its insured from overcharging by doctors, while the medical association replies that such bargains are a private matter between doctors and patients.

Doctor and Patient

One of the fears of critics of "socialized medicine" is change in doctor-patient relations, particularly by the entry of lay officials into medical questions. Such a possibility worries the medical association in each country, and as a result it insists that "socialized medicine" change pre-existing doctor-patient relations as little as possible. As a result, socialized medicine tends to freeze the pre-existing working conditions of doctors and simply changes the way they are paid. The Medicare statute is even more forceful than other national health insurance laws in drawing the line. Its introductory words say that "Nothing in this title shall be construed to authorize any Federal officer or employee to exercise any supervision or control over the practice of medicine or the manner in which medical services are provided."

The sites of doctor-patient contacts that are paid for under the official systems abroad are usually the traditional sites. In most countries—the

United States is one of the few exceptions in this respect—general practitioners traditionally do not treat patients in hospitals, and "socialized medicine" simply perpetuates this custom. Where general practitioners customarily have seen patients in their private offices and in the patients' homes (as in most of Europe), the insurance scheme or health service continues to pay for home and office visits; where private insurance funds and the government traditionally provided polyclinics for participating general practitioners (as in Eastern Europe, the U.S.S.R., and many underdeveloped countries), "socialized medicine" builds more polyclinics. Where specialists customarily have seen patients in the hospital (as in England, Holland, or Sweden), the insurance schemes and health services pay the specialists by methods tending to restrict treatment to the inpatient or outpatient facilities of hospitals; where some specialists traditionally worked in hospitals while other specialists had full-time or part-time private office practices (as in France and Germany), national health insurance usually pays specialists' fees for both hospital care and office care.

Under all European schemes, the patient may see any general practitioner who will accept him. There are the usual limitations found under private practice: if a doctor is very busy, he will be unable to accept new patients who present no emergencies, and getting an early appointment with a general practitioner is particularly difficult in countries with few physicians, such as Sweden. A few limitations arise out of the organization of certain programs: in order to guarantee that doctors give conscientious care and do not build up long lists of patients for mercenary reasons, England and Holland limit the number of patients for whom a G.P. will be paid under the official system, but any number of other patients may be taken privately; official schemes will not pay for patients who "shop around" among doctors for multiple opinions, although such patients may still enjoy this luxury by paying privately. In those European countries that pay fees to specialists for office visits, the patients may select any specialist of his own choice.

In several important ways, some patients may lack freedom of choice—but this tends to arise from traditional practices. In several countries with national health services—for example, in the U.S.S.R., in Poland, and in the rural areas of underdeveloped countries—all persons living in a district are automatically assigned to a general practitioner appointed for that district. When a patient is hospitalized under national health insurance or under national health service, he is treated by whichever specialists are assigned by the chief of service, and the patient and general practitioner usually have no say in designating the particular doctor. Similarly, when a patient seeks a specialist's care in the outpatient clinic of a hospital or in a community polyclinic, he must see whatever specialist is on duty at the time of his visit, although some countries allow him to schedule an appointment with a particular member of the duty rota.

The desire for the freedom to choose one's own specialist is one of the principal reasons for the survival of private practice in countries with "socialized medicine." In order to be treated by the chief of service and not by one of his young assistants, the patient must see the chief privately and pay personally. In order to avoid the crowded and unpleasant wards of public hospitals in Latin Europe and in underdeveloped countries, the patient must pay for one of the private rooms in the chief's public hospital or he may enter a private clinic where the chief has admitting privileges. In countries with "socialized medicine," private practice is less common among general practitioners than among specialists, but it survives for similar reasons. If paid privately, a G.P. may accept a patient whom he would be unable or unwilling to add to an already long list of insured patients. The private patient will get an appointment sooner and may get from the doctor more time and more emotional support.

The presence of private practice is one of the sources of conflict between the medical profession and the administrators of national health insurance and of national health services. Common accusations of the administrators are that doctors give more time and attention to their private patients, minimize time spent in the hospital and in other official work sites, and divert profitable patients from their public practices into their private practices. These complaints are particularly serious in Latin Europe and in underdeveloped countries, where low national incomes and poor tax collection result in low salaries for the public hospital doctors. Until salaries can be raised, the administrators and the medical association can do little except deplore neglect.

In practice, the sick funds and national health services have little say in the matter of how doctors treat patients. But the budgets of sick funds must be protected against the possibility that a few doctors may do medically unnecessary work for money. Detecting and disciplining such doctors is one of the more controversial problems of national health insurance. The sick funds get bills covering all patients, and statistical records of work norms are calculated. The funds become suspicious of a doctor's practice only if he performs far more acts than do all other physicians, a comparison also commonly made by American private health insurance firms when controlling abuse. Only if a doctor is flagrantly out of line will the sick funds send one of their employed physicians to discuss the problem. Usually the only sanction is a refusal to pay all the doctor's bills, but this is possible only in systems where the funds pay the doctor directly. The patients and the public almost never hear of any disputes between doctors and funds. The European funds no longer re-examine individual patients in order to evaluate a doctor's practice, since the medical association would react explosively, as it did in France during the 1930s.

One of the drawbacks of "socialized medicine" is that it freezes the existing structure of medical institutions and of doctor-patient relations. Improvements can be introduced only with difficulty. For example, the traditional practice of not allowing general practitioners to treat hospital inpatients is made permanent and is extended throughout the country by payment systems that give hospitalization fees or salaries only to members of hospital staffs. The establishment of the National Health Service in England widened this split by creating permanent staffs in numerous hospitals where local G.P.'s had practiced part of each day. Many reformers now urge that G.P.'s continue to see their patients during hospitalization in order to ensure continuity of care and provide the patient with a familiar face, but any such change would require revisions of the payment system, appeasement of the hospital specialists, and reorganization of the general practitioners' work schedules. It is equally difficult to modify the system of territorial assignment of general practitioners in Eastern Europe in order to give patients more free choice among doctors, since this would require changes in payment procedure, changes in work schedules, more personnel, better transportation, and more money. Alterations of any large structure usually raise the specter of higher costs and resistance by those doctors who are pleased by the *status quo;* administrators, therefore, let sleeping dogs lie.

The Quantity and Quality of Care

National health insurance or a national health service is sought because large social classes cannot afford medical care or because large regions of the country lack medical facilities. The result is always a mixture of successes and disappointments. "Socialized medicine" enables the poor to get medical care more easily, since financial barriers are reduced, but the quantity and quality of care are never altered as much as its creators had hoped.

The biggest difference is visible in underdeveloped countries, where governments build hospitals and clinics in rural areas and in urban slums that never had them before. The Soviet Union is the best example of a formerly underdeveloped country whose extensive medical services could not have been created without government planning and financing. However, adequate nationwide expansion of a government health service is limited by several factors: underdeveloped countries lack the tax resources to satisfy all needs; few doctors and nurses are willing to work outside the largest cities, and no government is willing or able to force them.

The effects on medical care in the somewhat more developed countries are more modest. Where quality depends on facilities, "socialized medicine" can lead to improvement because of the investment of public funds. In public hands, the hospitals for the poor may be financed far better than if private owners alone paid for buildings and equipment; improved financing was the principal motive for nationalization of private hospitals in Italy and in several other countries in recent centuries. National health insurance funds have built polyclinics in Spain, Italy, and Greece and have allowed participating doctors to see insured patients there, thus giving the doctors access to equipment that they could not afford to buy for their private offices.

In the highly developed countries, the quality of the private office practitioner's work is affected very little. The sick funds and the Ministries of Health leave the problem of quality primarily to the medical schools, to the profession as a whole, and to the consciences of individual doctors. The medical association would fight any close scrutiny of the work of doctors by these public bodies, which are perceived solely as agencies for the payment of medical care. The quality of office care has probably improved since the introduction of national health insurance and of national health services in Europe—but in large part the change is due to the universal tendency for medicine to improve over time. Perhaps better collection of bills has enabled some doctors to buy equipment that they could not have afforded under completely private conditions. A few ·sick funds affect the quality of care slightly by paying higher fees for professionally approved as opposed to professionally disapproved procedures; for example, surgical reduction of hernia is paid for under French national health insurance while hand reduction is not covered. A few funds affect quality by refusing to pay for the acts of a specialty, such as surgical operations, unless they are done by a fully qualified specialist. In general superior performance is not rewarded, except by appointment to the better posts and by referral of many private patients—forms of recognition that occur in all public and private systems. England's National Health Service awards higher salaries to specialists whose distinction is recognized by a committee of doctors, and leading Russian physicians receive medals and extra pay; but otherwise "socialized medicine" is compelled by the medical profession itself not to evaluate and discriminate among its members.

If the quality of medical care is not improved as much as one might expect, the same is true of the quantity. "Socialized medicine" probably reduces the number of people who would otherwise be inhibited by financial considerations from seeking medical care. But comparisons of statistics over time, and some recent surveys, suggest that the increased number of such patients is small. Some recent health surveys in England and elsewhere have turned up a surprising number of people who fail to take their medical problems to freely available health services, because of apathy or ignorance.

Thus, Americans should not expect spectacular increases in the quality and quantity of medical care under the new statute. The language of the law—previously quoted—prevents the government from regulating the quality of care directly (even assuming it were competent to do so), and

American doctors are already so well equipped on the average that increased public spending will not materially improve their facilities. Many of the aged are already heavy users of medical care through private payments, private health insurance, and charity. Medicare's principal effects may be economic and psychological: it will enable the aged to spend their money on other things, and it will enable some of the aged to get care without applying as indigents. Among the principal effects of Medicare may be small increases in the incomes of doctors and hospitals, as in the case of national health insurance abroad: doctors and hospitals will collect full payment for some aged patients who might otherwise have been charged little or nothing, particularly for long-term care.

"Socialized Medicine" Through Harmonious Evolution

After medical care for the aged is included under social security in the United States, probably there will be no immediate pressures for enactment of a more comprehensive national health insurance scheme or a national health service. The trade unions—the principal force behind "socialized medicine" abroad—are for the most part, satisfied with the private arrangements secured through collective bargaining here. However, a mixture of public and private solutions eventually may be sought for the problems of incomplete benefits, mounting premiums, and unstable financing of the present mélange of private insurance and public assistance programs. Perhaps some form of standardization may develop by voluntary agreement among all these programs, with the use of federal taxation to collect insurance premiums, with legal standards, with federal subsidies, all under a representative council possessing statutory authority. Thus national health insurance may ultimately come to America by evolution—not by government fiat but by the private parties themselves using government procedures and sanctions to carry out their public mission. This pattern occurred in Holland, and the harmony and efficiency of that country's health services recommend it as a model.

Such a harmonious collaboration between government and private health agencies seems far removed from the usual rhetoric about "socialized medicine" in America. But development of such a system already seems well under way in the United States. Despite the occasional political controversies that catch headlines, daily relations between medical organizations and government have long been harmonious in America. And in many activities, government already provides medical services or assists private efforts with subsidies and sanctions. For example, few voluntary hospitals and private medical schools could be constructed today without public grants; most of the funds for clinical research in America come from the federal Treasury, most medical students attend state-supported schools and many of the others are subsidized by government scholarships; the private practice of the health professions depends on government licensure administered by members of the professions; public hospitals owned by municipalities, states, the Veterans' Administration, and the United States Public Health Service relieve the voluntary and proprietary hospitals of much of the heavy burden of caring for the chronically ill and medically indigent. Thus the real issue in America—as in all other countries—is not *whether* government shall play a central role in medical care but *what* that role should be.

Medical Men in Practice

Thus far, the articles have dealt with medicine as a whole, that is, medicine as an occupation the organization of which may be looked at and compared with that of other occupations on a national or society-wide basis. However, while such broad occupational organization does indeed exist, within it there is a variety of suborganizations represented by such things as specialty societies and schools of opinion; and there are significant variations in the kind of work that members of the general profession perform. The nature of the work itself seems to be connected with systematic variation in the characteristics of the workers as well as in the way work is organized into medical practice. This section of papers concerns itself with the actual practice of medicine by individuals and with the way practice varies. Of great significance to the variety of practice is the setting in which individuals work and the influence of this social setting and the special kind of work on professional characteristics and performance. The papers are arranged to begin with the broadest level of historical variation, going through variation between specialties and within specialties, types of practice in an urban community, and variations of work and its organization within a single institution in the community.

The Bulloughs present a brief sketch of the development of Western medicine over the ages, including reference to some of the difficulties that medicine has had in developing its present-day professional organization. They also broadly sketch the problems of medical practice today which have been exacerbated by the rapid development of medical specialization over the past century. In the next paper, George Rosen addresses himself specifically to the rise of modern medical specialization in the nineteenth century and in the course of his analysis suggests what is surprising only at first thought—that in those years specialization constituted a threat to the profession because it implied (correctly) that individual members varied in their competence to perform specific procedures and make specific diagnoses. Professions are prone to assert that the basic standards they establish in training and for licensing allow the patient to assume that any properly certified man is competent. The development of specialties of course attacks this notion at least to the extent of saying that only the most general competence is assured by profession-wide standards. Beyond that some individuals are more competent than others in a particular area. Indeed, in present-day medicine the major structural source of differentiation is in fact the specialty.

Nonetheless, the specialty is not the ultimate, irreducible source of patterned variation in medical careers and performance. Within it there are various schools of opinion and interest which compete with one another for support. In her paper Bucher shows how, just as the notion of the "whole" profession underlay some of the resistance to specialization in the nineteenth century, so the notion of the "whole" specialty resists differentiation into subspecialties which may be the seeds of future, full-fledged specialties. Differentiation within specialties is seen as a function of "segments" which themselves are the outcome of processes of collective behavior. In the specialty of pathology that Bucher analyzes, two segments are seen to be in interaction, each struggling to reshape the focus of the general specialty.

But pathology is a relatively inconspicuous specialty in medicine. More conspicuous and more complex is psychiatry. The many broad currents of ideology, knowledge, practice, and patient care which are present in the various psychiatric "schools" are discussed by Schatzman and Strauss. Throughout, they insist that psychiatry, like every other specialty of medicine, should be an object of sociological study rather than something to be taken at face value as presented by psychiatrists themselves. An example of the kind of analysis Schatzman and Strauss call for is found in the next paper, where Daniels specifically devotes herself to one kind of practice in psychiatry. Comparing the private practice of psychotherapy with the practice of psychiatry in the military, she shows how the setting in which the military psychiatrist works is responsible for delineating many of his treatment goals, stimulating a very special kind of "theory" within psychiatry in general and shaping the kind of relationship he has to his patients.

Whereas Daniels takes private practice as a constant against which to compare military practice, Solomon presents evidence bearing on the way in which private practice itself varies. He shows how various careers in private practice, representing various kinds and degrees of success in the community, can be differentiated by the kinds of hospitals used. Hospitals themselves may be seen as stratified within the community. Those of high prestige serve one kind of practitioner and those of low prestige others. While there is no doubt that changes have been and are taking place in the use of religion and ethnicity as criteria by which hospitals select their medical staffs, the fact of stratification of medical institutions and careers in the community remains and is likely to remain a critical component of variation in the level and direction of physician performance. In a city as large as Chicago, of course, greater variation is likely to exist than in smaller communities. Solomon's sketch, however, stands as an indication of the dimensions of stratification which occur both among medical institutions in a community and among the careers and practices of its medical men.

Turning from varieties of medical institutions and practices in a community to variations within a single institution, the paper by Coser examines the different modes of organizing work to be found in different units of the same hospital. There she contrasts surgical with medical work, the former typically requiring more rapid and decisive activity than the latter. She shows how the requirements of surgery lead to a more flexible, less authoritarian atmosphere than those of medicine. This outcome is similar to that found in the military, which, while it is generally characterized by fairly rigid discipline both in peacetime and behind the combat lines, changes its organization markedly when men are in actual combat.

It should be clear from these papers that the idea that there is some standardized professional activity shared by all those in the profession of medicine is problematic. So is the idea of some single mode of organizing such activity. What the medical man does at work and how he does it seem to be at least a partial function of a variety of social factors, not the least of which is constituted by the nature of the community and the institutional setting within which his work is carried out. Since mere professional education and licensing do not seem to be adequate grounds for predicting and thus "controlling" medical work performance, it follows that it is of the greatest importance to understand how, in concrete work settings, the performance of medical work is controlled. This is the problem addressed in the final paper, which points to serious deficiencies in the way performance is controlled in a setting staffed by professionals with better-than-average training and organized in ways which permit more regulation than can take place in the average practitioner's private office. Thus, regulation of physician performance may also be seen as a variable rather than as a constant feature of professional organization in general.

BIBLIOGRAPHIC SUGGESTIONS

In reading about variations in the organization of medical work, the place to start is in the historical and anthropological record. But while there are many excellent histories of medical knowledge, few histories have focused on medical practice. The recent work by Vern L. Bullough, *The Development of Medicine as a Profession* (New York: Hafner, 1966), emphasizes the organization of the profession, but the analysis ends far short of modern times. The classic work by Richard H. Shryock, *The Development of Modern Medicine* (New York: Alfred A. Knopf, 1947) is oriented toward social analysis, and deals with more modern times, particularly in the United States. In the case of anthropological studies, no single source can be cited which is entirely satisfactory for the purpose of sociological analysis, though excellent materials are scattered from one monograph to another. A review article with a large bibliography of anthropological studies is S. Polgar, "Health and Human Behavior: Areas of Interest Common to the Social and Medical Sciences," *Current Anthropology* 3 (April, 1962), 159-205. However, a specialty known as "medical anthropology" is beginning to emerge, and bibliographic resources in the area are likely to be improved very shortly.

Three books may be cited which analyze the experience of medical men in other countries. For the Soviet Union, see Mark G. Field, *Soviet Socialized Medicine: An Introduction* (New York: The Free Press, 1967). For Israel, see Judith T. Shuval, *Social Functions of Medical Practice* (San Francisco: Jossey-Bass, 1970). For England, see Rosemary Stevens, *Medical Practice in Modern England, The Impact of Specialization and State Medicine* (New Haven: Yale University Press, 1966).

In the case of the medical specialties and subspecialties in the United States, there is in fact very little systematic and empirical data available, with but a few articles scattered here and there through the journals. The greatest attention has been paid to psychiatry, as our own selections in this book suggest. For psychiatry, the references in the Schatzman and Strauss article reprinted here will suffice.

There is also comparatively little available on the nature of medical practice. The classic work is by Oswald Hall and appeared in three articles: "The Informal Organization of the Medical Profession," *Canadian Journal of Economics and Political Science*, 12 (1946), 30-44; "The Stages of a Medical Career," *American Journal of Sociology* 53 (1948), 327-336; "Types of Medical Career," *American Journal of Sociology* 55 (1949), 243-253. A study of the diffusion of a new drug among 216 physicians in four Midwestern communities which is also quite revealing of many of the contingencies of community practice is James S. Coleman, Elihu Katz, and Herbert Menzel, *Medical Innovation, A Diffusion Study* (Indianapolis: Bobbs-Merrill, 1966). Finally may be cited a study of the way urban patients respond to various types of medical practice: Eliot Freidson, *Patients' Views of Medical Practice* (New York: Russell Sage Foundation, 1961).

A few representative studies of hospitals may also be cited here. A descriptive introduction to the hospital is provided in Temple Burling, et al, *The Give and Take in Hospitals* (New York: G. P. Putnam's Sons, 1956). A complex survey of twelve Michigan hospitals is reported in Basil S. Georgopolous and Floyd C. Mann, *The Community General Hospital* (New York: Macmillan, 1963). A number of different kinds of studies are reported in Eliot Freidson, ed., *The Hospital in Modern Society* (New York: The Free Press, 1963). A very revealing field study of community hospitals is reported in Ivan Belknap and John G. Steinle, *The Community and Its Hospitals* (Syracuse: Syracuse University Press, 1963). And finally may be mentioned the comparative study of mental hospitals by Anselm Strauss et al., *Psychiatric Ideologies and Institutions* (New York: The Free Press, 1964), a book which also deals with different schools of opinion and different careers and practices in psychiatry.

6

BONNIE BULLOUGH
VERN BULLOUGH

A Brief History of Medical Practice

Medicine has long served sociologists, either consciously or unconsciously, as the model profession, and in recent years medical sociology itself has emerged as a major field of research. The organizational structure, the work role, the socialization process, and the interpersonal relationships of the doctor as well as various paramedical groups have been studied. Considerable investigation has also been carried out in the hospital setting. Medicine, however, is rapidly changing, and very little attention has been given to how current American medical practices developed or to the variety of institutional arrangements under which medicine has operated in the past. Obviously, a brief paper is not the place to give the whole history of medicine. Our purpose here is not so much to give a step-by-step account of the origin and development of medicine or to list all the great names in the field but to make generalizations about the past that might give insight into current conditions and provoke further discussion among sociologists. Nevertheless, since the paper is historical, we can approach the subject chronologically.

Primitive and Ancient Medicine

Though there were great variations in culture between the many preliterate societies, just as there are differences in cultural patterns among contemporary primitives, medicine seems at first to have been closely allied with religion. In fact medicine as an occupation started with the shaman who was not only the physician but the priest, sorcerer, poet, storyteller, and even chief. In an unspecialized society, the shaman was the first specialist and encompassed most of what we now regard as the learned professions. Undoubtedly, the more sophisticated shamans incorporated empirical practices with their religious and magical methods, and many of these were passed on to their successors, so that gradually a store of medical knowledge was built up. Moreover, the union of medical and priestly functions

86

gave the treatments prescribed by the shaman more efficacy and authority than folk remedies which might lack such divine backing. This union in itself might have tended to help cure many people who might otherwise not have been cured.

By the time written history appears in the Tigris-Euphrates and Nile Valleys, a role separate from the priestly one had started to develop for the medical man, although ancient physicians still retained a close association with the gods. In the Tigris-Euphrates Valley, for example, illness was regarded as punishment for sins—for violating the norms of the society by stealing, killing, blaspheming, committing adultery, drinking from an impure vessel, etc. Such a conceptualization of disease had great influence upon medicine; it was carried over into the Old Testament, and from there into Christianity. Even today epidemics are sometimes thought of as plagues sent by God.

Since the victim of an illness or accident need not even have been aware of his sin, the necessary treatment first required an effort to find out in what ways the gods were offended, then to appease them through magical rites and incantations. Rational methods, however, were not entirely excluded since once the evil had been exorcised, it still might be necessary to remove the poison which it had left behind. This last aspect of treatment was left to the *asu,* a type of priest who, without abandoning the dominant beliefs of the culture, utilized drugs and surgery as well as incantations and charms to treat the afflicted. This use led to the more secular type of medicine evident in the surviving law codes, especially those of Hammurabi (1704-1662 B.C.). The punitive nature of many of these laws suggest that the *asu* had lost much of his religious sanctity and in fact was regarded with considerable suspicion. Gradually the *asu* assumed a distinctive appearance; he shaved his head and carried a bag of herbs, a libation jar (filled with water), as well as an incense burner, to indicate his calling as physician.

Egyptian society underwent much the same development, although the emerging physician probably retained a somewhat higher status than he did in Mesopotamia. This is indicated by the deification of Imhotep, the contemporary of Zoser, the third-dynasty pharoah who built the stepped pyramid. Imhotep not only served as physician but as pyramid builder, astrologer, and general all-purpose handyman, but after his death he became a folk hero, then a demigod, and ultimately the god and patron of the healing arts. With his protection Egyptian medical practitioners developed some independence from the regular priesthood and acquired as well considerable skill in the treatment of external wounds. Internal maladies, with less obvious etiology, were more likely to be treated by supplication to the gods or with charms, incantations, and other forms of magic. Though the Egyptians are known for their mortuary practices, the Egyptian physicians did not communicate with those who worked in the house of the dead so had only rather hazy ideas of internal anatomy and physiology. They did, however, acquire some useful knowledge about herbs and certain inorganic materials. Specialties of a sort also developed, until by the fifth century B.C., the Greek historian Herodotus described specialists for the belly, for the eyes, for the colon, and for other parts of the body.

At least some of the Egyptian and Mesopotamian physicians were literate, as there are numerous extant medical documents from these civilizations. The Egyptian physicians also went through a long period of training which closely paralleled that of some of the priests. It is quite possible that the physicians produced by this training limited their practice to the upper classes. The poor people and slaves undoubtedly relied on religious incantations, on folk remedies, and on home nursing care to meet their medical crises as the masses of people living in these areas still do.

Greek and Roman Medicine

Greek medicine borrowed from that of the other peoples of the ancient Near East, but the Greeks also made important contributions of their own. Medical practitioners worked under the divine patronage of Asclepius, a semilegendary physician who was deified. There was an actual cult of Asclepius that established healing temples throughout the Greco-Roman world where patients went for rest, nursing care, and cure. In addition, the Greeks developed more secular practitioners who had considerably more independence than their predecessors in the Tigris-Euphrates and Nile Valleys. This development was due in part to the fact that the Greeks lacked an overall religious cosmogony and were convinced that the gods had not revealed everything to men but instead left much for them to find out themselves. It has been argued that the earliest secular medical healers were members of certain families who guarded their medical secrets, passing them on from father to son. Whether this was the case or not, eventually several medical schools developed, and candidates other than sons of physicians became medical practitioners. These schools were not like modern ones but instead tended to be built around one man or a small group of men who taught their students by means of an apprenticeship program. The apprentice, in fact, often acted as an assistant to the physician, carrying out many of the more menial tasks until he had mastered the trade. Undoubtedly, many of the Greek physicians were illiterate, although those of higher status were literate.

The most famous of the Greek medical schools was that on the island of Cos associated with the name of Hippocrates. Little is known about this semilegendary physician, but a collection of medical writings was made at Alexandria in the third century B.C. and attributed to him. Probably he wrote few, if any, of the treatises that bear his name. Most of them were later assigned to him because he had such a great reputation as a physician and observer. The Hippocratic *corpus* not only includes much about

Greek medical concepts, but it also gives us invaluable insights into actual medical practice. In general it seems that education was by apprenticeship, and was more empirical than philosophical. There was no licensing or regulating of medical practitioners, and probably there was a tremendous variation in their abilities. Some of these physicians, who probably looked upon themselves as the leaders, tried to establish codes of ethics, the most famous of which is that associated with the name of Hippocrates. There was also a tendency for the medical practitioners to try to identify themselves with a particular school, such as that of Cos, that had a good reputation. Usually only the rich could afford the services of the best-trained medical practitioners, although some cities did support public physicians. Most of the poor and the slaves relied upon folk remedies, uneducated practitioners, or turned to the temples of Asclepius. The status of physicians varied greatly. In fact, it might be said that in the Greek world the physician's status was more dependent upon that of his client or patient than on his position as a medical healer.

It seems clear that the Greek physicians probably reached a higher level of competence than any other ancient practitioner. Greek medicine was exported to the rest of the Mediterranean world first by Greek conquests and then by those of Rome. Under the Greek Ptolemies in Egypt, medical education and research received royal patronage in the Museum at Alexandria. It was here that the Hippocratic *corpus* was compiled and that the first recorded anatomical investigations began. Other rulers such as the King of Pergamum also supported similar institutions, but with the Roman conquest, secular medicine began to lose some of the status that it had gained. This might be because the Greek physicians who first entered the Roman world did so as slaves or were regarded with suspicion because they were foreigners. Roman medicine, before the Greeks appeared on the scene, had been rather primitive, although Roman efforts on public-health-type projects were much more advanced. For the educated Roman, Greek medicine made its greatest impact as part of the basic liberal arts training instead of as a way to earn a living. As a result, medicine became more theoretical, less empirical, more a topic for conversation than a way of earning a living. Nevertheless, there were several outstanding physicians, most of them Greeks or Greek-trained. The most eminent of these was the Greek-speaking Galen, born in 130 A.D. He traveled around the Mediterranean world to study medicine under various famous men before settling in Rome, where eventually he became physician to the Emperor Marcus Aurelius. Galen wrote at least 100 treatises and today his surviving works fill some 22 volumes. Though Galen was the greatest medical experimentalist of the ancient world, his very ability and comprehensiveness tended to encourage system building and theoretical medicine rather than serving as a model for further experimentation. Galen and Hippocrates, as well as some lesser writers, tended to be regarded by their successors as com-

pilers of medical Bibles, books whose words were to be accepted as the
truth without further questioning.

The trend toward theoretical medicine so apparent in Rome was accentuated by the decline of western urban centers in the second and third centuries A.D. Specialization (and medicine was one of the early specialties)
more or less demands large centers of population. With the decline of
cities there were fewer opportunities for a trained physician to earn a living, although an emperor or king would still have his own medical adviser in attendance. Increasingly, the majority of the population, even
many of the noble class, had to rely upon folk remedies or their own
medical knowledge that they might have picked up in books. Even this
tended to decay as there was decline in schools (and in educational levels)
brought about by the growing ruralization and the disorientation caused by
the Germanic migrations into the western Roman Empire. Moreover, as
the Christian Church achieved dominance in the West, the chief purpose of
any kind of intensive education came to be to prepare the clergy. It was
the clergy, particularly those affiliated with monastic institutions, who preserved the theoretical knowledge of medicine, although few of them practiced it on any scale. Inevitably, much of the body of Greek medical knowledge, most of which had not been translated into Latin, was lost to the
West, much temporarily, some permanently.

Medieval Medicine

The Eastern Mediterranean, on the other hand, remained much more
urban-oriented. Occupational specialization, including medicine, continued
to exist at Constantinople and Alexandria, and then after the Arab conquest
of the seventh century, in various other parts of the new Islamic-controlled
areas. The Arabs did not force conversion to Islam and were particularly
tolerant of Jews and Christians. Moreover, since Islam in such a short
time changed from the religion of a desert people to the religion of the ruling class of comparatively sophisticated and urbanized people, it had to
either incorporate the higher intellectual standards or turn away from them.
During the period of its greatest expansion, Islam chose to incorporate the
philosophical and scientific learning of the conquered peoples, and Greek
and Persian scientific and medical treatises were translated into Arabic and
spread throughout the Arabic-speaking world. Arabic-speaking physicians,
many of whom were Christians or Jews, also wrote specialized treatises
of their own. Eventually this Arabic medical knowledge reached western
Europe, at first through Spain, and then through Sicily and southern Italy,
where many Greek-speaking peoples continued to reside. Finally, westerners began traveling to the Byzantine capital of Constantinople to seek out
Greek originals instead of Arab translations. One of the key groups in the
transmission of Arabic and Greek medical ideas and concepts to the Latin

West during the medieval period were the Jewish physicians who traveled in both Islamic and Christian lands. One explanation for the large number of Jewish physicians in the medieval period might be that rabbis were encouraged to earn a living outside of the synagogue. Medicine became one of the favorite alternative occupations. This union of rabbi and physician should not be looked upon as a return to priestly medicine, since the rabbi himself was not regarded as a priest; his curative abilities were due to his medical knowledge and not to his sacred position. Moreover, the rabbi had the education to acquire the various theoretical concepts about medicine and enough patients to develop effective empirical abilities.

The decline of Western educational institutions was halted during the reign of the Frankish Emperor Charlemagne (768-814), who ordered all monasteries and cathedrals to establish schools. Medicine became part of the curriculum in many of the schools, although it was primarily theoretically oriented and only a few students studied it very intensely. The first major center of Western medical training came to be at Salerno. Probably there were several places like Salerno which had traditions of being healing centers, but by the tenth century Salerno's reputation had eclipsed its rivals. Salernitan medicine was at first empirically oriented, but it was further strengthened in the eleventh century when it added the medical theory brought into Europe by the translations of Constantine the African. Constantine (c. 1020-1087), whose origins and background are somewhat obscure, traveled throughout the Mediterranean world before joining the service of a Norman duke who brought him to Italy. There he entered a monastery where he spent the rest of his life translating Arabic (and Arabic-Greek) medical works into Latin. These soon became part of the curriculum at Salerno and from there spread into other emerging medical schools, some of which soon became recognized as universities.

There was a rapid growth in population during the eleventh and twelfth centuries which in turn led to a number of new urban centers, and it was in these that the first universities appeared. Universities originally derived from corporate associations, guilds of teachers or of students, and the two archetypal ones appeared at Bologna in Italy and Paris in France. Both of these pioneering institutions soon incorporated medical universities and it was in the medieval setting that medicine first came to be recognized as a postgraduate course. Students first studied a liberal arts course leading to an A.M. degree, after which they went into the more specialized subjects of medicine, civil or canon law, or theology. Normally, graduation in medicine implied a three-step process of bachelor, licentiate (license to teach granted by ecclesiastical authorities), and the master's or doctor's degree (admission into the guild of masters or doctors). The main purpose of the advanced medical degree was not so much to enable the graduate to practice medicine but to teach it, hence the title doctor (from the Latin *docere*—to teach). In university cities, however, the local medical faculty soon acquired considerable say over who would practice medicine, too. Through their influence with ecclesiastical and royal authorities, the university trained physicians, in fact, influenced the whole development of medicine. Moreover, the development of medical universities gave a continuity of high standards by the establishment of effective codes of ethics. However, the development of these standards had some unexpected consequences, not all of them positive. The surgeons, for their part, attempted to draw a distinction between themselves and their rivals, the barbers or barber-surgeons, by adopting the methods of the physicians, even going so far as to establish their own college of surgery. Barber-surgeons also followed the same procedures, and this Parisian struggle between the various medical practitioners was one of the first major boundary disputes in medicine. In the struggle the surgeons tended to lose out to the physicians on one side and the barber-surgeons on the other, both of whom made an informal alliance against the surgeons. Still, the French kings were unwilling to give the university physicians the monopoly that they sought because the various monarchs held that the physicians restricted themselves to treating the upper classes, while the barber-surgeons alone were willing to deal with the masses of people. The struggle also demonstrated some of the same issues now present in the current rivalry between existing paramedical practitioners, since the physicians emphasized their high status by refusing to do certain tasks which they regarded as beneath them; the surgeons in turn did not carry out procedures that they regarded as suitable only for barbers. Even within the ranks of the barber-surgeons there came to be status divisions. The university-trained physicians, however, insisted on control over the apothecaries, the one group that they regarded as essential to the practice of medicine as they conceived it.

Early Modern Period

It is perhaps worthy of comment that most of the medical advances of the early modern period were not made by the Parisian physicians and surgeons who were so concerned with their status, but by Italian-trained physicians or by surgeons whose educational system was not so riddled by rivalries. In addition to the anatomical discoveries connected with the name of Andreas Vesalius (1514-1564) and centered in the Italian universities, there were also major advances in physiology such as the discovery of the circulation of the blood by William Harvey (1578-1657), who studied in Italy. The most important surgeon of the period was Ambroise Paré (1510-1590), who served his apprenticeship in the French Provincial city of Laval and made his reputation as an army surgeon.

In spite of a better understanding of anatomy and physiology, and some improvement in surgical techniques, the physician and surgeon even as late as the eighteenth century was not able to give very effective medical care. Though there were many forward-looking investigators at work such as

John Hunter (1728-1793), the problems of disease and health were so vast and complex, and the weight of past tradition so pressing, that the physician was probably no more able to cure his patients than he had been at the time of Hippocrates. Inevitably, many physicians became disillusioned when the new discoveries failed to lead to universal laws of healing, but only tended to lead to greater confusion. Anxious to find a single explanation for all disease, they tended to neglect the scientific method or to follow it only a short way. The result was the building of vast theoretical systems of medicine based upon speculative logic rather than a true understanding of the nature of illness. Though it is true that the various systems often had some scientific observation behind them, and occasionally led to valuable insights, the system-makers found favor primarily because they gave simple answers to complex problems. In extenuation of the physician it should be said that the medical practitioner usually had no real way of determining whether a proposed cure was effective, even if his patient recovered. This could only be done by experimenting with different kinds of treatment for the same illness, and most medical practitioners saw only a few cases of any type of illness, rarely enough to even be sure of the kind of disease they were treating. Specialization was considered unprofessional and institutionalized medical research had not yet developed.

The medical systems which resulted continued to exercise great influence almost up to the twentieth century. While a short paper is not the place to examine the systems in detail, a sample of some of the ideas should be indicative of the problem. One of the system-makers was Georg Ernst Stahl (1660-1734), who held that a sensitive soul or *anima* inhabited every part of the human organism and prevented its spontaneous putrefaction. Disease then became nothing else than the tendency of the *anima* to reestablish the normal order of tonic movement as quickly as possible. Friedrich Hoffman (1660-1742) regarded the body as a kind of hydraulic machine kept going by a "nervous ether" circulating through the nervous system. When the machine or *tonus* was normal, the body was healthy. When it was not normal, illness resulted, and treatment could be sedative, corroborant, tonic, or evacuant, according to the necessity of stimulating or quieting the *tonus* of the nerves. John Brown (1735-1788) held that disease was either *sthenia,* a result of overstimulation, or *asthenia,* an inability to respond to stimulation. Homeopathy, developed by Christian Friedrich Samuel Hahnemann (1755-1843), was based upon the principle of *similia similibus;* in effect, diseases could be cured by the administration of drugs or treatments which produce a condition similar to the disease. Thus hot compresses were prescribed for burns, opium to cure somnolence, and so forth. At the opposite extreme was allopathy, which adhered to *contraria contrariis* and required that sedatives be given in excited states and stimulants in depressed states. There were many others; the important thing about the systems is that they gave the medical practitioner an easy answer to almost any illness.

With the system-makers more or less dominating medical practice, there was also a rapid growth in quackery. In essence, the quacks proposed even faster cures than the licensed physicians. As a general rule they had no medical training. Multiplying rapidly in the eighteenth century were the nostrum-makers who invented salves or tonics which claimed to cure all ailments. Their growth, particularly in England, was in part due to the development of the patent system during the last part of the seventeenth and the first part of the eighteenth centuries. More important, however, was the increasing exclusiveness of the physicians and their unwillingness to increase their numbers to serve the growing population, particularly in metropolitan areas like London. At the beginning of the eighteenth century, for example, the College of Physicians in London had only 114 members, about 80 of whom actually practiced in the city. The obvious alternative for most people was the apothecary who dispensed medicines upon prescription. Technically, the apothecary did not diagnose, but obviously what was good for one man's cough seemed to him to be good for someone else's. Many apothecaries began to sell their medicines; and when the College of Physicians attempted to prevent such sale without a prescription, the House of Lords refused to allow this prohibition because of the shortage of physicians. The next step was for apothecaries (and physicians) as well as uneducated laymen to patent certain concoctions, or rather to copyright the name and to advertise heavily in medicine shows and in the penny press which was beginning to appear. Nostrum promotion achieved in the words of one scholar "the very perfection of extravagance" in eighteenth-century England. Patent medicines, in fact, became the mainstay of newspaper advertising until almost the twentieth century. In the United States, most of the patent medicines at first were English, although the Americans entered the field with great originality in 1796 after the U.S. Patent Office was established. Most of continental Europe adopted the same techniques. It was only after medical research itself began to show results that the nostrum-makers and the system-builders were effectively challenged. Even then it required direct government intervention to curtail many of the abuses; physicians also had to face up to their responsibility to treat the masses of people, since until the twentieth century, trained medical practitioners restricted themselves primarily to the upper classes.

The Hospital and Specialization

Closely allied with change in medicine was the appearance of the hospital. Hospitals were a medieval development that had originated through an effort to provide shelter for the traveler, the poor sick, the orphan, and others whose family could not take care of them. Most of the early hospitals had been staffed by monks or nuns who assumed caretaker responsibility, although the larger institutions often had a trained medical person attached. After the universities had appeared, the hospitals began to be used for clinical teaching, but it was not until the end of the eighteenth century that physicians recognized the tremendous potential present in the hospitals. In part, this was because hospitals themselves grew rapidly as Europe became ever more urbanized during the industrialization of the eighteenth and nineteenth centuries. Thousands of new immigrants moved into the city from the countryside, where they soon fell victim to typhoid fever, tuberculosis, or other illnesses endemic in the unsanitary cities. Since the new arrivals had no families or friends who were willing or able to take care of them, they ended up in hospitals, and these rapidly grew in number. To a research-minded physician the overcrowded hospitals offered unprecedented material for clinical observation—and for autopsies. France, particularly Paris, served as the starting point for a new type of medical research combining physical examination with autopsy to develop better diagnosis and treatment. The French Revolution abolished the old universities, academies, and traditional institutions, including the distinction between surgeons and physicians that had so long handicapped medicine in France. Hospitals in conjunction with the universities became the major training center for a new generation of doctors. Although this situation meant that the low-income people who ended up in the hospitals provided clinical examples that the physician later used to cure his more well-to-do private patients, the poor at least received some sort of medical treatment. In England the hospitals had little connection with the universities, and this led to a separation of medicine from the university and to a concentration in the city hospitals. The result was to ghettoize medicine in England by cutting it off from the cross-fertilization with other disciplines present in the university. In Scotland, however, the university and hospitals were combined. Both methods came to be imitated in the United States, but it was not until the twentieth century that the university-hospital system won out. Throughout the nineteenth century, hospitals, both in Europe and in America, were primarily for the poor and were more caretaker institutions than treatment centers. The contemporary hospital is primarily a development of the last 40 years.

As hospitals became more important in the development of medicine, so did specialization. Specialism was strongly opposed by the medical profession, in part because in the past it had been associated with quackery, but also because of the traditional conservatism so inherent in medicine. Usually, the budding specialist began by opening special dispensaries where he treated the poor without fee, thereby provoking less resistance from the profession. Once a specialty had been established, clinics were opened. The next step was to establish special chairs in the university medical schools, found a specialist society, and begin publication of a journal. During the nineteenth century such specialties as orthopedics, ophthalmology, pediatrics, dermatology, neurology, and others developed. Some fields such as dentistry, at least in the United States, became so special-ized that they broke off entirely from the mainstream of medicine. On the continent in particular, but also in Scotland, the medical school came to be closely associated with the university. In the last part of the nineteenth century the German university model with medicine as a graduate specialty came to have great influence through the Western world.

Public Health and Scientific Discoveries

The eighteenth century also saw the beginning of a change in attitudes toward illness that is associated with the Enlightenment, a philosophical movement which shifted the center of interest from preoccupation with the fate of the soul in another world to improvement of conditions in this one. It was at this time that the words "social science" first appeared. The result of this shift in attitude was a public campaign by concerned individ-uals about the atrocious health conditions in armies, navies, prisons, and hospitals. One of the first results was the introduction of an effective pre-ventive measure against smallpox, first by variolation and then by vaccina-tion perfected by Edward Jenner (1749-1823). The development of accurate medical statistics made it possible to determine the differences between urban and rural disease rates and to differentiate causes of deaths. Improve-ments in sewers, water supplies, and housing, all brought noticeable progress. England took the lead in many of these early public health ef-forts, but Germany in the last part of the nineteenth century became pre-eminent. Rudolf Virchow (1821-1902), the most influential physician of his time, created the dictum "medicine is a social science." Max von Pet-tenkofer (1818-1901) was also important; his Institute of Hygiene founded in Munich in 1866 was the first scientific center to rigorously investigate hy-gienic problems.

Medicine also benefited from scientific discoveries which finally enabled the physicians of the twentieth century to actually cure people for perhaps the first time in history. The theory of contagion was confirmed by the efforts of the chemist Louis Pasteur (1822-1895). The bacteriological theories of Pasteur were applied to surgery by Joseph Lister (1827-1912), who devel-oped an efficacious antiseptic surgical method. Effective methods of anes-thetizing patients were also developed through the work of American den-tists and later by obstetricians. Surgery was revolutionized as surgeons were able to do major operative procedures that they had never before dared to attempt. The gulf between the speculative and empirical practitioner no longer existed, and the search for grand theories lost out. It was replaced by a disease-centered approach to the treatment of illness. Although medical men were still often able to treat only symptoms, research was aimed at improving the differential diagnoses and finding the specific causes and treatments of morbid conditions. With the work of Sigmund Freud (1856-

1939) and those who followed him, the disease-centered approach was also applied to mental illness. There is now, however, an ongoing controversy among psychotherapists (encouraged by medical sociologists) over the efficacy of nosography in understanding mental illness.

American Medical Developments

The United States for much of its history was a colonial outpost of European medicine. As a general rule, people with high status in Europe did not immigrate to the new world, so that most of the early American medical men were ship's surgeons or similar types of practitioners who had learned their craft in an apprenticeship program or had no training. Once they arrived in the United States, the newly settled medical practitioners were expected to care for all types of illness, perform surgery, mix drugs, and even pull teeth. Undoubtedly many of them even treated cows, horses, or pet dogs. Regardless of their own inadequate training, these early medical practitioners soon found it advantageous to take on apprentices. This meant that the level of medical skill in America was very low, although some Americans did go to Europe for training, particularly to Edinburgh, the leading British medical school of the day. By the time of the American Revolution only about five percent of the total medical practitioners held university degrees. In spite of this, everyone who practiced medicine assumed the title "doctor," which in Europe was reserved for university teachers or university-trained persons.

It was not until 1765 that the first American medical college was established in the College of Philadelphia, and this was soon followed by schools in New York, and at Harvard, Dartmouth, and Yale. Though these schools were called colleges, they were little more than apprenticeship training centers with the addition of lectures by university professors. It might have been possible for these schools to have raised the level of medical practice if the United States had not suddenly begun expanding westward. The opening up of the west, coupled with the influx of vast numbers of immigrants, created a shortage of medical personnel. Anyone could claim to be a doctor and even establish a medical school. More than 400 medical schools were founded in the nineteenth century. Few had any connection with institutions of higher learning or even any recognized educational standards. Instead, they were proprietary institutions, run on students' fees, and designed to show a profit; the more students, the more profit. Few of them required a high-school degree, let alone any college work, for admission; and the student, regardless of qualification, usually graduated at the end of two or three years without any real practical experience. Of course, there were some medical schools that were better than others, but the general level was not very high. All awarded the title of doctor, so that all kinds of practitioners from natural healers to graduates of Edinburgh claimed the title of doctor.

It was to bring some sort of standards to medicine that the American Medical Association was formed in 1847. The early years of the association were spent in trying to reform medical education, but they had little success until they began a campaign to secure state licensing laws with AMA-approved examiners. The first such board was established in Texas in 1875 and by the end of the nineteenth century this aspect of the struggle had been won. Licensing laws eliminated some of the most inadequate of the medical schools, but the standards of American medicine were still not very high. The best-trained physicians still received their education in Europe, and American-trained physicians contributed very little to advances in medicine. It was not until the founding of the medical school of Johns Hopkins University in 1893 that medicine was established as a graduate discipline on the German model and that medical teachers were regarded as full-time professors instead of voluntary lecturers who earned their living from private practice. Other medical schools, such as Harvard, had pioneered some aspects of the Johns Hopkins program, and soon adopted the remainder.

The very lack of medical standards in nineteenth-century American medicine resulted in the United States becoming a haven for new systems of medicine such as osteopathy, chiropractry, naturopathy, systems that Europe was finally beginning to discard or had not even heard about. The United States also became the center for all kinds of nostrum promoters. It was not until 1906 with the passage of the Pure Food and Drug Act that some effective control appeared. Thus the efforts of the AMA to raise medical standards through the establishment of state licensing and the abolition of proprietary medical schools seem justified. In the process, medical schools in the United States became part of the university as older university medical schools renewed their ties and others sought university ties. It was not until the University of Chicago medical school was founded in the 1920's, however, that medical school professors became fully integrated into the university faculties. The result of the abolition of the proprietary medical school was a rapid decline in the total number of schools as well as the number of medical graduates. Today there are fewer physicians in relation to the population than there were before the first World War. One of the effects of the reforms of the AMA was to make an artificial scarcity of doctors in the United States, something that does not exist in most other highly developed countries. The result was to increase both the salary and the status of the physician beyond that in most other countries. The AMA, however, cannot bear sole responsibility for this lack of medical schools, since various states have been slow to establish medical schools, and state governments as a whole have only recently begun to bear the responsibility for financing the education of medical and paramedical practitioners to the same extent that, for example, they supported agricultural education or veterinary science.

Socialized Medicine

An inevitable outgrowth of the concern over the health of the poor was the realization that they received very inadequate medical care. Public health measures such as inoculation or vaccination and the isolation of infected persons benefited the poor as much as they did the upper classes. Other than this, however, medical advances mostly seemed to benefit the upper classes, since they were the ones that could afford adequate care. Charity hospitals had been the usual method of treatment for the poor, but with the growth of medical knowledge, it was realized that preventative medical measures could also be taken. The most effective action was taken in Germany, one of the most industrialized countries and the one with the most advanced medical techniques. In 1883 a national sickness insurance was enacted giving free medical care to workers. These benefits were later extended to include the families of workers. The German example was soon followed by other European countries with high medical standards, including Austria in 1888, Sweden in 1891, Denmark in 1892, Belgium in 1894, and Switzerland in 1912. England was somewhat slower to act. Limited compensation for some workers was established in 1880 and this was gradually extended until in the 1940's there was comprehensive medical care for everyone. The Soviet Union, though not particularly advanced medically at the time, put all medical and health care under state control after the revolution of 1917.

The United States, in part because of the federal government structure, and in part because of the very backwardness of its own medicine, was slow to act. Traditionally, county governments provided welfare service for the sick, and though state governments did enter the public health field, they did so gradually and with great hesitation. The federal government was even more hesitant and it was not until the aftermath of the First World War and the Great Depression that it entered the social welfare field in any force. By that time the AMA itself had emerged as the leading opponent of any governmental intervention. Because of this opposition the federal government entered only indirectly, first through funds for hospital construction, for medical research, for medical education, and finally a limited form of Medicare. Much of the opposition of the AMA was undoubtedly due to the fact that partly through the efforts of the organization the American physicians as a group had attained a higher status than any other group of physicians in the world. Though the country doctor has always had a warm spot in American mythology, the ordinary practitioner did not have high status or income in nineteenth-century America. With the reforms initiated by the AMA, both his income and status began to rise until today he is the best paid member of any professional group. Ordinary physicians, even in advanced countries, lack this status, although the university medical teacher ranks equal to his American contemporaries. While this paper is not the place to analyze the medical opposition to government-sponsored medical care, the net result has been that, though American medicine is the best in the world, not all segments of the population benefit from it. As far as mortality and morbidity statistics are concerned, the United States fares rather poorly when compared with other industrialized countries.

Paramedical Practitioners

One of the effects of the new discoveries in medicine which seem to appear in almost geometric progression was a continued growth in specialization. This, as was indicated, took place in the continental countries long before it appeared in the United States, but once it reached the United States it forced a radical change in medicine by moving it into the hospital. Today American medicine, perhaps more than that in any other country, is hospital-centered. The importance of the hospital to modern medicine is in part dependent upon the emergence of modern nursing. Nursing reforms are usually associated with the name of Florence Nightingale (1820-1910), but she was just one among many who were responsible. With the trained nurse at the bedside of the patient, the physician could delegate responsibilities to her, yet maintain control of the case. At first nursing, like medicine itself, was primarily restricted to the benefit of upper-income groups, although student nurses, like student physicians, received their training in hospitals established for charity cases. With the development of better aseptic techniques, the nature of hospitals began to change, and trained nurses began to move into the hospital. Physicians soon found that they could treat patients more effectively in hospitals than in homes. The growth of insurance programs in the United States, both governmental and private, also brought more people into the hospital. Moreover, as new diagnostic techniques were developed and new kinds of treatment were discovered, it became impossible for the physican to treat the patient in his home or even to do so in his office. The hospital increasingly came to be used for short-term patients instead of for the poor and hopeless as it had been.

The proliferation of medical discoveries also changed the nature of medicine, since the general practitioner no longer could deal with all types of medical problems. Even the general practitioner tended to become a specialist, usually in internal medicine, with preparation beyond the M. D. degree. Where 100 years ago the average physician was not even a high-school graduate and spent only a couple of years in medical study, he now had to devote years of his life beyond the bachelor's degree and even beyond the M. D. This fact has tended to restrict the recruitment into medicine to only those students from the higher socioeconomic levels since only the well-to-do can afford to send their children to medical schools and support them during the years of postdoctoral study. This situation in itself affects the ideas and concepts of the medical school.

Specialization in medicine has also encouraged the growth of hospitals since they became the meeting ground for various specialties. Matching the specialization among the doctors has been the growth of paramedical personnel. Nursing, for example, developed a number of auxiliary helpers while other new occupations such as X-ray technicians, laboratory technicians and medical secretaries emerged, most of them centered in and around the hospital. Instead of being able to establish a one-to-one relationship between himself and his patient, the physician now finds himself the supervisor of a number of paramedical practitioners and only one among several medical specialists. If he is a general practitioner or internist, his role often seems to be that of referee between the various specialists he consults and the paramedical personnel who carry out the care of the patient. It is inevitable that many physicians long for a role conceived in an earlier age when the doctor had fewer patients and did much of the actual care himself. The result has been a growing tension between the physician and the paramedical practitioner as well as almost impossible demands on his own time. Moreover, the paramedical practitioners are themselves demanding individual autonomy and power so that there are growing tensions between various occupational groups. Physicians, by their scarcity, and by their long educational training, have also priced themselves out of many of the jobs that they would like to perform. In effect, the physician finds himself a victim of his own ideology of the past in a new age of scientific medicine. Though in earlier times the doctor often served the king or great nobles and combined the roles of all of today's specialists and paramedical practitioners, he was not able to do as much for his patient as he can today, but it is now done in a fragmented way by many people on the medical team.

In summary, although the role of the physician has always been to treat the sick, many aspects of that role have changed through the centuries. It has been influenced by events external to the profession as well as internal ones. The structure and culture of the society in which the physician operates has also influenced the role of the doctor. At the present time medicine, not only in America but throughout the world, is changing rapidly. This makes medical occupations a fertile research field for sociologists, while the hospital presents a controlled social environment which can facilitate investigation.

FURTHER READING

Much of this paper is based upon our own research into primary source materials, which are not cited here. The following books will be helpful to readers who wish to pursue the subject.

Ackerknecht, Erwin H. *Medicine at the Paris Hospital, 1794-1848* (Baltimore: The Johns Hopkins Press, 1967).

Bullough, Bonnie and Vern Bullough. *The Emergence of Modern Nursing* (New York; Macmillan, 1964).

Bullough, Vern. *The Development of Medicine as a Profession* (Basle, Switzerland: Karger Books, 1966).

Puschmann, Theodor. *A History of Medical Education* (New York: Hafner, 1966. Facsimile of 1891 Edition).

Sigerist, Henry E. *American Medicine* (New York: W. W. Norton, 1934).

_____.*A History of Medicine—Primitive and Archaic Medicine* (New York: Oxford University Press, 1951).

Shryock, Richard Harrison. *Medical Licensing in American, 1650-1965* (Baltimore: The Johns Hopkins Press, 1967).

_____.*Medicine and Society in America, 1660-1860* (New York: New York University Press, 1960).

_____.*The Development of Modern Medicine*, rev. (New York Knopf, 1947).

Young, James Harvey. *The Toadstool Millionaires, a Social History of Patent Medicines in America before Federal Regulation* (Princeton: University Press, 1961).

7

GEORGE ROSEN

Changing Attitudes of the Medical Profession to Specialization

Specialism is an essential feature of modern medical practice and a considerable proportion of all physicians limit their work to one field. But specialization of function in the recognition and treatment of disease is not restricted to modern times, or to social and economic systems of a high degree of complexity. Vocational specialism is widespread in primitive groups, and specialization in the practice of leechcraft is by no means uncommon among them.[1] However, such forms of specialization follow other cultural laws than does the modern type, and need therefore not be considered here.

Medical specialism in its modern form is a product of the nineteenth century, so that this study will be limited almost exclusively to this period, except for occasional references to the present century. The purpose of this report is to present an analysis of the varying reactions of physicians to the rise and development of an innovating form of medical practice, namely, medical specialization, and to investigate the social, economic, and psychological factors involved therein.

Specialization in Europe dates back to the beginning of the nineteenth century, and it did not become prominent on the American medical scene until after 1850. Nevertheless, the reception accorded to this form of practice both here and abroad was practically the same. The mass of the profession responded to this new tendency with open hostility, or at best, viewed it with suspicion. Opposition to innovation in a given situation

Reprinted from the *Bulletin of the History of Medicine*, 12 (July, 1942), pp. 343-354, © The Johns Hopkins Press, by permission of the author and the publisher. This article is a condensed version of a chapter in George Rosen, *The Specialization of Medicine with Particular Reference to Ophthalmology* (New York: Froben, 1944).

1. For specialization among primitive groups see: Willard Z. Park, *Shamanism in Western North America, A Study in Cultural Relationships* (Northwestern University Studies in the Social Sciences, no. 2, 1938), p. 97 ff.; Robert Redfield. *The Folk Culture of Yucatan* (1941), chap. XI; E. E. Evans-Pritchard, *Witchcraft, Oracles and Magic among the Azande* (1937), Parts II, IV; and W. H. R. Rivers, *Social Organization* (1932), p. 148.

arises from the intimate interaction of cultural and psychological factors, the cultural providing the historical and social setting which arouses specific psychological attitudes in the participating individuals.[2] Consequently, if we wish to explain this attitude of antagonism, we must analyze the socio-historical circumstances that engendered it.

Ophthalmology was one of the first medical specialties; and the earlier ophthalmic literature, especially in England, contains much that is relevant to our subject. An examination of the sentiments expressed by both the opponents and the advocates of ophthalmic specialization reveals some of the basic factors involved in the antagonism and suspicion evoked by the appearance of this type of practice.

Until the eighteenth century the diseases of the eye had received almost no attention from the regular medical profession, with the result that this field of medical activity had been preempted by quacks. In his *Great Surgery* published in the fifteenth century, Guy de Chauliac told his readers that because of the uncertainty of the outcome, all discreet practitioners ought to leave cataract operations to itinerant healers, and similar sentiments were expressed by other medieval physicians.[3] One of the largest groups among these itinerant empirics were the "oculists" and "cataract couchers," of whom Georg Bartisch, in his book on the care of the eyes published in 1583, says: "Nor is there a lack of old women, vagrant hags, theriac sellers, teeth pullers, ruined shopkeepers, rat-and-mouse catchers, knaves, tinkers, hog butchers, hangmen, bum-bailiffs, and other wanton, insolent, good for nothing vagabonds, all of whom boldly try to perform this noble cure. Some of them, and they are by no means few in number, make their appearance at certain times and attract attention to themselves by means of magnificent clothing, precious gold and silver, many servants and horses, excessive ostentation, and by creating a great stir, so that many good folk have not only been shamefully and evilly swindled, but also excessively overcharged, and, in addition, even ruined and caused to lose their lives." Finally Bartisch admonishes the authorities not to allow patients having eye diseases "to fall into the hands of such irresponsible destroyers and murderers of eyes."[4] Similar accusations are made by Richard Banister, an English contemporary of Bartisch. In his *One Hundred and Thirteen Diseases of the Eyes and Eye-Liddes* published at London in 1622, he also holds up to ridicule and contempt these itinerant practitioners and their ways. "They take their patients," he says, "into open markets and there for vain glories sake, make them see, hurting the patient only to make the people

---

2. Bernhard J. Stern, "Resistance to the Adoption of Technological Innovations," in *Technological Trends and National Policy* (1937), p. 59.

3. Hermann Peters, *Der Art und die Heilkunst in der deutschen Vergangenheit,* 2te Auflage, (1924), p. 42.

4. Cited by Peters, *ibid.*, pp. 84-85.

wonder at their rare skill. Some others make scaffolds on purpose to execute their skill upon, as the French-men and the Irish-man did in the Strand, making a trumpet to be blown before they went about their work."[5] The eighteenth century produced the most notorious of these gentry, the self-styled Chevalier Taylor, who traveled about Europe extolling his merits and accumulating patients and wealth.[6]

These conditions persisted throughout the seventeenth and eighteenth centuries in England and on the Continent, and references to disreputable oculists who went from town to town practicing their art are not uncommon during the first decades of the nineteenth century.[7] In the United States such itinerant charlatans continued their activities until well into the latter part of the century.[8]

The disrepute of these peripatetic oculists and of other practitioners of the same ilk was so great that when certain men within the medical profession itself began to devote themselves to the diseases of some organ such as the eye, or a particular class of diseases, they did so at the risk of inviting aspersions upon their professional integrity and of being ostracized by their colleagues. There can be little doubt that group pressure, operating in the form of specific social sanctions such as ostracism, was indeed effective in retarding the rise of specialties. Benjamin Travers, one of the early English practitioners of ophthalmology, asserted in 1821: "In this country, I believe no one before myself, who designed to practice general surgery, ventured to give more than a cursory attention to the diseases of the eye. A fear of being disqualified in public opinion, by a reputation acquired in these, for the treatment of other diseases, was a motive, however groundless, sufficient to deter surgeons from the cultivation of a large and legitimate field of observation and practice."[9]

5. Cited in Casey A. Wood, "Address on an Exhibit of Early (Prior to 1860) British and American Ophthalmic Literature," *Journal American Medical Association*, (November 8 and 15, 1902)

6. For some accounts of Chevalier Taylor's travel in Germany see Eberhard Buchner, *Aerzte und Kurpfuscher. Kulturhistorisch interessant Dokumente aus alten deutschen Zeitungen (17. und 18. Jahrhundert)* (1922), pp. 73-74; 75-87.

7. See *Lancet* 11 (1827), 423, for reference to John Williams, itinerant oculist; his book, *Traite des Maladies des Yeux* (Paris 1815), is a good example of the literature produced by such men.

8. Wyndham B. Blanton, *Medicine in Virginia in the Nineteenth Century* (1933), p. 194; Indiana State Medical Society, "Report of Dr. Parvin of Indianapolis on Diseases of the Eye and Ear," *Cincinnati Medical Observer*, 2 (1857), 413; W. H. Byford, "Specialties and Specialists," *Cincinnati Medical Observer*, 2 (1857), 213; E. Williams, "Kyklitis or Inflammation of the Corpus Ciliare," *Cincinnati Medical Observer*, 2 (1857), 14; "Specialists and Specialism," *St. Louis, Courier of Medicine*, I (1879), p. 435; Louis Bauer, "On the Declining Relations of the Medical Profession to the Public," *Cincinnati Medical Observer*, 2 (1857), 101-105.

9. Benjamin Travers: *A Synopsis of the Diseases of the Eye and their Treatment* (London, 1821), pp. V-XIII. For a typical expression of opposition to specialization in Great Britain see *Edinburgh Medical and Surgical Journal*, 8 (1812), 362-364.

Furthermore, opposition to specialization was frequently justified on the ground that since medical science is unique and indivisible, the practice of medicine should be the same. Thus in 1812 the *Edinburgh Medical and Surgical Journal* reviewed a book by John Stevenson entitled *On the Morbid Sensibility of the Eye, commonly called Weakness of Sight.* In the introduction to this work Stevenson clearly dissociated himself from the quacks, and informed the reader that he had "for some time past, altogether relinquished *general* practice (*in the exercise* of which I have been for many years extensively engaged) for the express purpose of devoting my attention exclusively to the management of the eye and ear."[10] The reviewer, however, rebuked Stevenson for his temerity, remarking that if he had been "acquainted with the history of medicine, and of those men who have contributed most to its improvement, he surely could not have ventured to intrude such sentiments before the public. We have always conceived, and our opinion is not a singular one, that the practice of the medical art, and the study of the science of medicine, were one and the same, and that diseases of any particular organ could not be treated with ability and skill, but by those who had acquired an excessive knowledge of the diseases of the whole body. Upon these general principles we have always condemned those who have pretended that any knowledge could be obtained in the diseases and treatment of a particular organ, by practising on that organ alone, which the general practitioner might not acquire."[11]

It should be noted that ophthalmology during the eighteenth and early nineteenth centuries was almost exclusively ophtalmic surgery and was practiced by general surgeons, such as William Cheselden, Lorenz Heister, A. G. Richter, Antonio Scarpa, and Astley Paston Cooper. The conviction prevailed that no one could treat eye diseases successfully unless he practiced general surgery. As Samuel Cooper put it in 1815: "No one, except the thorough surgeon, can make the complete oculist. . .,"[12] a sentiment which we find echoed with approval by Travers, Middlemore, and others. In 1832 William Lawrence asserted that not only was the study of ophthalmology inseparable from general medicine, but that also the practical treatment of the eye diseases was best handled by those who regularly treated diseases of the entire body.[13] This attitude likewise finds expres-

A., "Observations on Specialties in Medicine," *Peninsular and Independent Medical Journal,* 2 (1859), 1-5; and Ashbel Woodward, "Specialism in Medicine," *Proceedings and Medical Communications of the Connecticut Medical Society* 2 (1867), 264-268.

10. John Stevenson, *On the Morbid Sensibility of the Eye, commonly called Weakness of Sight* (1810), p. 3.

11. *Edinburgh Medical and Surgical Journal,* 8 (1812), 362-364.

12. Cited by Travers, *op. cit.,* pp. V ff.

13. Richard Middlemore, *A Treatise on the Disease of the Eye and its Appendages,* 2 vols. (1835); John Vetch, *Practical Treatise on the Diseases of the Eye* (1820),

sion in the rules of the Royal Westminster Eye Infirmary, which required "that every surgeon belonging to it shall 'also be the surgeon or assistant surgeon of an hospital for the treatment of diseases generally.'"[14] Further indications of this attitude are evident in the reluctance with which men, such as William Bowman, became specialists, as well as the actions of Benjamin Travers and William Lawrence, who severed their connections with the London Eye Infirmary after seven and twelve years respectively, while continuing to maintain their connections with general hospitals for many years.[15]

Economic competition was undoubtedly an extremely important, if not a basic factor in the hostility evinced by the general practitioner to the appearance and multiplication of specialists. At a time when the economic situation of the medical profession was, on the whole, a difficult one, and the average practitioner often had a hard time of it, the success of the specialist was bound to arouse professional suspicion and resentment.[16] The general practitioner felt that the specialist's activities tended to degrade him in public opinion, and by narrowing his sphere of action to injure him pecuniarily. The conflict situation created by this intraprofessional competition appears most openly in the American discussions of specialization and its problems. In 1869 the Committee on Specialties of the American Medical Association in its report at the annual meeting pointed out that: "The chief objection brought against specialities is that they operate unfairly toward the general practitioner, in implying that he is incompetent to properly treat certain classes of diseases, and narrowing his field of practice."[17] At about the same time an editorial in a New York medical journal made it clear that: "The profession cannot be expected to listen to aspersions upon their judgment and skill, without imbibing a prejudice against the source from which they spring."[18] Several years later, in 1875, at the annual meeting of the New York State Medical Society, the report of the Committee on the President's Address, as presented by Abraham Jacobi, maintained that the tendency to specialization tended "to degrade

pp. VII ff.; Wardrop, "Lectures on Surgery etc.," *Lancet* (1833), 456.

14. "Intercepted Letters," *Lancet* 1 (1833-34), 188.

15. J. Hirschberg, *Geshichte der Augenheilkunde*, in Handbuch der gesamten Augenheilkunde (2te Auflage), Band 14, Abteil. 4, Kap. XXIII (England's Augenaerzte, von 1800 bis 1850), pp. 10-14.

16. On the economic situation of the medical profession: Richard H. Shryock, *The Development of Modern Medicine* (1936), pp. 257-258; Richard H. Shryock, ed., The *Arnold Letters* (Papers of the Trinity College Historical Society, XVIII-XIX, 1929), p. 164; and George Rosen, *Some Economic Aspects of Medical Practice in 19th-century America* (unpublished manuscript).

17. "Report of the Committee on Specialties, and on the Propriety of Specialists Advertising," *Transactions American Medical Association*, 20 (1869), 111-113.

18. "Specialties and Specialists," *The Medical Record*, 1 (1866-67), 525. See also "Advertisements by Physicians," *Boston Medical and Surgical Journal*, 71 (1864-65), 484.

the general practitioner in the estimation of the public."[19] Nevertheless, by this time it was becoming increasingly obvious that the opponents of specialization were fighting a hopeless rearguard action which could have but one result.

Before leaving our analysis of the opposition to specialization, consideration must be given to one other retarding factor which was operative, especially in the fields of practice dealing with venereal and genito-urinary diseases. The moral sanctions and the concepts of sin with which Western society, particularly in England and America, surrounded sex relations exerted a definite influence on the attitudes of the medical profession as well as of the lay public to practitioners devoting themselves to diseases of the genito-urinary organs. The social disapprobation which was the lot of the unfortunate victims of syphilis and gonorrhea was extended in greater or lesser degree to the physicians to whom they turned for treatment. The result was that a great many men refused in their private practices to treat such patients, driving them into the hands of quacks and unscrupulous practitioners. An editorial in the *Lancet* for 1857 informs us: "It has been tacitly agreed, that syphilis and cognate diseases were not exactly the most desirable to treat; that it was all very well in a foul ward at a hospital but that a large reputation for skill in such cases was rather to be eschewed as being not quite gentlemanly, and smacking somewhat of immorality. When sufferers look about them for relief, the result is that very few men are recognizable as specially skilled in this department of practice. Their attention is thus diverted from legitimate practitioners, and the advertising columns of the lay press are consulted with a view of selecting one from amongst those who, although obviously not of us, at all events assert loudly enough their qualifications for the cure of disease, with the concomitant little *agreements of secrecy, speedy cure, contract,* and so on. By dint of long usage, a blot has at last fixed itself upon the branch of practice which, above all others, requires the devotion to it of men of the highest character."[20]

A typical example of the consequences resulting from the situation described by the Lancet may be seen in the following advertisement from the Washington *Evening Star* of March 12, 1863:

Secret Diseases

Dr. H. E. Forrest Cures all Diseases of Imprudence, no matter how long contracted, or will receive no pay. He has now had several years experience in military hospitals in Europe, and warrants to cure any of the above diseases. Office hours, 12 to 4 and 6 to 10. Private rooms for consultations with ladies. Consultations free. Ist. north, between 7th and 8th sts. (3 story brick, name on the door).[21]

19. Annual Meeting of the Medical Society of the State of New York, *Medical Recorder*, 10 (1875), 108
20. *Lancet*, 2 (Saturday, Sept. 12), 1857.
21. Washington *Evening Star* (March 12, 1863), p. 3, column 4 (Personal).

The persistence of such attitudes until very recently, and their retarding influence on the development of a specialty such as urology are strikingly presented in remarks made in 1911 by members of the American Urological Association at the tenth annual meeting of the organization. At this meeting Hugh Cabot of Boston defended the right of urology to be considered a specialty.[22] In the discussion following Cabot's address, the urologists "let their hair down," and a number of very illuminating comments were voiced. Dr. Ernst G. Mark of Kansas City asserted "that we men who are making a specialty of urology should discountenance the old idea of the 'clap doctor.' That is where urology first got its black eye." [23] Dr. G. Frank Lydston of Chicago commented along similar lines. "It is not very long," he said, "since the term 'urology' was not known; and the genito-urinary surgeon was regarded as a 'clap doctor.' At the beginning, my own college clinic was largely devoted to entomological researches in crab lice. Strictures occasionally strayed in to be operated. With the competition of half a dozen general surgeons it was very difficult to build up a clinic."[24] To the remarks of his colleagues Dr. Granville MacGowan of Los Angeles added the following: "I think my friend Mark has hit the keynote in regard to the other thing. We treat the clap. You know how the public regard the question of gonorrhea, a shameful disease which anybody should cure easily, while it really is probably the most serious disease which affects mankind. . . . The public do not know this, they do not appreciate this, they have no idea of it, and so if a large proportion of a man's practice is taken up in treating what appears to them a trivial disease, they judge him accordingly. And if it were possible for us to cut it out of our practice, I think that our standing with them would be different."[25]

Although our analysis of the factors underlying medical hostility and opposition to specialization is by no means complete, yet enough evidence has been presented to show that such attitudes were due in large part to reactions implicit in group behavor.[26] Innovations in medical activity, just as in other forms of human behavior, arouse resentment because they upset established ways of thought and action, and disrupt stable relationships, in short, the mores of the group. The resultant psychological response evoked in most of the members of the group is a feeling of impropriety, since dissent from the mores is considered detrimental to the welfare of the whole group. Furthermore, within a given social milieu a process of social evaluation is constantly at work as a result of which values become attached to individuals and groups carrying on certain activities and operations. The product of this process is a prestige scale, in terms of

22. Hugh Cabot, "Is Urology Entitled To Be Regarded as a Specialty?" *Transactions American Urological Association*, 5 (1911), 1-10.

23. *Transactions American Urological Association*, 5 (1911), 14.

24. *Ibid.*, p. 15.

25. *Ibid.*, p. 17.

26. Stern, *op. cit.*, pp. 59-62; William G. Sumner, *Folkways* (1913), pp. 75-118.

which individuals or groups are given a particular status. As a result, "any person who has achieved a certain rank in the prestige scale regards anything real or imaginery which tends to alter his status adversely" with latent or manifest hostility.[27] This self-interest of the individual or the group in the maintenance of status is most consciously involved and expressed in the economic field. Finally, as we have seen, the social pressure exerted upon innovators in endeavoring to coerce them to uniformity with the rest of the group takes the forms of ridicule, disparagement, social ostracism, and often economic discrimination.[28]

Nevertheless, despite the vehemence of its exponents opposition to specialization was doomed to defeat. By the forties of the nineteenth century medical specialism, particularly in ophthalmology and otology, had already achieved a certain degree of respectability in Great Britain. In evidence of this fact we have the statement made in 1845 by William R. W. Wilde, one of the greatest otologists of the century, "that highly-educated medical men now apply themselves to the study and treatment of eye diseases solely."[29] Indications that the attitude of the American medical profession was becoming more favorable toward specialization were already prevalent throughout the decade of the sixties, yet this type of medical activity did not achieve official recognition until 1869 when the American Medical Association resolved "that this Association recognizes specialties as proper and legitimate fields of practice."[30] Not quite a decade later specialism was already regarded as inevitable.[31]

While we cannot enter into a detailed analysis of the factors which brought about this change in the attitude of the medical profession in Britain and America, a brief survey of the more important forces that were active in effecting this transformation will undoubtedly throw some light upon the entire process. In 1886 William Brodie, president of the American Medical Association, stated very frankly that the members of the profession "began to realize that by devoting themselves to one branch instead of working up a general practice, they could often do more good, earn more money, and have less arduous work to perform."[32] The great significance of the economic factor in bringing about a change

27. F. J. Roethlisberger, and William J. Dickson, *Management and the Worker* (1941), p. 556, also see all of chap. XXIV.

28. Stern, *op. cit.*, p. 62.

29. W. R. Wilde, Introductory Address delivered at the School of Medicine, Park-Street, Dublin, 1845, *Lancet*, 1 (1845), 434; for an early instance of the recognition of certain specialties ("diseases of the chest, eye, ear, in practice, and orthopedy in surgery") in the United States see Byford, *op. cit.*, p. 212.

30. *Transactions American Medical Association*, 20 (1869), 28-29.

31. Richard M'Sherry, "Notes on Relations between General Practice and Specialties in Medicine," *Maryland Medical Journal*, 2 (1877), 278; John S. Apperson, "Report on Advances in Practice of Medicine," *Transactions of the Medical Society of Virginia* (1886), 88-91.

32. Apperson, *op. cit.*, pp. 88-91.

in the attitude of the profession to specialization is attested by many writers on the subject.[33]

Specialism was profitable because patients were willing to pay for the services of men who were able to relieve conditions which general practitioners did not know how to treat.[34] The active role of the public in furthering the growth of specialization is amply confirmed by British, American, and European writers.[35] Typical is the statement of Sir William Bowman in a letter to his friend T. Pridgin Teale. "The ophthalmic field," he wrote, "was entered on gradually. . . . The public found me out. I could not have long followed both departments."[36]

A third factor making for specialization, and one which has been so generally accepted that we need but mention it here, was the tremendous expansion of medical knowledge and technique.

Furthermore, it is apparent that the social climate of opinion within which innovating factors and forces act will tend to retard or to expedite their operation depending on whether they are in accord with or in opposition to this climate of opinion. It should be recalled that throughout the greater part of the nineteenth century there prevailed a profound faith in progress as a result of the division of labor. The identification of medical specialization with this belief in progress and the beneficial effects of a division of labor made for a readier acceptance of this type of practice.[37]

Finally, it should be pointed out that the readiness with which innovation is accepted depends also on how closely the new resembles the old.[38] Recog-

33. *Medical Record*, 10 (1875), pp. 105, 158, 255, 489; E. D. Force, "Specialism in Medicine," *American Practitioner* (1876), 260; "Specialists, their Relations to General Practitioners," *St. Louis Courier of Medicine*, 1 (1879), 324-329; Wilde, *op. cit.*, p. 434; *Lancet*, 2 (Saturday, Sept. 12), 1857.

34. George Hunter, "The Place of Specialism in General Practice . . ." *Transactions of the Medico-Chirurgical Society of Edinburgh*, 4 (1885). 232 ff.; 7 (1887-88), 76 ff.; *Cincinnati Medical Observer*. 2 (1857), 413, 104-105; *Virginia Medical Monthly* 2 (1875-76), 419-422; *Toledo Medical and Surgical Journal*, 3 (1879), 449-455.

35. For an early recognition of this fact see Wilde, *op. cit.*, p. 434.

36. T. Pridgin Teale, "Abandonment of Iridectomy in the Extraction of Hard Cataract," *Transactions of the Ophthalmological Society of the United Kingdom*, 13 (1893), 2-4. Although no attention has been given in the present study to developments on the Continent, yet many of the factors and processes involved in the recognition of medical specialization were the same as in Britian and America. For the rôle of the public in France in 1853 see Dr. O. Heyfelder, "Reisebericht. Die Specialitäten in Paris," *Deutsche Klinik* (1853), pp. 391-392, also pp. 35-36; a similar picture is presented in a report published a decade later, see Heinrich Rohlfs, "Ueber den Specialismus in der Medizin," *Deutsche Klinik* (1862), p. 84.

37. Gudmund J. Gislason: "Specialization in Medicine," *Journal-Lancet*, 40 (1920), 545-546; Ross R. Bunting, "Specialism in Medicine," *Maryland Medical Journal* (1887). 413-415; "The Position of the Speicalist in Respect to the General Practitioner," *St. Louis Courier of Medicine*, 1 (1879), 588; Joseph Sandek, "The Relative Position existing between the General Practitioner and the Specialist," *Virginia Medical Monthly*, 2 (1875-76), 419; *Transactions American Medical Association*, 20 (1869), 111.

38. Stern, *op. cit.*, p. 61.

nition of innovation is made easier by the existence of transitional forms that permit the process of habituation to operate. Medical specialism was rendered more acceptable to the profession through the mediation of the type of practice known as partial specialization, which made it possible for the general practitioner to meet the competition of the full specialist on more equal terms.[39]

39. *Virginia Clinical Record*, 3 (1879), 189; Walter Rivington, "The Medical Profession (1879), 53-54; *Boston Medical and Surgical Journal*, 71 (1864-65), 485.

8

RUE BUCHER

Pathology: A Study of Social Movements within a Profession

Pathologists share with other specialists in medicine and the scientific disciplines the necessity of coping with rapidly changing conditions in their work life, changes which are dramatic even within one generation. A middle-aged pathologist interviewed for this study reflected the sentiments of his peers when he remarked of the present shape of the specialty, "I wouldn't know it anymore." We can expect that specialization and rapid change will increasingly characterize professions, insofar as they are based upon an expanding body of scientific knowledge and the sources of change from a more complex social organization of professional endeavor multiply. Yet, so far the sociology of occupations and professions has not been systematically concerned with processes of specialization and change in occupations.

A previous paper presented the beginnings of a "process" or "emergent" approach to the study of professions.[1] Its aim was to develop a theoretical framework which would focus more pointedly upon diversity and change in occupations, and provide some initial formulations of the main processes involved. The present study attempts to specify further the social processes involved in the development of professional groups. Briefly, the model with which we began posits the existence of a number of emergent groups within a profession. There are many identities, many values, and many interests to be found within the same profession, which tend to become patterned and shared. Coalitions develop and organize, both in opposition to older entrenched groups and for the furtherance of

Reprinted from *Social Problems*, 10, No. 1 (1962), pp. 40-51, by permission of the author and The Society for the Study of Social Problems.

I am highly indebted to Anselm Strauss and Everett C. Hughes, without whose encouragement and stimulating discussion this research would not have been conceived or concluded.

1. Rue Bucher and Anselm Strauss, "Professions in Process," *The American Journal of Sociology*, 66 (January, 1961), 325-334.

their own interests. We called these coalitions *segments*. We suggested, further, that segments tend to take on the character of social movements. They develop distinctive identities, a sense of the past, and goals for the future; they organize activities and tactics which will secure an institutional position and implement their distinctive mission. Our thesis is that such emergent groups and movements exist in even the most established professions and are the focal points of social change.

This study of pathology utilizes several kinds of data. First, there are intensive, unstructured interviews with forty-one pathologists in the Chicago metropolitan area. The respondents were selected to provide a range of points of view within the field and of the institutional settings in which pathologists work. Second, there are field observations made in each of the types of instutition sampled. The investigator followed a half dozen of the respondents through their work days, attended Clinical Pathology Conferences, teaching conferences, autopsies, and other routines involved in the work life of the pathologist. Third, various kinds of documentary evidence was scrutinized, especially discussions of professional matters appearing in the journals of the specialty.[2] In addition, other documents privately circulated in the specialty were brought to my attention by respondents when they seemed to bear upon the interests of the study. The results lean most heavily upon the interviews, although the other types of data were used for background and supplementary purposes.

Segments and the Changing Professional Milieu

We cannot begin our discussion of pathology conventionally, by defining the nature of the field, because our data consists in good part of the struggles of pathologists to identify themselves, and of conflicting identifications which have emerged. Pathologists are physicians, most of whom are certified by the American Board of Pathology, one of nineteen specialty boards organized within the medical profession. But pathology is a medical specialty which in some respects is closer to the basic sciences than to medicine. In the medical school curriculum, most of pathology is taught in the second year, grouped with the preclinical sciences of anatomy, physiology, and biochemistry. In hospitals, on the other hand, pathology is a clinical service. All pathologists would probably agree that path-

2. The interested reader will find that many journals in medicine and its specialties are rich in material bearing upon professional identity, values, and issues. The distinctive missions of the various specialities come through quite clearly in this literature. For a bibliography of such literature in pathology, see the author's Ph.D. thesis, "Conflicts and Transformations of Identity: A Study of Medical Specialists," (Unpublished Ph.D. dissertation, University of Chicago, 1961).

A note of caution, however. Interviewing pathologists revealed that this literature predominantly represented the viewpoints of one segment in pathology. Although it gave an accurate reflection of this position, it gave little indication of the existence of other positions, unless the reader was already alerted to them.

ology has attributes of the "basic" sciences, and also has attributes of a medical specialty, but they differ considerably among themselves in which aspects they emphasize and elaborate. A brief historical review will place the situation in developmental context.

Until relatively recently, pathology was principally an academic discipline. Termed the "basic science of medicine," it commanded great prestige in the medical schools. Nineteenth-century pathology, dominated by Virchow, had changed the whole face of medicine. Present-day pathologists are fond of pointing out that pathology "put medicine on a scientific basis." The image of the pathologist contained in this heritage is the investigator and teacher. Before the turn of the century, however, the possibilities for applying pathology to diagnostic problems in the living patient began to be exploited. This applied area, though, compared to the others, was relatively undeveloped for many years to come. The institutional bastion of the pathologist was still the medical school. Pathologists outside of the medical schools and major hospitals were few in number, and low in status among their medical colleagues.

In recent years, and particularly since World War II, several things have happened to alter this picture drastically. First, theories and methods of studying disease have changed, so that the traditional methods of pathology no longer lead the way; other fields, such as biochemistry, are "hot" areas. Pathology does not have the undisputed leadership in the medical sciences it possessed fifty years ago. Second, there has been a tremendous spurt in the application of laboratory methods to patient care. New techniques in applied pathology accumulated gradually throughout this century, but pathologists recognize a more dramatic acceleration since World War II. Third, medical practice has been reorganized so that there is great demand for these laboratory services. Physicians are becoming more and more dependent upon the services of a modern clinical laboratory in order to practice, and the services provided by the pathologist are increasingly defined as prerequisite to good practice.

Taking an overview of the field as a whole, pathology has lost its former position of scientific preeminence in medicine. At the same time, pathology has acquired the possibility of moving into a closer relationship to the mainstream of medical practice. It could become predominantly a practicing field, like other medical specialties. The central question for the specialty, thus, is which road should it take. Should pathologists maintain their scientific identity and attempt to regain their former position? Or should they exploit the possibilities of becoming a clinical specialty to the full?

Within pathology, two segments can be delineated which represent different solutions to this dilemma of professional development, and which are focal points of ferment and change. Segments are here defined as *groupings of professionals that share both an organized identity and a common pro-*

fessional fate. The delineation of two segments in the one specialty of pathology reflects the multiple perspectives on the field and differences in working conditions revealed in the interviews. Respondents differed in whether they saw pathology more as a "medical specialty" or more as a "science." Connected with such imagery of placement was the sense of mission held by respondents. If they saw pathology as a medical specialty, they related its mission to its role in the practice of medicine. If they saw pathology as a science, then its mission was investigation and communication of knowledge. Likewise, the way respondents organized their own work activities, and their models of what a pathologist's work life should be like, reflected these polar concepts. Those who saw pathology as a medical specialty tended to spend most of their work life in clinical diagnostic activities. Some pathologists attempted to steer a middle course between these two discrepant identifications of pathology, but the vast majority of respondents (35 out of 41) were committed primarily to one model or another.[3]

Pathologists who were interviewed recognized these differences in perspectives within the specialty, and they tended to distinguish themselves from other pathologists whose perspectives they did not share. Thus, they recognized closer colleagueship, actual and potential, with some fellow pathologists than with others. It is in this sense that we can speak of a professional identity shared by some portions of the specialty, and distinguished from other portions of the specialty. Further, pathologists who shared most aspects of professional identity tended to see the same things as "problems" or issues facing the field, and to respond to them similarly. This phenomenon was conceptualized as *shared fate.* Members of a specialty—or a whole profession—who share a fate see similar consequences for themselves ensuing from the same conditions. Those who do not share a fate do not see the same conditions as relevant to their fate, or do not believe that those conditions have the same consequences for them.[4]

When shared fate was taken into account, respondents clearly fell into two segments, which rallied around distinctive issues. One of these will

3. Following Becker, it should be pointed out that the use of the term commitment in this context involves, not only investment or involvement in a type of career, but a series of "side bets" which have the effect of channeling a person in a given direction. For example, some of these pathologists during residency training were making side bets when they concentrated upon gaining research experience at the expense of certain kinds of clinical experience. Howard S. Becker, "Notes on the Concept of Commitment," *American Journal of Sociology,* 66 (1960), 32-40.

The writer is also indebted to Becker and Carper for elucidation of the concept of professional identity. See Howard S. Becker and James W. Carper, "The Elements of Identification with an Occupation," *American Sociological Review,* 21 (1956), 289-298.

4. What is called "shared fate" here, Harvey Smith has referred to as differential sensitivity to professional contingencies. He says of a profession, "Each level and group may be sensitive to contingencies not shared by the profession as a whole. Thus, different parts of the profession may 'metabolize' at different rates, and any single action may have many diverse, and often conflicting effects within the professional institution." Harvey L. Smith, "Contingencies of Professional Differentiation," *American Journal of Sociology,* 63 (1958), 410-414, p. 410.

be called the *scientific segment*, whose members were united by concern over maintaining the scientific position of the specialty. The second segment, the *practitioner segment,* consisted of pathologists who made common cause in promoting the relationship between pathology and medical practice. As our definition of segment implies, members of both segments tended to be ill-informed about, and disinterested in, the problems which concerned the other segment.[5]

Regarded historically, each segment may be seen as a movement in different stages of development. Members of the scientific segment are the inheritors of the original movement which established pathology as a respected academic discipline and "put medicine on a scientific basis." The practitioners are a relatively newly emergent group. As one wise old scientist in pathology described them, these pathologists are "evangelistic." Like other social movements, these professional movements have an ideology, in the form of a professional identity. The shared definitions and values which comprise their professional identity guide the activity of those identified with the segment and influence the assessments they make of events. In line with the way the segment assesses their situation, they organize tactics for implementing their goals. Further, the methods the segment evolves for coping with their members' problems have important implications for the formation and alteration of professional identity. New identifications are forged as men deal with changing conditions.

In the following pages, the above ideas will be illustrated through analysis of the assessments the two segments in pathology made of their present position, and the tactics with which they cope with their position.

The Emerging Practitioner Movement

In the practitioner movement, we have something akin to the development of a new specialty. A new area of practice has appeared on the medical scene, just as the discovery of the X-ray led to the development of a new area of practice and a formally recognized specialty, roentgenology. The issues, as the practitioner in pathology sees them, are: We have new laboratory methods for the diagnosis and control of disease. Who is going to perform these functions? What field is responsible for them and what division of labor should be attained?

These issues have a familiar ring to anyone interested in the study of occupations and professions. They may lead to claims and counterclaims on the part of existing disciplines, cries of encroachment, and the emer-

5. Close to the same number of respondents fell into each segment, 20 in the scientific segment, and 17 in the practitioner segment. Because of the nature of the sampling procedure, these numbers are in no way indicative of the actual numerical strength of either segment. Comparing the sample with the distribution of pathologists by institutional affiliation recorded in the *Directory of Medical Specialists* suggests that the practitioner segment is by far the largest group. See Bucher, *op. cit.*, pp. 12-13, 36-37.

gence of new disciplines.[6] The practitioner pathologists maintain that pathology is the logical discipline to take over control of the techniques in question. In this case, then, rather than an entirely new discipline or specialty arising to claim the new area of practice, a segment from an older, established specialty has moved in to stake its claim. How does such a group, an offshot from a parent specialty, go about establishing its claim, and in the process, establish an emergent professional identity?

First, however, a few words about the roots of the practitioner movement. Small numbers of pathologists had been engaged in practice utilizing rudimentary laboratory diagnostic methods since the early years of this century. This new area of practice was first formally distinguished in 1922, when the American Society of Clinical Pathologists was formed. It appears that those who came together in forming this society included physicians who were originally trained in other clinical specialties, as well as pathologists.[7] For years, the group barely hung on, much less grew, and for a period in the 1930's was not recruiting enough young people to reproduce itself. Its members were underprivileged economically and low in prestige in relation to the rest of the medical community. The deviance of the early clinical pathologist is reflected in the belief, spontaneously expressed by all practitioner respondents, that these early practitioners were medical "misfits." The contemporary practitioner sees his forerunners as "maladjusted people who fled from medical practice," and who were "afraid to meet the public." These pathologists are still smarting under the sense of an inglorious past. And, as we will see, they are still at pains to dispel any remnants of this imagery which may remain in the medical community.

All this has changed dramatically since World War II. With the tremendous expansion of laboratory methods in medical practice, clinical pathologists are prospering. Their services are in great demand, highly respected, and the extent and character of their work has been revolutionized. Older men in the field are amazed and delighted by what has happened to them, but all age groups see themselves as riding the crest of technological advancement, continually expanding their sphere of operations.

But in such a booming field, it is all the more of a problem for pathologists to meet the demand for services, and protect their claims against encroachment. Practitioner pathologists find themselves vigorously pressing their claim against competitors both within and without medicine. From one side, they are threatened by people trained in the natural sciences, biochemists, bacteriologists, and others, who have entered medical laboratories in specialized positions and devise new techniques faster than the patholo-

6. See, as a recent example, William J. Goode, "Encroachment, Charlatanism, and the Emerging Profession: Psychology, Sociology, and Medicine," *American Sociological Review*, 25 (1960), 902-914.

7. Israel Davidsohn, M.D., "What's Past is Prologue," *The American Journal of Clinical Pathology*, 23 (January, 1953), 1-14.

gists can keep up with them. On the other side, there have always been men in other specialties, such as internal medicine and gynecology, with a special interest in laboratory methods, and who organize laboratories to carry out the work for their own departments. This situation, of multiple clinical laboratories under the control of other specialties, exists in many large medical centers today.

The practitioner pathologists have formulated a justification of their claim which involves demonstrating that they can make a distinctive contribution to this area of practice, and that they can do the job better than any other group. The usual battle cry sounded against the counterclaims of nonmedical professions to portions of laboratory medicine is that "pathology is the practice of medicine." By this pathologists mean that only persons with medical degrees are capable of properly interpreting and correlating laboratory findings in clinical cases. They lay stress upon clinical interpretation, and knowledge of disease in clinical settings which the nonmedical specialist is not prepared to contest. This kind of rhetoric is to no avail when the competitors are other physicians, however. In that case, the pathologist stresses elements of his training which distinguish him from other physicians—his extensive training in tissue diagnosis, broad knowledge of disease processes, and greater experience in laboratories—which he argues are essential to the task at hand.

In general strategy, the practioner movement is in a phase of expansion, and *territory-claiming*. The consequences of this position were very evident in the picture of pathology respondents endeavored to draw for the investigator. One group of tactics consisted of creating and promulgating a professional identity congruent with territory-claiming, while other tactics were concerned with securing their institutional position. First, let us take up the series of images practitioners utilized in promulgating their professional identity.

(1) Practitioners redefine the boundaries of pathology in such a way as to encompass their emergent activities. Pathologists of the scientific segment, following traditional lines, usually define their field as the "study of disease," and proceed to elaborate on the nature of the pathologist's interest in disease. If they define the field as including teaching and diagnosis of disease, they do not dwell upon these aspects, but place them in a more subsidiary position. Practitioners take just the opposite tack. They are not satisfied to say that pathology is the study of disease. If they use this phraseology at all, it is a prelude to further elaboration of the applied functions of pathology. The change in the conception of their discipline which all respondents emphasized is its part in medical practice. They place pathology squarely in medicine, as an integral part of medical practice. Most practitioners, in fact, defined pathology as "laboratory medicine." The laboratory medicine image seems to be currently the most satisfying one in expressing for these pathologists what they really do.

(2) Practitioners have developed, and proclaim, a new mission which expresses the unique contribution that they can make to medical practice. Medical specialties have their own specialized missions, which distill out the meaning of the many separate activities which they perform and serve as reference points in evaluating situations and guiding activities. The mission of the practitioner pathologist is twofold.

First, he emphasizes his service to the clinician. The practitioner pathologist feels that his real work centers upon the services that he provides to other physicians. This is his link to patient care. All of the routine services of the laboratory constitute a service to clinicians, but the pathologist of this orientation is most pleased when the attending physician comes to him with a problem, and he can discuss a particular immediate case with the clinician. As one respondent put it, "there is no reason for the pathologist to exist unless he serves the clinicians." The consultant role is the highest expression of this mission of service. All the practitioners considered it mandatory both to make themselves available to clinicians, and to present their knowledge in such a way that it will be most useful to a physician of another specialty. They consider themselves successful when the clinicians of their hospital have learned how to utilize their services, but they clearly state that the responsibility for initiating this relationship rests with the pathologist.

Second, he emphasizes the image of the pathologist as the educator of the clinician. He is the physician who takes on the mission of maintaining and improving standards of practice in his hospital. Both his training and his position in the hospital fit him for this task, according to the practitioner. The pathologist is one of the few full-time men on the hospital staff, and his orientation is far broader than that of other primarily hospital physicians, like radiologists and anesthesiologists. The pathologist plays a vital role in maintaining hospital standards through such activitivies as the autopsy, reviewing tissues taken out in surgery, and Clinical Pathology Conferences. Further, he contributes to the learning of the clinician in his consultant role. It is then that he can lead the clinician to think in terms of applying laboratory methods to solving his problems, and can advise the clinician from the perspective of his wide experience in diseases.

(3) Practitioners dissociate themselves from older images of the pathologist and put forward new images. Dissociation from older images has been observed in other occupations bent upon getting ahead. But dissociation is probably also an integral part of the process of identity formation. In a group like these pathologists, setting up counterimages—what they are *not*—is extremely important in defining the limits of the group and leading to a demarcation of what they *are*.[8]

8. This use of counterimages by professional groups—which can also be clearly detected in specialty literature—can be compared with the boundary defining functions of

As pathologists move more directly into the arena of patient care, they present themselves as physicians, capable of entering into and understanding the problems of other physicians. This image of the contemporary pathologist is strongly contrasted with images of the pathologist of previous generations. The old pathologist, a "lab rat" with little interest in clinical problems, was not a proper colleague to other medical practitioners. The contemporary pathologist, however, is a new breed who participates in the medical fraternity as an equal and who is interested in patients. One respondent reported that he quells the doubts of other physicians over whether he is one of them by telling them that he has a narcotic license and writes prescriptions. Thus, the practitioner flashes signals of his physician status as much as possible. Along the same line, many of them proudly reported that they see patients and their relatives themselves, and are fully capable of carrying out a physical examination.

In addition to creating and presenting a professional identity appropriate to the claims they make, practitioners are concerned with building institutional relationships and protecting their position within institutions. Two main types of activity meet this latter concern.

First, practitioners create associations which define appropriate institutional arrangements for pathologists and represent their interests. There are two such organizations, the American Society of Clinical Pathologists and the College of American Pathologists. The former is more concerned with continued education and scientific advancement, and the latter with socioeconomic problems, but they overlap in both areas. Spokesmen for both proclaim the ideology of the practitioner. In general, the policy of the organized practitioner movement is to embrace the model of entrepeneur-style practice held up by organized medicine, and attempt to bring the institutional conditions of pathologists into some approximation of this ideal. They engage in a number of tactics, including alliance with similarly placed specialties like radiology, negotiation with opposing organizations and, finally, litigation over such issues as whether pathology services are defined as professional services or hospital services, and the proper contractual relations between hospitals and pathologists.

While only a few of the practitioner respondents were involved or particularly interested in these national organizational activities, they were all very much involved in hewing out a position for themselves within their own institutions. They were engaged in establishing and maintaining relationships with the clinicians for whom they provide service, working out administrative problems of their own service, and juggling relationships with hospital administration and competing services within the hospital. The new practitioner pathologist encounters whole new sets of working relationships and institutional problems which are peculiar to his situation,

---

deviancy posited by Dentler and Erikson. Robert A. Dentler and Kai T. Erikson, "The Functions of Deviance in Groups," *Social Problems*, 7 (1959), 98-107.

and not shared with other specialties or other segments of his specialty.

Second, practitioners become concerned with recruitment to the segment and the proper training of those recruited. The practitioner pathologists define the "shortage" of pathologists as their major problem. Recruitment is particularly vital to them because, if they are to effectively establish their claim to continually expanding techniques, they must provide enough pathologists to take over the new positions which are opening up. As they point out themselves, wherever pathologists have not been present and pressing their claim, their competitors have moved in. Recruitment, thus, protects them from invasion of their territory.

In recruitment, practitioners find themselves in competition, not only with other specialties, but with the other segment in pathology. They want to recruit people into the practice of pathology, not just into pathology. In seeking to recruit students, they utilize an imagery of pathology which expresses their own segmental identification. They particularly emphasize the role that pathologists play in patient care. However, they consider themselves at a disadvantage in recruiting and training, because they do not have the access to potential recruits academic pathology does, and complain that students do not gain a proper image of pathology from academic pathologists. Nor can they control the training programs as readily. One of the chief sources of friction between the two segments is the residency training program, in which practitioners want more time and effort put into preparing young men for practice, while scientists want to reserve the time for research training.

The Scientific Segment and Revitalization

We have said that the scientific segment represents a professional movement in its later stages of development. Pathology claims many of the great discoveries in medical science of the past, but the issue for contemporary pathologists is how to continue to substantiate this claim. The course of events has thrown scientifically oriented pathologists on the defensive, and they find themselves having to cope with threats on two major fronts, with considerable consequence to their professional identity.

First, the emergence of the practitioner movement has created a number of problems for scientifically oriented pathologists. Practitioners promulgate an alternative identification of pathology, and insofar as the practitioners succeed in identifying pathology as a service specialty, and gather more and more services under the auspices of pathology, it becomes increasingly difficult for the scientists to fulfill their traditional mission of research. The majority of scientifically oriented pathologists have worked in departments which carried out service functions. As long as those functions were few in number, and did not require great specialization in training, it was quite possible for the pathologist to fulfill service responsibilities to his and his insitution's satisfaction, and still carry out a heavy research program. As departments take on more service functions, greater proportions of time are snatched away from research. Thus, the scientific segment is caught in a *conflict of fateful interest* with the practitioners. It is a conflict of interest in the sense that the pursuance of one segment's interests interferes with the other segment's interests. Each segment has its own requirements of the work situation, but cannot achieve them without detriment to the other segment.

Hence, scientifically oriented pathologists are very much concerned with the issue of how much service, if any, their departments should take on. So far, no common assessment of the problem has taken hold. Assessments are local, and solutions are not only local, but highly fluid. Much of the difficulty in achieving a concerted policy appears to flow from ambiguities in the scientific pathologist's own identity. He too, considers himself basically a physician, which means that he incurs some responsibility for the application of his knowledge to patient care. Many respondents felt strongly that the pathologist's research was enriched by contact with clinical problems. These conceptions leave the scientific pathologist vulnerable to the kind of appeal the practitioner segment makes, and complicate the problem of just where a line should be drawn against the expansion of service functions. In this sample, departments which succeeded in drawing a strong line were those that had a particularly strong and locally supported research ideology.

The scientific segment also encounters conflict of interest with the practitioners on the fronts of recruitment, training, and certification of the next generation. The scientists claim that practice is draining off many able young pathologists from research careers. Practice offers opportunities and immediate financial rewards which did not exist for the previous generation of pathologists. Certification further complicates the problem. Board certification—increasingly controlled by practitioners—has gradually required wider knowledge of applied pathology than the young research-oriented pathologist is prepared for. Leading research men in the sample were concerned that the young men who take the time and trouble to prepare themselves for certification will be lost to research. On the other hand, those who do not gain certification will be at a severe career disadvantage. If the trend continues, certification could become a deadly squeeze upon the recruitment of young people into research careers.

The scientists are just beginning to develop some concerted tactics for handling these latter problems, principally through the channel of federal support for research careers. The current interest of government in supporting research is considerably strengthening the position of academic careers in medicine. The number of people entering full-time academic research careers is increasing in all of the specialties. Pathology will certainly benefit from this movement. But it also seems likely that support for research careers will further a division between practice careers and research careers, an outcome which most pathologists prefer to avoid. Despite the segmentalization of the specialty, pathologists have maintained an idealistic investment in the integrity of the "whole" of the specialty.

The second source of threat to the scientific segment is the loss of the former prestige of pathology as a scientific discipline. Changes in the problems and methods of the medical sciences have forced pathologists to re-evaluate their own discipline. In the face of the practitioner movement—a group which claims that pathology is primarily a practicing specialty—it is all the more necessary for the scientists to reaffirm their scientific claim. From the near unanimity of responses among the scientists in the sample, it appears that the movement to rejuvenate pathology as a science is well underway, and involves the following tactics.

(1) They attempt to break the identification of pathology with a traditional, declining methodology. Morphological techniques (the techniques of anatomical pathology) have long been the dominant, core method of pathology, to the point where, now that these techniques are not as fruitful as they once were, pathologists find it necessary to assert that pathology and morphology are not synonymous. They want to get away from an image of the pathologist as a man who "looks down the barrel of a microscope." Instead, they draw attention to new methods coming into pathology, and stress that pathology is not *just* morphology. The pathologist is not limited by the past. Here again, we have dissociation from older images.

(2) At the same time that they dissociate themselves from total identification with morphology, they defend a morphological background. Morphology is what pathologists are trained to do. Like psychotherapy, it is a skill which requires many years of preparation and practice before a man is considered competent. But pathologists are the only group with this kind of training. So morphology is what pathologists can do that no one else can do. Further, respondents point out examples of research that has failed because the investigators were not morphologically skilled. They conclude that although the value of morphology is limited as a principal technique, it is still useful in relating experimental data to human disease.

(3) They evolve new conceptions of an appropriate method for pathology. The conception of method espoused by the scientifically oriented respondents is that pathologists are not limited to any one set of techniques, but can use the techniques and methods of any of the sciences in pursuit of their problems. Pathology "brings together the tools and methods of many fields in the study of disease." However, most respondents favored, and exemplified in their own research, utilizing their morphological background in conjunction with other methods, usually biochemical. The conjunction of morphology with clinical methods was less valued by many of the pathologists in this sample. As one respondent put it, he would be promoted for

his experimental research. Thus, these pathologists were moving in the direction of a synthesis of traditional with newer methods borrowed from the basic sciences.

(4) There is a reformulation of the traditional research mission, so that the sense of mission takes into account both traditional elements and the shifts in method in defining the special contribution the pathologist can make to the scientific community. The contemporary pathologist may use any of the methods of the basic sciences in studying disease, but there are two things the pathologist has which makes his contribution to medical science unique, according to respondents. First, he has a broad knowledge of disease and familiarity with clinical entities, which basic scientists do not have. Second, he has background in morphology. The combination of this dual background with basic science techniques allows the pathologists to do research no one else can do. As one respondent put it, they can combine structure and function in ways that have never been done before.

Thus, with the scientific segment of pathology, we have a case of a scientific discipline built up around a core methodology facing the problem of survival as that methodology is progressively exhausted. The pathologists have found a formula—we might call it a "revitalization formula"—which allows them to preserve what they consider unique to pathology at the same time they transform their methods. They can point to their special perspective. The anatomists, who have been in a similar position for a longer period of time, apparently have still not succeeded in defining what is uniquely anatomy, although they have long since gone through a great diversification of methods and problems.[9] By contrast, the pathologists will probably escape the fate of becoming a collection of people gathered together by the necessity of teaching a basic subject matter in the medical curriculum.

Discussion

In pathology, we have found two distinct segments which are focal points of social change within the specialty, and which are in different stages of development. It seems reasonable to hypothesize that the tactics of these groups will be found in other occupational movements in comparable phases of development. The newly emerging segment characteristically develops a claim to its work area, proclaims a mission, defines work roles and relationships, and creates associations to forward its interests. This pattern may also be clearly seen in the new specialty.[10] What happens to the older segment when changing conditions undermine its original claims is

9. For an example of the discussion going on in and around anatomy, see Joseph Brozek, "Body Composition: A Challenge to Human Anatomists, *AIBS Bulletin* (Published by the American Institute of Biological Sciences), 11 (June, 1961), 10-11.

10. Dan C. Lortie, "Doctors Without Patients. The Anesthesiologist—A New Medical Specialty" (Unpublished M.A. thesis, University of Chicago, 1949).

less clear. In pathology, the more traditional segment reiterated the value of the older mission, and maintained what they considered unique to their approach by a synthesis of new methods with traditional methods, which we call a *revitalization formula*. It may be, then, that most segments that survive have hit upon such a revitalization formula. But an alternative pattern of survival probably also occurs, and that is survival by virtue of fulfilling a continuing institutional requirement.[11]

Further, it appears that the pattern we have found in pathology, an expansive, territory-claiming segment, and an older, traditional segment thrown into a defensive posture, is not at all unusual among the professions. A similar relationship between segments exists in American psychiatry, with the older, somatically-oriented segment losing ground before the increasingly popular psychodynamic approach.[12] The emergence of clinical psychology and the response of experimentalists to this development presents another illustration of this general pattern.[13] But the case of psychology, which has also spawned a dramatic expansion of social psychology, suggests that the pattern can be more complexly woven, with more than two segments involved. These observations point to the need for comparative studies of patterns of occupational development which focus upon relationships between segments.

In general, this research suggests that our concepts of professional and occupational organization should more systematically take into account the existence of segments, and their developmental character. Segments, as we have analyzed them, involve much more than "types" within a profession. They are another, albeit loose, form of organization within the profession, and they are continually in movement, their character at any point in time reflecting their historical development and their relationships to a shifting professional millieu. Since segments have their own requirements of the professional milieu, and attempt to control their surroundings so as to implement their own specialized goals, studies of institutions where professionals work would profit by consideration of the particular segments involved. This kind of analysis would also provide a powerful tool in the study of professional politics. Finally, it should be recognized that careers, and recruitment and socialization into a profession, are patterned by segments. The areas of recruitment and socialization typically engender and reflect competition and conflict between segments, and types of careers repre-

---

11. As mentioned above, this seems to be the case with anatomy. The Townsend movement presents an analogous type of resolution on the part of a nonoccupational movement, in that the emphasis has shifted away from the original mission toward maintaining the institutionalization of the movement. See Sheldon Messinger, "Organizational Transformation: A Case Study of a Declining Social Movement," *American Sociological Review*, 20 (February, 1955), 3-10.

12. Bucher and Strauss, *op. cit.* See also a forthcoming article by Danuta Ehrlich and Melvin Sabshin "Psychiatric Ideologies: The Relation of the Structure of Attitudes to Self Designation."

13. See Goode, *op. cit.*

sent commitment to particular segments within a profession.

In conclusion, some comments may be made on the relevance of this analysis of professional movements to collective behavior theory. One of the most difficult problems that has faced workers in the area of collective behavior is delineating the phenomena with which they are concerned. Attempts to distinguish collective behavior as dealing with unstructured versus structured behavior, or noninstitutionalized as against institutionalized behavior, inevitably are confronted with the tendency of the phenomena to slip in and out of these categories. Research and theory on social movements has reflected this ambiguity. For the most part, social movements have been thought of as occurring outside of the major institutions of society. Yet, social movements become institutionalized, and enter into a variety of relationships with established institutions. The occupational movements described in this paper play out their destiny totally within the framework of some of the most respected and conventionalized institutions of our society. Although there are important differences between these occupational movements and the more "classic" social movement—for example, in occupational movements the leadership usually consists of people of high status in institutions, and recruitment and socialization occurs through institutional channels—the parallels are sufficiently striking to make comparisons between these movements and others feasible. This suggests that a great deal of behavior usually subsumed under the rubric of "institutional" may be studied from a collective behavior point of view. If this position is followed through, collective behavior might realize its potentialities of providing the tools of analysis of process and change in social organizations.

9

LEONARD SCHATZMAN
ANSELM STRAUSS

A Sociology of Psychiatry: A Perspective and Some Organizing Foci

This paper is concerned with a conceptual structure that would give sociological shape to the field of psychiatry. Its more ambitious purposes are to
suggest several sociological models as organizing principles for viewing
that field and other professional practice fields like it; also, to suggest a
number of research problems of value to sociology. Behind these purposes
is a concern for some questionable benefits accruing to sociology from its
association with, and application to, professional practice and service fields.
Social scientists generally may well feel flattered by the demand for their
skills and products. Yet much work being done constitutes a service to
these practice fields, answering to practical problems suggested by practitioners rather than to problems of fundamental importance to social
science itself.

In psychiatry, much of what goes by the name of sociological research
contributes little toward developing theory essential to an exclusive sociological position—a position which carries no notable concern for the legitimacy, efficacy, efficiency, or morality of psychiatric practice. For several
decades now, sociologists have dealt with problems of mental illness,
psychiatric practice, and psychiatric institutions.[1] Many, and perhaps most
of them, have come to accept both the legitimacy of psychiatric practice
and its supporting assumptions, though not necessarily its underlying theories. They tend to accept the "facts" of mental illness, and concern themselves with applying their expertise to "problems" of etiology, ecology,
treatment, administrative structures and processes; hence the many studies
on social factors productive of "disturbance," the prevalence and incidence
of "mental illness" among varied populations, professional and patient

Reprinted from *Social Problems*, 14, No. 1 (1966), pp. 3-16, by permission of the
authors and The Society for the Study of Social Problems.
We wish to acknowledge the helpful criticisms and useful suggestions given by Howard
S. Becker and Barney G. Glaser; also historical materials provided by Melvin Sabshin.
    1. A representative list of such writings might include the following publications: Ivan
Belknap, *Human Problems of a State Mental Hospital* (New York: McGraw-Hill, 1956);

roles, ward organization, and the consequences of these for patient health and control. Many of these sociologists want to help psychiatrists understand how social events impinge upon psychiatric events or, intrigued with mental illness as a phenomenon, want to learn for themselves how "it" occurs. Some have collaborated with psychiatrists on such matters and have come to share concepts—indeed, whole frameworks—with them. Of course, not all are so accepting of psychiatric assumptions and practices. There are a few who tend to picture the psychiatrists' relationships with patients less as treatment than as work in the interest of the psychiatric establishment. Given this critical perspective, there is little interest in certain standard "problems"—for example, in studies of prevalence and incidence—since the search for mental disturbance is not viewed as independent of the "production" of it.

The assumption behind this paper is that it would be much more fruitful for sociology if more research were done about psychiatry than in it or for it. A more comprehensive and sociologically oriented model, providing a new perspective for the study of practice fields such as psychiatry, would offer some protection against being led into taking sides, willy-nilly, in internal battles. It would offer protection also against taking for granted many matters that the practitioners themselves take for granted. Most important, a more sociologically oriented model forces a much larger range of relevant questions about the field of study.

Our own position stems from a dual tradition: sociological social psychology with its emphasis upon the perspectives of actors within delimited kinds of "worlds," and a later tradition of the sociology of work with its special focus upon occupations and careers.[2] The focus on psychiatry in this paper is as much an attempt to provide a scheme with wide implications for the study of social order as it is to provide a more limited one for the study of psychiatry.[3]

John A. Clausen, *Sociology and the Field of Mental Health* (New York: Russell Sage Foundation, 1956); Elaine and John Cumming, *Closed Ranks* (Cambridge: Harvard University Press, 1957); H. Warren Dunham, and S. Kirson Weinberg, *The Culture of the State Mental Hospital* (Detroit: Wayne State University Press, 1960); H. Warren Dunham, *Sociological Theory and Mental Disorder* (Detroit: Wayne State University Press, 1959); Joseph W. Eaton and Robert J. Weil, *Culture and Mental Disorders* (New York: The Free Press, 1955); Robert E. L. Faris and H. Warren Dunham, *Mental Disorders in Urban Areas* (Chicago: University of Chicago Press, 1939); Erving Goffman, *Asylums* (Garden City, N.Y.: Doubleday, 1961); Herbert Goldhamer and Andrew Marshall, *Psychosis and Civilization* (New York: The Free Press, 1953); August B. Hollingshead and Frederick C. Redlich, *Social Class and Mental Illness* (New York: John Wiley, 1958); E. Gartley Jaco, "Social Factors in Mental Disorders in Texas," *Social Problems*, 4 (April, 1957), 322-328; Henry L. Lennard and Arnold Bernstein, *The Anatomy of Psychotherapy* (New York: Columbia University Press, 1960); J. Myers and B. Roberts, *Family and Class Dynamics in Mental Illness* (New York: John Wiley, 1959); Arnold M. Rose, ed., *Mental Health and Mental Disorder* (New York: W. W. Norton, 1957); Leo Srole et. at., *Mental Health in the Metropolis* (New York: McGraw-Hill, 1962); Alfred H. Stanton and Morris S. Schwartz, *The Mental Hospital* (New York: Basic Books, 1954).

2. See E. C. Hughes, *Men and Their Work* (New York: The Free Press, 1958).

3. The same remark can be made about our earlier publications: A. Strauss, L.

Interprofessional Process

Some years ago we and our colleagues developed a model for studying
certain psychiatric events.[4] This was a logical outgrowth of our research
on mental institutions. Our framework was applied mainly to the properties
of certain specific hospitals and to the professional training, careers, and practices found there. *We viewed the modern psychiatric institution as a professional
"arena"—a work locale to which different professionals come, with varying
career patterns, treatment ideologies, differing conceptions of each other as
professional, and varying degrees of commitment to the institution of which
they were part.* This model led to a view of social order in the modern
psychiatric institution as a process and consequence of negotiation. Using
the model, we were able to study how the professionals negotiate their respective tasks and adjust (or fail to adjust) their professional and ideological requirements to each other. The model was adequate for our more limited purposes: the study of psychiatric, interprofessional processes in face-
to-face situations within given settings, where the professionals have a mandate for forging working relationships with mental patients.

A considerable number of questions worthy of investigation are raised by
that model. Broadly put, these questions bear on how professionals representing different disciplines manage to forge a division of labor—indeed,
how they manage to "survive" each other in the context of a given institutional situation, particularly when the professionals hold divergent ideological views. Also, there are questions concerning ways in which emergent
operations, developing operational philosophies, and styles of work modify
professional, institutional, and ideological commitments. More specific questions can also be raised and investigated: what are the different kinds of
claims being made according to discipline, according to dominant treatment
ideology, or in the absence of notable ideological content? What kinds of
professional claims find no grounds for negotiation in given settings or in
given ideological contexts? Conversely, what claims are negotiable in given
situations? Are there characteristic or patterned strategies of negotiation? The
interprofessional model offers many questions worthy of translation into
researchable problems.

Since the development of that model, our conceptual horizons have broad-
ened. We have looked at psychiatric practices not directly related to specific
hospitals and have found that our "old" model falls short of encompassing
the richer textures of experience which impinge upon psychiatry as a whole
and which, in the broadest sense, constitute the contemporary psychiatric

---

Schatzman, R. Bucher, D. Ehrlich, and M. Sabshin, *Psychiatric Ideologies and Institutions* (New York: The Free Press, 1964); L. Schatzman and R. Bucher, "The Logic
of the State Mental Hospital," *Social Problems,* 9 (1962), 337-349; Schatzman and
Bucher, "Negotiating a Division of Labor Among Professionals in the State Mental
Hospital," *Psychiatry,* 27 (1964), 266-277.

4. *Ibid.*

scene in urban America. Although we shall endeavor here to present additional models for the large task, our general framework is substantially the same.

Turning now to other interprofessional processes, we pose two closely related questions as a starting point. What do people of an urban community understand about mental illness and psychiatric practices? How do these understandings enter into their daily lives? If we assume that "the community" is a fiction or hypothetical construct, then, since there are many modes of understanding as well as of participating and consuming, we are dealing with many groups or aggregates of people who stand in different relationships to psychiatry—including those within and those without the commonly understood province of psychiatry.

Within psychiatry itself there are relatively wide differences in understanding about the nature of mental illness, the therapeutic process, and about professional roles. In fact, one striking feature of modern psychiatry is the widespread disagreement over very fundamental problems. Psychiatric practitioners on all levels often find it difficult to agree on what behavior is sick and what is sick about the behavior; what to name it, including whether it needs to be named. If, indeed, they come to agree on these points, they may become involved in controversy over the etiology of the behavior or its seriousness. When and if they reach agreement here, they may engage each other in argument over where treatment is to be conducted, whether in inpatient or outpatient systems, or in day care centers. But decisions of this kind require prior agreement as to the urgency of intervention. At the next point in the decision process, we find considerable and fundamental disagreement over treatment, broadly as well as specifically: psychotherapy, milieutherapy, somatotherapies—or combinations of these, and how much of each.

In addition, treatment decisions lead to problems in patient management (including whether management and treatment are separable). Here there is a welter of decisions over permissiveness and control, over the kinds of privileges the patient will enjoy, and whether such privileges must be earned or given at the discretion of some person or group. Who makes the decision is a matter of increasing difficulty and complexity in contemporary hospital psychiatry. Professionals become embroiled in debate over who controls all or portions of the treatment and management process: the doctor, other professionals, all the professionals together, the patient himself, all the patients themselves, or everyone in the institutional community. Professionals get deeply involved in discussions of how well the patient is doing, how much longer treatment is required, including whether anyone ever gets well enough to conclude treatment. The near disappearance of the word "cure" stands as mute testimony to an issue lost through rhetorical and functional exhaustion.

To think in terms of a single psychiatric community is to stretch one's imagination beyond credulity.[5] It is far more plausible, logically and empirically, to think in terms of clusters of psychiatric thinking and practice, with cluster formations (representing people both inside and outside of psychiatry) shifting in terms of specific issues and problems. In part, the clustering is a function of commitments by practitioners to their respective professions. Many clues to questions about the interprofessional process can be found in events governing the professions themselves, for every professional is something of an embodiment of a special training process—one which gives him not only practice skills, but ideology and career patterns, all of which command his loyalties.

Professional Process

It is not our intention here to focus upon the training of the professional, but to utilize a more inclusive framework, one which has to do with the relationship of a profession to social movements. In their "Professions in Process," Bucher and Strauss have posed a model of the way in which professions evolve through a study of a medical specialty, pathology.[6] Already separated from the "medical profession," pathology itself becomes divided, not so much as a result of a "natural" division of labor, but in terms of a social movement within the specialty.

Hypothetically, *we can posit a process of segmenting or branching for all the professions, indeed for all large human groups sustained over time— through divisions of labor, through social movements within segments which come to espouse "unorthodox" missions, and through attractions toward segments evolving from still other groups and movements.* This model of professions in process is a piece of history itself, of ideas as well as of groupings—twisting and turning, splintering and branching, combining and recombining. (One may think immediately of an analogy between the growth of a profession and the growth of a tree. However, the analogy is necessarily incomplete because the assumed historical "core" or "trunk" of a profession, unlike that of a tree, is a fiction. What we have in mind is that branches from one trunk move toward those from another, become entwined, bend earthwards and reroot themselves, forming new trunks "in their own right," and then develop their own branches of systems in endless process. Perhaps a better analogy in this context would be that of a stream or river, where the larger body is found later rather than earlier in the process, resulting from many small tributaries merging to constitute the river itself, which finally branches off into estuaries as it finds its way to the sea.)

5. Strauss *et al., op. cit.,* chap. 3, pp. 38-50. For an excellent theoretical statement, see also Norton Long, "The Local Community as an Ecology of Games," *American Journal of Sociology,* 64 (1958), 251-261.

6. R. Bucher and A. L. Strauss, "Professions in Process," *American Journal of Sociology,* 66 (1961), 325-334.

Every historian of social thought and of sociology comes to grips with problems posed by this professional process. Working them out involves the working out of history. Is sociology itself a trunk, or is it a limb grown out of philosophy ? Then which portion of philosophy would be the trunk? To answer such questions requires taking some perspective on history, in given time and space. How we attack these problems and others like them reflects the model we have in mind. The model is not new. We use it systematically or casually when we ponder, for example, movements within social work which led it in the direction of neo-Freudian psychiatry; similarly, when we consider movements within segments of cultural anthropology and psychoanalysis, and the subsequent birth of the school of culture and personality. Schools and groups do not come from whole cloth; they are woven by specific people in a given time and place, when social-cultural events provide conditions for their emergence. The sociology of knowledge and history of philosophy and science provide ample evidence for the viability of this model.

Implicit here is a sociological dynamics productive of dynamism within psychiatry. Strands of change within psychiatry not only underlie current confusions but enhance them. We have reference to the growth of the recent milieutherapeutic and community psychiatry movements, already significantly altering interprofessional relations and institutions. Simultaneous with these movements is a growing ascendance of the psychodynamic orientation over the older somatic perspective; but also looming on the horizon are developments in biochemistry and genetics which portend perhaps further profound changes within psychiatry. Such emergent movements have important implications for defining and discovering illness, as well as for treating it and for reordering relations among professionals working within psychiatric institutions. Sociologists may well concern themselves with the way in which the many segments of psychiatry have emerged. Looking ahead, they may be able to predict the courses or directions yet to be taken. Looking at psychiatry today with its many segments, ideologies, and practice models, they may find that study useful for understanding professions in general. Such study may help reveal some unwarranted assumptions being made about the boundaries and characteristics of modern professions; for example, their presumed unity, stability, and continuity; also, by implication, the modes and extent of control by professions over its membership, and the influence of institutions and other professions on them.

The professional process model not only helps us trace the directions taken by professions and their segments and specialties, but also helps us understand, and even predict, the kind of career being fashioned by persons moving along any particular branch line. Psychiatrists-to-be, for example, having come up through medicine and branching off into psychiatry, are very soon confronted with critical choices, since the psychiatric limb itself is many-branched. Detailed examination of a career requires more than dealing with "a" residency; what kind of psychiatric residency is the question, and with what consequences?[7] Are there comparable choices for occupational therapists, or for nurses? If so, do these choices have the same sorts of consequences for these professionals? By following one branch line rather than another, a psychiatric professional determines the kinds of interprofessional situations he will later select as appropriate for himself. He determines what situations he will be able to work in comfortably, or at all, for some clinical settings may not, for structural or ideological reasons, allow him to express his professional mission.

The psychiatric resident, for instance, trained in "one to one" psychotherapy, may find it most difficult to develop a career in community psychiatry, or in institutions ideologically committed to the idea of therapeutic community. His residency may in fact predispose him to a career in office psychiatry or psychoanalysis and prejudice him against accepting any milieu as having significant therapeutic value for patients. The predisposition is not mechanical; it refers to a process within the residency—or any formal program undertaken by any psychiatric professional—of learning about, and becoming committed to, specialized thought about mental illness, about care and treatment, and about one's central task as a professional. Sociological inquiry may well focus on the kinds of practice models to be found in the welter of training programs, how learning one or another of them affects practitioner choices, and also how such models constitute or affect the perspectives of their carriers on the task structures of their co-professionals.

Public Process

As a field of study, psychiatry does not end with histories of professions and professionals; it begins there. Within psychiatry proper we find many special "worlds."[8] However, these worlds are continuous and interrelated with other and equally complex worlds. *On the periphery and further out are many publics which stand in many different relationships to psychiatry—consequently having members who comprehend, consume, and participate in psychiatric practice in many different ways.* A sociology of psychiatry would in the last analysis be concerned with who understands what about mental disturbance—and with what consequences for the discovery, the handling and treatment of disturbance by those within psychiatry as well as by all those who might avail themselves of psychiatric practice. Indeed, we should be studying who says what behavior is disturbed or sick, and what is thought to be sick about the behavior in the eyes of the observer, whoever he might be.

7. R. Bucher, "The Psychiatric Residency and Professional Socialization," *Journal of Health and Human Behavior*, 6 (1965), 197-206.

8. Tomatsu Shibutani, "Reference Groups as Perspectives," *American Journal of Sociology*, 60 (1955), 565-567; and his "Reference Groups and Social Control" in

Earlier we expressed dissatisfaction with the concept of community, precisely because it could not, as currently used, help us conceptualize the many "communities" and aggregates which view or use psychiatry. For this reason we turn now to the concept of "public" for help in sorting out and identifying the many groupings. Introduced by Herbert Blumer, in the context of "Collective Behavior," it will, with modification, serve us here; for interactionists and process-oriented sociologists are accustomed to viewing apparently "stable" features of the contemporary urban scene in that context.[9]

Blumer used the term to apply to groups or aggregates who engage in controversy about issues. By ignoring controversy as a necessary condition, we may simply view a public as an aggregate or group whose understandings and actions *vis-a-vis* psychiatry are patterned and therefore constitute a distinct universe of people and behavior. Each universe may be lasting or ephemeral, but its identification would be determined by its patterned relationship to psychiatry.

On the periphery of psychiatry "proper" lies a relatively broad network of quasi-psychiatric persons, often serving as a filtering system. We refer to police, the clergy, teachers, general medical practitioners, personnel officers, vocational guidance personnel, and so on—people who regularly, intermittently, casually, or formally accept or assign themselves responsibility for ferreting out illness, for treating it, for referring it on to others, or for various combinations of these actions.[10] Questions here have to do with how these people—within or outside of agencies—interpret their own licenses to act.[11] What characteristic judgment do they make about behavior? What are their conceptual thresholds for recognizing mental disturbance? How competent do they think they are in these matters relative to their evaluation of the competence of professional persons or facilities within psychiatry? It would appear possible and most fruitful to sort out patterns of comprehension and action among the dozens of occupational and professional classes along the borders of psychiatry.

Still further removed from the professional psychiatric province is a larger hinterland of laymen—some almost professional in their comprehension, and some so far removed in their conceptual grasp of psychiatry as to be practically oblivious of a professional realm.[12] In between, presumably, are aggregates of persons who entertain a wide variety of understandings and

A. Rose, ed., *Human Behavior and Social Processes* (Boston: Houghton, Mifflin, 1962); also Anselm Strauss, *Mirrors and Masks* (New York: The Free Press, 1959, pp. 161-164).

9. Herbert Blumer, "Collective Behavior," in R. E. Park, ed., *An Outline of the Principles of Sociology* (New York: Barnes and Noble, 1939), pp. 221-280.

10. See Elaine Cumming, Ian M. Cumming, and Laura Bell, "Policeman as Philosopher, Guide, and Friend," *Social Problems*, 12 (Winter, 1965), 276-286.

11. See Kai Erikson's monograph on deviancy and mental illness in seventeenth-century New England, *Wayward Puritans* (New York: John Wiley, 1966).

12. See Charlotte Schwartz, "Perspectives on Deviance—Wives' Definitions of Their Husbands' Mental Illness," *Psychiatry*, 20 (1957), 275-291.

whose actions with respect to psychiatry and mental illness are at least as varied as their understandings. Our interest here is wider than that ordinarily given the public province which most readily leads to demographic studies. Our questions go beyond what various sex, age, educational, or economic aggregates think about mental illness. We need this information too, but we need more; for example, we need data and concepts on specific occupational groups and aggregates: lawyers, engineers, social scientists. What do people prominent in the various news media, particularly newspapers, think about psychiatry and its practices? How do they represent psychiatry to their audiences—through editorials, health and education columns, cartoons, and through periodic mental health crusades? Are there, in other words, characteristic modes of thought about psychiatry flowing either from occupation specifically or social structure generally?

The importance of this sort of inquiry becomes evident when publics emerge around specific issues bearing upon psychiatry, the resolution of which affects the advocates of existing positions.[13] Publics emerge in response to issues, disperse when these issues are resolved or no longer serve as issues, and then re-form when still other issues arise. Also, publics emerge in response to social movements which in one way or another affect psychiatry.[14] Publics can become the precursors of social movements, which directly or indirectly impinge upon psychiatry; for example, civil rights, antipoverty, social medicine, and the mental health movement itself. The questions here are: What specialized groups and occupations engage in dialogues and other actions that affect psychiatry? What characterizes their thinking about psychiatry?

The concept of public also helps us focus on ways in which groups and aggregates consume psychiatric services. Segments of lay and quasi-psychiatric populations are becoming increasingly sophisticated about psychiatry, particularly the psychodynamic varieties. Shifting modes of understanding and action pose exciting sociological research problems. Thresholds for recognizing or naming behavior as "disturbed" are changing as ever increasing numbers of persons are being exposed to the language of disturbance as well as to availability and possibility of psychiatric help.[15] The popularization of psychodynamic vocabularies and the increasing acceptance of disturbance as natural, inevitable, and treatable enhance participation in the psychiatric universe of discourse and in the consumption of psychiatric goods and services. Among certain lay groups, this has proceeded to the point where nearly everyone is involved in some kind of clinical operation: as patient, as lay diagnostician or therapist,

13. With regard to issues other than the psychiatric, see Howard S. Becker, *Outsiders* (New York: The Free Press, 1964); and Alfred Lindesmith, *The Addict and the Law* (Bloomington, Ind.: Indiana University Press, 1965).

14. Kingsley Davis, "Mental Hygiene and the Class Structure," *Psychiatry*, 1 (1938), 55-65.

15. See Kai Erikson, "Patient Role and Social Uncertainty: A Dilemma of the Mentally Ill," *Psychiatry*, 20 (1957), 263-274.

as referral agent, or as general psychodynamic interpreter—for themselves as well as for others, often whether requested or not.[16]

The popular understanding and concern for such matters as "personality development," "interpsychic relations," "the unconscious," and "defense mechanisms" make increasingly complex social structures; they alter ways of viewing oneself and others. What are the implications of this phenomenon for the often asserted "increasing" incidence of mental illness and for the concurrently increasing importance of psychiatry? How does this approach compare, theoretically and empirically, with one that accepts reports of an increase in incidence and attributes it to the increasing complexity of life, to fears of "the bomb," and so on? Sociologists interested in this area might find it most fruitful to trace the implications of this psychiatric "conceptual explosion" for modes of participation and consumption, whether the persons affected are patients or simply part of the milieu.

On the other hand, some groups and aggregates are relatively untouched by such a broad movement. One can detect this insularity among persons of lower socio-economic levels, particularly among certain ethnic groups.[17] Substantial pockets of people still apply folk vocabularies and folk remedies to the apprehension and handling of their ailments, both fancied and real. No doubt urban centers will be plagued for years by people who do not enter the psychiatric universe of discourse and thereby offer many problems for civic communities and psychiatric agencies. Problems suitable for research are numerous in this area, having to do mainly with tolerance levels, the vocabularies applied, and characteristic remedies for assorted deviant behavior. Our own continuing interest in such problems has revealed, for example, marked differences in mutual understanding between Mexican-American patients and "Anglo" psychiatric personnel over the meaning of normal behavior, mental illness, and psychiatric practices. Studies of personal and interpersonal dialogues arising out of such contexts between subcultures would throw considerable light upon cross-class and cross-ethnic interaction.[18]

While the relevance of this focus to clinical problems is apparent, we would caution against that relevance as a primary reason for research. Sociological research into the thinking of ethnic groups about "mental illness" should be done without using the perspective of psychiatry. A principal sociological issue here has to do with the conditions and the characteristics of social order and action as they pertain to deviancy, whether the order and action occur within relatively closed communities, or arise when elements of different communities deal with each other. Research might well proceed at two levels: one having to do with the ebb and flow of publics and social movements on specific or general issues relevant to psychiatry; the other dealing

16. Eliot Freidson, "Client Control and Medical Practice" *American Journal of Sociology*, 65 (1960), 374-382.

17. Frank Riessman and Sylvia Scribner, "The Under-Utilization of Mental Health Services by Workers and Low Income Groups—Causes and Cures," *American Journal of Psychiatry*, 121 (1965), 798-801.

18. Marvin K. Opler, ed., *Culture and Mental Health* (New York: Macmillan, 1959).

with characteristic patient careers within the context of special groups, where these groups are defined by modes of understanding and dealing with deviancy and psychiatric practice.

Just as the interprofessional model provides a reasonable basis for study in careers as they flow through specific work settings, the public process model provides the basis for examining how illness careers are conditioned by the milieu from which mental patients enter various psychiatric settings. Since patients do in fact negotiate their fates in the psychiatric settings, it may be seen that the two models merge; patient and professional careers develop in arenas characterized by confrontation and negotiation, with the patient actively bargaining on his own behalf, but also influencing professional decisions and careers.[19] In our earlier work we were able to depict four relatively distinct modes of patients' thinking about their illnesses and about treatment and care. We suggested the possibility of many patient career types, with distinct consequences for their management in hospitals. Many of these careers are short and special. On the other hand, the world of psychiatry seems well endowed with persons who have made long-term commitments to "illness" and who fashion careers from patient-hood itself. Research questions here bear on the role of the institutional process as a factor in the development of such careers. In what ways is this process perhaps like a residency in psychiatry, replete with the learning of a special language and sets of strategies which contribute to making a career?

Sociocultural Processes

Sociocultural changes in American life account both for much of what is claimed that the mentally ill need and for the kinds of institutions and practices being fashioned for them. Institutions, like people, have historical and social loci; therefore, what obtains within given institutions may well be best understood or explained in terms of conditions having no necessary relationship to their intended work. For example, Americans may be developing certain forms of institutional practice, not so much because they are designed for better psychiatric treatment but because they are less expensive than other forms of practice, or meet the requirements of some special public, or answer to certain historical imperatives in the life of a modern society. Design for psychiatric treatment may be a rationalization of ideological sentiment, itself an historical product.[20] This statement bears some brief elaboration, for behind mental institutions are social and philosophical trends which give rise to ideas about appropriate institutional forms.

19. Strauss *et al.*, *op. cit.*, pp 262-291; see also William Caudill, *The Mental Hospital as a Small Society* (Cambridge: Harvard University Press, 1958); and W. Caudill, F. Redlich, H. Gilmore, and E. Brody, "Social Structure and Interaction Processes on a Psychiatric Ward," *American Journal of Orthopsychiatry*, 22 (1952), 314-334.
20. For an extended discussion of ideology and practice in another area (industry),

During the latter half of the nineteenth century, the United States developed the state mental hospital. We are all familiar with this form of hospital; there are some still remaining, seemingly unchanged over the years. Today they are widely regarded as medieval, cruel, or totally unsuitable for the treatment of the mentally ill. Yet they were once regarded as suitable. Strauss and Sabshin tell us exactly how suitable they were; the state hospitals siphoned off many of the poor, the indigent, and the unassimilated immigrants, and effectively hid them from public view and concern.[21] They relieved the cities and states of special welfare and protection problems and saved whole families from the threat of downward mobility. All this they did with a minimum of cost to the nation, allowing expansion of its frontiers and development of its resources. We would say that this institutional form was appropriate simply because at that time it reflected the needs, ideas, and character of American life. Sociologically, it fit. Today it no longer fits. Now we are developing new institutional forms and practices appropriate to the needs, ideas, and character of American life today—and not necessarily appropriate to the needs of the mentally ill. This assertion should not be construed as an attack upon psychiatry; it simply reflects our observation on the state of psychiatry as a science, and of the collective uncertainty within psychiatry today over what the mentally ill in fact need.

Since the heyday of the state hospital, America has become remarkably urban and industrialized, a nation of great wealth, capable of new allocations of its resources. A number of changes in ways of living and thinking have allowed important groups to define mental illness as a grave social problem—a primary problem rather than a subsidiary one, heretofore dealt with at a distance and in the cheapest way. What social and philosophical changes have made this possible or even mandatory?

Between the two world wars, America chose social welfare over social Darwinism which meant, in part, that it chose to engineer a social order marked by upgraded and equalized participation in political democracy, material consumption, and multiple styles of urbanity. To accomplish this, it insisted upon guaranteeing the requisite means for individual and group participation and pushed for maximum individual achievements. America pours its wealth into vast numbers of opportunity programs to achieve its goals and names almost any conceivable group, event, or thing a social problem if it can be seen as threatening the achievement of these goals. Hence, its concern for the "culturally deprived," the underachievers, the school dropouts, the job displaced, the aged, the ill, the retarded, and mentally disturbed. This concern goes beyond that of the nineteenth-century humanitarians

---

see Reinhard Bendix, *Work and Authority in Industry* (New York: Harper & Row, 1963).

21. Anselm Strauss and Melvin Sabshin, "Large State Mental Hospitals," *Archives of General Psychiatry*, 5 (1961), 565-577.

who involved themselves with underprivileged out-groups on moral grounds. Now all these aggregates are seen as special in-groups whose conditions are intolerable to society, if not actual threats, in light of today's social and economic requirements. Other categories, such as those containing addicts and homosexuals, have their special advocates bidding to add them to the list of those who should be helped. The student protest movement will probably result in still more being added. In one sense, American pragmatism is in full bloom, having converted most personal-social events into "problem solving" or clinical situations.

These material, social, and philosophical developments have undoubtedly had their effect upon psychiatric practice. Sociologists would do well to look at current and projected patterns of practice in these terms. For instance, to what is the "open door" practice related? Why are patients increasingly being brought into institutional decision-making processes? Why do they sit in groups and engage in public and secular treatments? We do not believe psychiatric practitioners invented or currently use these ideas independently of changes in the national scene. This assertion is not meant to deprive the Freudian movement of its just deserts; rather, we would treat and study this intellectual movement as one among many which have altered the life of Americans. The Freudian movement, followed closely by developments in the social sciences, has induced parallel effects in areas and institutions other than the psychiatric, *e.g.*, child rearing, education, and even the training for professional work (as in nursing and social work). On the other hand, other sectors and institutions have induced parallel developments within psychiatry. Examples are economic institutional developments in expanding "consumer markets," in rapid mass-production, in quality control, and in the expansion of corporate leadership and responsibility. Our own recent observations in several well known, experimentally minded psychiatric settings have set us to thinking about these parallels.

Most psychiatric practice today can thus be faithfully conceived of as a social movement that serves to return the mental patient physically and conceptually to the mainstream of society—a society geared to mass production and consumption, a society which increasingly regards mental illness as a primary social problem and mental health as a mandatory condition to participation in the good life. *In sum, an important aspect of the sociological endeavor should aim at relating ideologies of psychiatric practice and institutions to other movements which are organized around political, economic, social, and psychological ideologies, including conceptions of freedom, equality, humanitarianism, and pragmatism.* This, then, is another guiding model for the sociological study of psychiatry.

Institutional Processes

So much psychiatric work goes on within institutions that sociologists can hardly fail to note developments in institutional form and wonder about their implications for professional career, practice forms, and treatment ideology. *Institutions impose limitations upon practices and ideas, but in truth are modified by them. The precise ways in which these are related is an important aspect of sociological inquiry.*

In view of what we have been saying about trends in American life, the sociological question might well be: Whither psychiatry? Psychiatry today is undergoing a veritable revolution in institutional form and practice. Americans have moved beyond state hospitals for the poor and beyond sanitaria or one-to-one treatments for the economically well-to-do. These systems are by no means gone from the scene but have been bypassed or modified beyond recognition. Psychiatric professionals are dealing today with very different populations than formerly. These populations are educationally upgraded, demanding more and new forms of psychiatric goods and services. Psychiatry has thus developed forms that are sociologically, and perhaps even psychiatrically, suitable for these populations and their newly conceptualized needs. Ideas and development in preventive medicine, in vocational counseling, and in rehabilitation have also had their impact upon psychiatry. Sentiments generated by economic and social movements—buttressed by tranquilizing drugs and by wealth which demands expenditure to satisfy these sentiments—provide the ideas which have led to mental health "centers" as against hospitals and clinics, as well as to "therapeutic community" and community psychiatry. These are rapidly becoming standard modes of institutional practice.

In addition, sociologists will note the emergence and proliferation of centers where treatment is conducted in the context of research. Like anthropologists confronted with the disappearance of primitive societies, sociologists may find themselves hard-pressed to find "pure" treatment centers. We suspect many sociologists are mistaken in their belief that they are studying treatment systems, when in fact their data are better analyzed in terms of psychiatric research organizations. Those who ponder consequences to the patient of professional, institutional, and ideological requirements might well add research requirements to the list. And certainly the patient is not the only one affected; professionals themselves have to face up to a growing imperative to "do research." This suggests a series of researchable problems on modifications in structured and developing requirements among these several important attributes of psychiatric practice, and upon relations among professionals themselves: nurses and doctors, clinical and research staff, administration and research, etc. Since research is tied up with money and sponsorship, a series of questions may be suggested about the facts and effects of the flow of federal and state money through institutions, their uneven distribution between and within institutions, and the pressures and strategies for getting money and using it. We are familiar enough with ways in which institutions handle problems posed by lack of funds. But are there institutions threatened by a flow of funds in amounts which exceed their ability to consume them efficiently and legally?

Another question is: What institutional models are emerging? We have seen how "therapeutic community" swept into prominence in American psychiatric life. Yet one can also see some psychiatric centers which doctrinally imitate the form, while others creatively misread its directions or change them to suit local requirements. Some clinical chiefs are in opposition to therapeutic community, severely restricting its influence, and particularly the variation of patient government; consequently they restrict the roles of coprofessionals. On the other hand, many clinical chiefs, because of an eclectic or pragmatic disposition, are responsive to these new ideas, but are thereby rendered defenseless against the encroachment of coprofessionals upon their prerogatives. Authorities in some institutions adopt a monolithic ideological position and severely restrict the prerogatives of entire team wards, creating professional deviancy along the way; in other institutions, each ward develops sharp differences and thus poses problems for institutional control since there are consequences flowing from this variety of approaches. How do these situations impinge upon— even create—professional as well as patient careers? How do various treatment programs affect professional task structures: for example, programs involving large and small group therapies; age, sex, and diagnostic groups; psychodrama; occupational therapy; recreational therapy patient government?

With the introduction of interprofessional teams to inpatient units, and the proliferation of "night hospitals," "day hospitals" or day care centers, half-way houses, family care settings, and clinics which offer individual or group therapy, we are witnessing two increasingly important developments. First, there are decisive alterations occurring in the structure of a team leadership. Secondly, there is a vast increase in interinstitutional distribution of patients. Since our purpose here is only to focus attention upon problems, we shall merely raise further pertinent questions. Are the new institutional forms and practices—group and community therapies especially—altering the nature of medical leadership in psychiatric work? If so, what do various professionals stand to gain or lose, and how do they define gain or loss?

With respect to the second point noted above, we can ask one more important question. We are literally and figuratively tearing down the walls of hospitals, opening their doors, decreasing the duration of inpatient status and, at the same time, ideologically accepting the currently viable assessment that patients are rarely cured, and thus developing a vast complex of state and local institutions which become increasingly specialized and which provide screening and shuttle services, as well as treatment for patients. As the two groups—patients and professionals—make their ways through this institutional labyrinth, we may ask: What are the implications for their respective careers in illness and profession?

Sociological Endeavor

In the foregoing pages we have criticized sociologists (more by implication than by documentation) for not consistently and broadly developing their own sociology of psychiatry. We have pointed to several important processes which together suggest ways in which the sociological endeavor might be systematically directed. We have also suggested a number of research questions relevant to each process. The overall framework, or set of models, points to quite a large-scale undertaking directed toward the enrichment of sociological theory rather than one so closely tied to the service of psychiatry. Briefly, the models related to: 1) *Interprofessional Process*—a view of the psychiatric institution as a professional arena, involving confrontation and negotiation; 2) *Professional Process*—a perspective on professions emphasizing organizational and ideological segmentation and branching over time; 3) *Public Process*—a view of public rhetorics in terms of who (groups) understands what about mental disturbance and psychiatry, and with what consequences to psychiatric practice; 4) *Sociocultural Processes*—a perspective on changes in psychiatry as affected by social, cultural, and historical imperatives; 5) *Institutional Processes*—a perspective on institutional forms as affecting professional practice, treatment ideologies, and careers. We believe these models are fully as useful for the study of other professional practice fields (*e.g.*, nursing, medicine, education, social work, city planning) as for the study of psychiatric practice. When sociologists address themselves to such fields, they tend to become embroiled in the struggles within these fields, or at least to accept a number of assumptions made by practitioners. This species of going native is in striking contrast to the considerable distance researchers maintain about such matters as religious sects, political behavior, and even social class. One hazard of studying—not to say affiliating with— professional practice fields is that they not only seem important to society, but that the direction of their development is subject to considerable internal debate. When a sociologist accepts the terms of the debate, his contribution to it, however couched, is the essentially rhetorical one of an interested citizen.[22] (Writings on urbanization, race, and delinquency are especially clear examples of rhetorical devotion).[23] A powerful aid in freeing oneself of any practice field is to adopt the kinds of models suggested in this paper.

The reader may claim that we are eschewing contributions to these practice fields, perhaps even that we are advocating abandonment of a moral responsibility to help. Yet attention to sociological problems does not pre-

22. See Kenneth Burke, *A Rhetoric of Motives* (Englewood Cliffs, N.J.: Prentice-1950).

23. See "A Note on Imagery in Urban Sociology" in Anselm Strauss, *Images of the American City* (New York: The Free Press, 1961), pp. 255-258; Tomatsu Shibutani and Kian Kwan, *Ethnic Stratification* (New York: Macmillan, 1965); and David Matza, *Delinquency and Drift* (New York: John Wiley, 1965).

clude contributions to these fields. Good research and writing are public endeavors, available to theoreticians and practitioners. The latter will, in any event, make their own interpretation of sociological writings, and will judge the discussions and findings in terms of their relevance to issues pertinent to themselves. We may, in fact, make the best contribution to practice by examining, defining, explaining, and predicting issues and problems within a strict sociological framework and with sociological problems in mind.

10

ARLENE K. DANIELS

Military Psychiatry: The Emergence of a Subspecialty

The problem faced by psychiatrists in the military is similar to that of any group of professionals in that they are expected to maintain ethical and technical standards in their work no matter how alien, indifferent, or antagonistic the setting. Independent of any supervision, they may have to overcome indifference and hostility. They may have to resist temptations to exploit or neglect their clients. Presumably, socialization or training in their profession will prepare members to resist pressures toward unethical behavior once they leave the parent community.[1]

This paper is a by-product of various studies in military psychiatry. Research began in 1962-64 while the author was principal investigator of a study entitled "A Study of Social Factors Affecting Acceptable and Unacceptable Responses to Army Life in the Trainee Population," U.S. Army Research and Development Command, Contract DA-DM-49-193-66-G181. In the following years the specific formulation of this paper was made possible by an NIMH postdoctoral fellowship to study the relationship between military psychiatry and military legal procedures, 1F3-8885-01. Systematic review of these data and some additional data collection were aided by two further small grants from the Army (66-G-9209) and (2212). The paper was completed under the auspices of an NIH grant HD02776-02 to study Problems of Social Change and Control in Professions for which the author is a co-investigator.

I should like to thank my associate and friend, Rachel Kahn-Hut, for her help in rewriting, and also the helpful informants and technical experts in military psychiatry who contributed to my education, especially Colonels Roy Clausen, Ralph Morgan, and Vincent Sweeney. In addition, I should like to express my gratitude to Sherri Cavan, Joan Emerson, Dorothy Miller, Robert Sommer, and Thomas Scheff for their suggestions on the development of the argument. Richard Daniels, Neil Friedman, and Edwin Lemert made heroic efforts to reduce or clarify the military jargon sprinkled throughout the text. I wish to thank Eliot Freidson for general editorial advice and encouragement. Finally, thanks to Lauren Banks for research and technical assistance above and beyond any reasonable expectations.

1. A rationale and explanation for the argument that professional communities exert strong controls on members is presented by W. Goode, "Community Within a Community: The Professions," *American Sociological Review*, 22 (April, 1957), 194-200. For a view which questions the efficacy of general professional controls to influence the behavior of practitioners see J. E. Carlin, *Lawyers' Ethics* (New York: Russell Sage Foundation, 1966).

The public expects, in return for licensing and autonomy, that professionals will be independent and reliable under adverse conditions. But it may be difficult to adhere to this strictly "professional" stance for those who are employed in bureaucratic organizations: And the difficulties may become even more marked within authoritarian, coercive organizations. The main difficulty arises when the professional edict to put the clients' needs first comes into conflict with the bureaucratic understanding that first loyalty is owed to the organization.

The thesis of this paper is that military psychiatrists have responded to organizational pressures not only by an adjustment in their professional behavior to organizational requirements, but also by creating a new definition of their appropriate function and a new identity as community psychiatrists. In this view, there has been a change in techniques of practice and also a change in approach and theory. Professionals who practice in this area develop a skill and a theory about their professional activity which makes them unfit in many ways for practice in the traditional, private practice setting. At the same time their new definition of standards and functions unites them with the growing number of psychiatrists working in areas where similar organizational pressures exist—in hospitals, prisons, and schools.

Community psychiatry is not a subspecialty in the same sense as, for example, child psychiatry.[2] There is no formal training period nor any special certification requirements beyond those for general psychiatric practice. Nevertheless, professionals who practice in this area develop a skill and a theory about their professional activity which would be quite uncongenial in many ways to the pattern of practice in the traditional setting. Yet the general public as well as the parent profession consider all psychiatric training equivalent, and a single license to practice covers the entire field.

Civilian and Military Practice

What are the chief differences between civilian and military psychiatry? In the traditional private practice of psychiatry, the practitioner uses some form of analytically oriented long-term therapy with a limited number of patients. Usually patients are seen individually and privately in a quiet office which is tastefully and comfortably appointed. The psychiatrist is a "free" professional offering service to a patient who comes voluntarily to

2. For a discussion of the development of a subspecialty see R. Bucher and A. Strauss, "Professions in Process," *American Journal of Sociology*, 65 (January, 1961), 325-334. For a discussion of the divisions between psychiatry and the rest of medicine, see H. L. Smith, "Psychiatry in Medicine: Intra or Interprofessional Relationships?" *American Journal of Sociology*, 63 (November, 1957), 285-289. See also H. L. Smith, "Psychiatry: A Social Institution in Process," *Social Forces*, 33 (1954), 310-316.

receive it. Although difficulties such as "transference" and "resistance" are likely to occur, these are issues within the therapeutic situation. The therapist and patient are not in serious conflict over "real life" matters as, for example, a patient's wish to leave the Army, the hospital, or to remain in school. For traditionally the psychiatrist is loath to interfere in the patient's life in any way, to make judgments, or even to appear to moralize. Ideally, the patient becomes motivated to help himself and to meet his own ethical standards. He alone explains to the psychiatrist the circumstances of his life and how he "feels" about them. The psychiatrist then interprets these feelings to the patient. While relatives or interested parties sometimes volunteer additional information, it is usually of secondary importance. Psychiatrists often explicitly reject such "outside" information, indicating that their relationship exists solely with the patient. While the nature of *all* private practice may not be caught in this characterization of the field, the range of variation within the field is much smaller than the range suggested by a comparison with psychiatry in other settings.

What happens when psychiatry as it is generally known in private practice moves to other settings? Within the mental hospital as total institution, structural arrangements and goals have quite decisive effects on what we "know" psychiatric treatment should involve.[3] The physician-psychiatrist easily becomes an impersonal administrator, responsible for the welfare of patients, rather than to the patient himself. The actual psychiatric care of patients is delegated to nurses, technicians, or—in cases of severe overcrowding—no one. Far from finding the ideal relationship with a wise and kindly doctor, the patient may find himself in a "custodial warehouse" where he is more or less filed away and forgotten. Such problems are exacerbated in large state or veterans' hospitals obliged to accept all those needing asylum. These hospitals are often the end of a transmittal line for persons with no place else to go. Even when it is recognized that no real psychiatric care can be provided, persons may "stack up" in these institutions if all alternative resources have been exhausted. While the problems of the military are quite different, nevertheless the military establishment, which is also a total institution, faces the problem of what to do with certain kinds of recalcitrant, odd, or mentally ill persons in its midst. Further, it must deal with these difficult persons despite the fact that military priorities and values limit the use of many expensive facilities and psychiatric personnel considered desirable in civilian hospitals. These priorities and values in the military system become the crucial factor differentiating civilian from military psychiatry.

3. For a discussion of the drastic rearrangements which occur in institutional psychiatry see E. Goffman, "The Medical Model and Mental Hospitalization," in *Asylums* (New York: Anchor Books, 1961), pp. 321-386.

The Military Mission[4]

The broadest goals of the military machine, in order of importance, are generally considered to be crippling the enemy in war, protecting our fighting strength, and maintaining the force in preparedness during peace.[5] The first responsibility of the medical corps derives from the second "mission" of the military: maintaining the fighting strength. This goal, translated into medical terms, is repairing the wounded so they may fight again. The "professional myth"[6] of the medical corps is based on this combat function—heroism under fire and extreme pressure of work while ministering to battle casualties. Working with wounded persons also fulfills the second military goal of caring for the seriously wounded who may be repaired but not returned to battle. Those who will not fight again are entitled to care for injuries incurred in the line of duty.[7] Similarly, luckless bystanders receive care.

A less dramatic but extremely important function of the medical corps is

4. The data for this paper were gathered from interviews, military documents, and a limited amount of nonparticipant observation. The interviews were collected in 1964-68. They include interviews with all (15) supervisors and (48) residents in psychiatry at two large military training hospitals. Regular and reserve officers at a variety of other posts (approximately 35) were also interviewed. Supplementary interviews (approximately 60) were gathered during this same time period with ancillary or related personnel such as other military medical specialists, social workers, psychologists, technicians, Judge Advocate General Officers, Red Cross and financial assistance workers, chaplains, members of the Adjutant General's and the Inspector General's staff, provost marshals, secretaries, hospital registrars, patients, and "line" commanders from the company level to the brigade level.

A summary of the research on military documents and related materials is available as "Selected Bibliography for the Military Psychiatrist," Defense Documentation Center (unclassified), AD 616 624. The problems of observation and field work in the military community are presented in "The Low Caste Stranger in Social Research," in *Ethics, Politics and Social Research*, ed. Gideon Sjoberg (Cambridge: Schenkman Publishing, Co., 1967), pp. 267-296.

Throughout this paper, references to military psychiatry are primarily to Army military psychiatry. The great majority of interviews and observations were located in Army contexts. However, interviews, research into published materials, and the observations suggest that the conditions of practice in other branches of military psychiatry are substantially similar even though minor variations exist. Army military psychiatry was chosen as the focus for study because the Army is the largest branch of the Armed Forces. Its services, including those pertaining to military psychiatry, are the most elaborated and extensive of the three major branches of the Armed Forces.

5. H. Russell, "The Army Psychologist as a Mental Health Consultant: Mental Health Consultation," presented at the February 5, 1962, Session, *Current Trends in Psychology in the Army Medical Service*, Second Bi-Annual Conference (Washington, D. C.: Walter Reed Army Institute of Research 1962).

6. H. L. Smith, "Contingencies of Professional Differentiation," *American Journal of Sociology*, 63 (January, 1958), 410-414. Smith points out how important professional fictions can be in symbolizing and stabilizing occupational groups. These fictions help define and organize the work for group members. They are also the source of the myths which attract and inspire new recruits.

7. Treating the seriously wounded also has a morale function by creating the general expectation that wounded soldiers will be cared for; therefore a soldier risks less by engaging in battle. I am indebted to Joan P. Emerson for this observation.

helping to maintain the fighting force in preparedness. This involves maintaining the health and fitness of the military community in noncombat areas, in peace as well as war. In addition to the regular medical activities required to maintain the fitness of the troops, responsibility extends to medical care for the dependent families which are clustered around most permanent posts. Beyond this, large military hospital centers give care to the retired and disabled soldiers and *their* families.

Psychiatry in Combat

Psychiatrists as part of the medical group are expected to help repair the wounded so they can return to fight again. They also give psychiatric care to noncombatants and to the military community just as other types of physicians give medical care. Although psychiatrists enter combat settings like their medical colleagues, their duties and problems are different. From the military point of view, a major problem develops when the diagnosis of combat exhaustion leads to a mushroom growth of casualties. In World War I, when men broke down with hysterical or psychiatric symptoms considered "illness," they were evacuated to hospitals in the interior as medically, that is, psychiatrically ill. Others then became "ill" in the same manner. A contagion of psychiatric symptoms would often decimate the ranks of a unit. These cases were never able to return to active duty. In more recent wars, the nature of military concerns required that the psychiatric profession provide some theoretical interpretation of illness which would permit humane treatment while holding the line against "permissive" diagnoses which appeared likely to encourage the spread of symptomatology. In short, something between classical permissive theory (where symptoms provide an excuse to avoid performance of duty) and a blanket refusal to recognize the reality of mental illness was required. This requirement provoked new research assessing the performance of men under stress.

In the developing view, classical psychoanalytic theory and the "out" it might provide was not only disadvantageous for the Army, but also harmful for the individual. It was argued that evacuating a man with a mental illness label might make a permanent neurotic cripple of him by "fixing" the temporary symptoms. "Fixing" occurred when the expression of symptoms was rewarded by removal from the stressful situation. The reward in combat settings, of course, is hospitalization away from the combat zone. First the patient is trapped by "secondary gain"—his escape from the stressful situation and the eventual disability pension creates a lifetime dependency on his psychiatric category. In addition, a man may be injured by guilt and remorse feelings at leaving his comrades in those difficulties from which he has escaped through an ambiguous "mental breakdown." As a consequence of the application of this theory by psychiatrists, soldiers were aided in adjusting to their military responsibilities. The psychiatrists became responsible for on-the-spot treatment by which they could minimize the risks to the man and support the military mission at the same time. By permitting time for the spontaneous remission of stress-induced disorders, the psychiatrist encouraged fortitude among the soldiers.

These theoretical ideas were conceptualized as the theory of practice known as "combat psychiatry." This practice included such techniques as "command consultation," "denial of symptomatology," and "supportive therapy", and by it, psychiatrists were able to reduce drastically the numbers of soldiers incapacitated by "combat exhaustion" (or "shell shock").[8] When soldiers exhibited symptoms of combat exhaustion, psychiatrists interviewed the officers and buddies of the victim (command consultation) in order to discover the circumstance surrounding the breakdown. They minimized the seriousness of the symptoms to the man whenever possible (denial) in order to prevent him as well as others from defining the problem as one of mental illness. When men were screaming, weeping, vomiting, hallucinating, or engaging in other forms of extreme or bizarre behavior, they were "supported" rather than "treated." They were told that they had experienced a normal "stress reaction." They were offered sedatives on the spot and told that with twenty-four to forty-eight hours of sleep, rest, quiet, hot food, and other such comforts, they would be all right. They were assured that they could return to performing their duties without fear of "going crazy." The success of this treatment procedure was that it enabled many "casualties" to return to the field.

Unfortunately, follow-up studies under combat conditions have not been systematic. It is not known, therefore, what percentage of those declared in a state of remission were able to function effectively upon return to combat. Comparisons of survival rates for soldiers who have and have not been treated for combat exhaustion and returned to duty, for example, have never been made.[9]

Since the success of this approach depends upon early, firm, and consistent "denial" of the psychiatric significance of symptoms manifested under stress, the psychiatrist requires help to support and reaffirm this point of view. Military psychiatrists have assumed responsibility for teaching the value and techniques of this form of treatment both to other physicians and to commanders of units who might refer persons whom they assume are in distress. The psychiatrist has to convince commanding officers that the symptoms are not as serious as they seem, that men can endure a great deal more when they are absolutely convinced, and by the commander himself, that they

8. The foremost proponent of this view is Col. Albert Glass (Ret.). See A. Glass, "Psychotherapy in the Combat Zone," *Symposium on Stress* (Washington, D. C.: Army Medical Service Graduate School, 1953), pp. 284-294, and A. Glass et al., "The Current Status of Army Psychiatry," *American Journal of Psychiatry,* 113 (February, 1961), 673-683.

9. For a discussion of the problems connected with gathering data on this area see A. J. Glass, "Effectiveness of Forward Neuropsychiatric Treatment," *Bulletin U. S. Army Medical Department,* 7 (December, 1947), 1034-1041.

have to do so. From this viewpoint, helping the soldier face his responsibilities for his own sake also helps to maintain the fighting strength. As one reserve officer explained it:

> You put someone in a difficult situation and say to them, "What would you say if I said to you, 'The requirements are you are to drive a racing car next week at 100 miles an hour and you may be killed. But you have to do it or be shot.'" If I then say to you, "You might get out of it," your motivation lessens quite a bit for attempting the task.

As a consequence of this theoretical perspective the psychiatrist enforces the official policy required of line officers. The military psychiatric perspective is additional support for the line officer to help him hold the line. Ultimately the use of the psychiatric label is sharply curtailed to those extreme cases where the psychiatrist finds it applicable.[10]

Psychiatry in the Garrison Post

The theories and techniques developed to meet combat responsibilities are generalized and made applicable to other aspects of military psychiatry practice.[11] For example, psychiatrists are required to evaluate soldiers who are "not making it" in the service. They screen out those who should be discharged and also "screen in" any who just might be persuaded to "shape up." When making recommendations regarding disposition for treatment, transfer, or release from the service, in these cases, the military system encourages psychiatrists to make them on the cautious side militarily: when in doubt, diagnose as healthy, recommend a "further trial of duty." While the regulations governing such discharges contain provisions covering men who for personal reasons cannot, or will not, perform their duties, they are made possible "for the convenience of the military" as well as for the best interests of the individual. But, there is some of the same ambivalence in the military bureaucracy about this channel of release as there is about removing people from combat.[12] The problem before the military

10. The following articles present a descriptive and philosophical elaboration, necessarily oversimplified here. B. L. Bushard, "The U.S. Army's Mental Hygiene Consultation Service," *Symposium on Preventive and Social Psychiatry* (Washington, D. C.: Walter Reed Army Institute of Research, 1957), pp. 431-443, and H. W. Brosin, "Panic States and their Treatment," *American Journal of Psychiatry* 100 (July, 1943), 54-61.
11. As of June, 1968, for example there were 18 U.S. Army psychiatrists in Vietnam —out of approximately 282 (the official number permitted to the U.S. Army under the terms of the doctors' draft as of June, 1968). Figures supplied by Col. R. E. Clausen, M. C., Director of Personnel and Training, Office of the Surgeon General, Dept. of the Army, Washington, D. C.
12. The history of the administrative discharge in the U.S. Army, for example, has been dogged by a certain indecision about whether or not this discharge should or does contain any punitive elements. An effort to make the discharge less stigmatizing was made by dividing the discharge into two parts of which one part would be clearly less disapproving. The Army regulations have undergone many changes in number; but they have always had two types of administrative discharge, of which one is gen-

authorities in using the administrative discharge is reflected in the following joke:

> An eccentric inductee made his training squad apprehensive and unsettled by his inveterate habit of picking up scraps of paper, turning them over, then shaking his head sorrowfully while saying: "No, that's not the one." As his habit became more and more compulsive, it came to the attention of his officers. After several mental and physical examinations, the authorities decided to give him an administrative separation. On the day the final recommendations were approved and signed, his first sergeant sought him out to give him his discharge. The man showed no sign of attending. He continued turning over scraps of paper and muttering disappointedly to himself: "No, that's not the one." The sergeant tugged at his sleeve and forced the paper into his hand. The soldier absent-mindedly turned it over and then his eyes lighted. "Ah, yes," he said. "That's the one." [13]

The psychiatrist must take this ambivalence into account in making his decisions. By turning to the theory developed in battlefield experience, the psychiatrist tends to support one side of the ambivalence through his professional decisions. With the benefit of the soldier in mind, the psychiatrist encourages him to continue his attempts to succeed in the service. It is seen as psychiatrically beneficial to give the soldier a second chance. It also keeps the psychiatrist from coming into direct conflict with military authority, for by taking the military psychiatry view, he is also helping to "hold the line."

Often, the affairs of the soldier are already substantially settled and the decision of the psychiatrist that no mental disease or defect is present does little to alter the outcome of administrative processing. But the tendency to deny mental illness, irrespective of its theoretical relevance, may have considerable effect on the career of the soldier whom the psychiatrist examines. The psychiatrist provides an essential element in many administrative procedures; but he provides little protection against the bureaucratic pressures of the system. The significance that the judgments of a psychiatrist sometimes have can be seen in the assistance given to the legal branch of the military, the Judge Advocate General Corps (JAG). Psychiatrists provide the kind of advice and recommendations to JAG that forensic psychiatrists offer in the civilian courts. They provide expert testimony for defense and prosecution. But most commonly what the psychiatrist does is to provide the clearance to proceed with a trial by his finding that there is no mental illness. In this respect he resembles the State Psychiatrist in a civilian trial. Consequently, the psychiatrist primarily limits the possibility that an accused may enter

erally recognized to be somewhat more disapproving or punitive than the other. The intent seems to be to provide punitively minded commanders with an administrative alternative which somewhat favors their perspective. Norman Brill documents the difficulties of the Army in its vacillation between a liberal and a more stringent discharge policy in Chapter IX, "Hospitalization and Disposition," *Neuropsychiatry in World War II*, Vol. I. (Office of the Surgeon General, Washington, D. C., 1966), pp. 199-203.

13. I am indebted to Thomas Scheff for this antique jest.

a plea of not guilty by reason of insanity. The definition of mental illness permitted within the military framework is somewhat restrictive. Such problems as alcoholism and homosexuality, for example, are specifically exempted from the illness classification. Accordingly, in many legal actions the psychiatrist inevitably becomes a better witness for the prosecution than for the defense.[14] In this respect he differs from the specially retained, privately practicing psychiatrist who may support the defendant.

From Therapy to Diagnosis

One important difference in the two types of practice concerns the importance of treatment as opposed to screening, diagnosis, and evaluation. Private practitioners in the ordinary course of treating patients who come voluntarily have no need to name the type of complaint from which a patient suffers. In private practice it is important to work with a patient, rather than to diagnose him. In this context, diagnostic skill is related mainly to such questions as recognizing the types of patients who can be treated successfully and those that cannot. However, military requirements focus on screening, diagnosis, and evaluation rather than treatment. Or rather, "treatment" is redefined in terms of group processes and requirements. The military psychiatrist "treats" the organization rather than the individual patient.

What does treatment of the organization involve? In private practice, the usual procedure is to follow the fifty-minute-hour schedule with each patient. Each patient is seen for brief therapy (one hour a week for about a year) or for analytic therapy (three to five hours a week for up to five years or more) in the doctor's private office. In the military setting, a course of therapy is generally much shorter than either of these alternatives. The therapy may be restricted to such matters as prescribing medications and giving advice. The patient may be seen for ten or fifteen minutes rather than fifty minutes.[15] The average time period for a course of therapy for each patient may fall in the one-month range.[16] In this approach, great emphasis is placed upon behavioral change as distinguished from the personality change anticipated in analysis. In accordance with this emphasis, situational adaptability is encouraged rather than the development of self-awareness and "personality growth." Of course, these goals are not necessarily mutually exclusive. But, as has been noted, should one inhibit the other, in the military it is the situational adaptability which must take precedence.

14. See J. J. Gibbs, "The Role of the Psychiatrist in Military Justice," *Military Law Review* (DA Pamphlet 27-100-7) (January, 1960), 51-59.

15. There are, of course, many psychiatrists in civilian life who prescribe medications as the main form of therapy, and who see patients in very brief interviews. See A. Strauss et al., *Psychiatric Ideologies and Institutions* (New York: The Free Press, 1964).

16. This impression is drawn from interviews with military psychiatrists, observations of appointment books at clinics, and military psychiatry literature.

An example of the professional implication of these differences in civilian and military practice can be seen in the psychiatric approaches to a "social" problem: homosexuality. There is considerable disagreement in psychiatry as to just what this problem represents: is it a symptom of a character and personality disorder or of a more serious psychotic disorder? Can homosexuality be either or both of these disorders? Is homosexuality really an emotional problem amenable to analysis in terms of psychiatric theory? Or is it a general social problem to which psychiatry might sometimes be applicable and sometimes not? Does it involve a "problem" or a moral judgment?

Such questions about homosexuality are more likely to arise in the civilian than in the military practice of psychiatry. In private practice, if homosexuality is a presenting problem, it is generally seen as a severe personality disturbance which requires lengthy treatment and for which there is a poor prognosis. In the military practice of psychiatry, the problem is viewed from a rather different perspective. Many military psychiatrists do not see homosexuality as necessarily a serious problem if it does not lead to disruption of the military organization. The issue of basic personality disturbance thus is sidestepped and the focus of attention becomes situational adjustment. Thus military psychiatric theory eliminates an interest in treating this type of patient.

From Patient Welfare to the Good of the Service

Perhaps the most striking difference between the civilian and the military psychiatrist lies in the relationship of each to his patient. The private psychiatrist is traditionally a "free professional" who offers his talents and expertise on a fee-for-service basis. The central feature of this relationship is one of free choice and trust. The military psychiatrist and his patient are both employees of the same system. They each have bureaucratic commitments and responsibilities irrespective of personal predilections. For example, neither psychiatrist nor patient may be seeing the other voluntarily. Some screening requirements (as for security risks or for an accused awaiting trial) may be obligatory for the patient. And some consultation requests to see a patient from other medical corps officers or from high-ranking commanding officers may be mandatory for the psychiatrist in his role as a military officer. What may be peripheral responsibilities for the private practitioner (as when he testifies in court or makes an evaluation for an insurance company or an employing organization) become core responsibilities of the military psychiatrist.

Within the military context, the psychiatrist becomes an agent of the bureaucracy.[17] The patient becomes a referral whom the psychiatrist sees in

17. The works of Szasz contain many searching criticisms of psychiatry when its practitioners become agents of other parties and when they become responsible to par-

his capacity as an agent of the establishment, not as the patient's agent. Therefore, when problems of conflicting interests arise, the psychiatrist may be placed in a quandary. What is best for the patient may be the opposite of what is best for the system. Such problems arise most dramatically in time of combat. In order to maintain the fighting strength the psychiatrist is expected to keep men "on the line." Accordingly, he tells the patient whom he judges able to recover what he thinks best for the patient: that he must ignore his symptoms and return to his duties. If the psychiatrist does not use good judgment (and there is no way to be infallible) he may be sending a dangerously shattered man back to almost certain death.[18] Despite the development and elaboration of military psychiatric theory, such problems are not entirely resolved.

These problems also arise in a host of less gravely serious but still difficult situations.[19] One such problem is the lack of privileged communication. This problem is solved by identifying the psychiatrist as therapist to the organization. This identification permits the military psychiatrist to make his own decisions about how the best interests of the organization and the individual are to be accommodated. Thus the psychiatrist may decide that it is really in the best interests of all concerned to collect no incriminating material for the official record. Before developing this position about the limitation and priority of their responsibilities, psychiatrists often worry about a Criminal Investigation Division (CID) agent's request to see their private files on a patient. And they worry about how best to avoid entrapping a referred patient into admission of criminal activity when the patient mistakenly sees the psychiatrist as a confessor, instead of as the agent of the military. The precaution of reading the terms of Article 31 of the Uniform Code of Military Justice to the patient really does not settle the problem of the psychiatrist's ethical responsibilities in every case.[20] While such dilemmas do have their parallels in occasional situations facing a psychiatrist in any type of practice, they are an intrinsic concern in the military practice of psychiatry because of the psychiatrist's dual loyalties.

The Practice of Therapy in Military Settings

The array of expectations about the psychiatrist's expertise differs in other ways from the ideal expectations in civilian practice. The psychiatrist must

---

ties other than the direct patient. See especially "Classification in Psychiatry," in T. S. Szasz, *Law, Liberty, and Psychiatry* (New York: Macmillan, 1963).

18. Grinker and Spiegel discuss the moral uncertainties and agonizings that psychiatrists may feel when they are in such a position. R. Grinker and J. Spiegel, *Men Under Stress* (Philadelphia: Blakiston, 1945).

19. See R. Clausen, Jr., and A. K. Daniels, "Role Conflicts and Their Ideological Resolution in Military Psychiatric Practice," *American Journal of Psychiatry*, 123 (September, 1966), 280-287.

20. Article 31 is the general statement warning an accused that anything he says may be held against him during legal proceedings.

coordinate or conciliate the expectations of the patients and the third parties to whom both psychiatrist and patient are responsible. The kind and extent of treatment and attention a patient receives are quite different from the treatment a voluntary, paying patient is likely to receive in civilian life. Primarily, in the traditional analytic framework available in the civilian setting the patient may be encouraged by the psychiatrist to talk about and develop his feelings about his problems, but in the military setting he may be required to deny or minimize such problems. Further differences are introduced, even in those areas where the military psychiatrist expects to conduct therapy along the lines of his civilian counterpart. These differences are introduced by the military value system in which all military responsibilities have priority over the conducting of therapy.

Psychiatrists and their patients are transferred to other posts often enough so that long-term analysis is generally out of the question. Even during the time they can meet, bureaucratic responsibilities of both psychiatrist and patient make it impossible to maintain regular hours without interruptions and cancellations. In private practice, for example, the psychiatrist and the patient may arrange simultaneous vacations to minimize the interruption of therapy. Such arrangements are not possible in a military setting where annual leave must be taken at the convenience of the particular segments of the organization to which one is assigned. Further, since patients and psychiatrist are on different assignment schedules, their total time in residence at a particular location will rarely coincide. Finally, the daily schedules of both patients and psychiatrists are difficult to make regular; either may be called to special meetings, assignments, or even short tours of duty at other locations which will disrupt the scheduling of appointments in a way not usually found in private practice.

For these reasons, the regular formal practice of psychiatric therapy is relegated to special doctors with special patients in special places. What do these elaborate qualifications mean? Psychiatric therapy defined as a series of vis à vis sessions in a private office is largely confined to major military medical centers. This technique is practiced mainly by residents as part of their training. The patients, for reasons related to their convenience, the convenience of the military establishment, and the convenience of the psychiatrists themselves, are mainly dependents of the military or retired personnel rather than military personnel on active duty. The paradox of this arrangement is that military psychiatry becomes most like civilian practice when it turns away from the active duty personnel. The "best" care available, when it is defined as care like that available in private practice, is not offered to the troops.

In choosing from the potential population, residents and their supervisors are guided by many of the same considerations which might apply in other psychiatric settings. The most desirable patients are those with hopeful prognoses, amenable to or eager for treatment, and geographically stable enough to stay for an entire course of treatment. In the private practice of psychiatry, such patients would probably be the wives and children of professionals and others who are "well to do." In the military such patients are the wives and children (the "dependents") of military personnel.[21] And the military experience provides a new example of the special conditions required for the application of traditional analytic theory. In this area then, theory and practice retain many similarities to the traditional ideas surrounding the private practice of psychiatry. The new theories are reserved for a different population. Where the psychiatrist serves as an agent of the organization, he can use the theory and techniques of military psychiatry even where the patient is somewhat reluctant to participate. Traditional psychoanalytically oriented therapy depends upon the willingness of the patient to continue in therapy, to try to understand and accept a new perspective on personal problems. Such a method is powerless if the patient resists and terminates.

The compartmentalization of these theoretical perspectives illustrates two problems facing military psychiatry. First, it must meet the professional and public expectation that psychiatry within the military organization can offer the equivalent of what is available through modern psychiatry in other contexts. In order to do this, the patient's interests must be given the first priority. (In this way the assertion that military-trained psychiatrists have the right to the same licensure as any other trained psychiatrist can be legitimated.) Second, it must face the organizational priority that group interests be served before individual interests, should the two conflict.

Where the patient is to any extent controlled by the organization which employs the psychiatrist to help him, methods of evasion and resistance are more restricted. Consequently, more directive and even coercive therapeutic tactics become possible. Such methods are more likely to be available in community psychiatry than they are in psychoanalytically oriented practices. Community or Social Psychiatrists are more likely to find a somewhat vulnerable population in their practice (the poor, the defendants in various types of court actions, students, the residents of a disintegrating ghetto). This population may be faced by a formidable array of social services interested in their betterment in addition to the psychiatrist. Even where the psychiatrist is not himself coercive, his activities may be tied to services (parole officers, welfare departments, legal authorities, school officials) which are.[22] Consequently, the main similarities between the military

21. Seventeen of a sample of twenty-five psychiatrists and residents at a large Army hospital stated that they preferred to treat feminine dependents to servicemen because "motivation is better," "they are more stable," "they are available for longer periods of time," "it is nice to have a motivated patient rather than someone who is there because he is ordered," "the psychiatrist is absolved of any sort of administrative responsibility for the patient," and "such patients are more cooperative."

22. Some of the coercive possibilities inherent in community psychiatry are presented in a satirical vein. See K. Keniston, "How Community Mental Health Stamped Out the Riots (1968-78)," *Trans-Action,* 5 (July/August, 1968), 21-29. For a discussion

and civilian practices appear in considering the developing practice of community psychiatry.

Community Psychiatric and Command Consultation

Community (social) psychiatry differs from traditional ideas in psychoanalysis by its emphasis on environmental context and social rehabilitation.[23] In community psychiatry, adjustment to the setting and manipulation of the setting in order to help an individual adjust is of prime importance. The aim of major importance to psychoanalysis—change in basic personality effected through a long-term relationship with a therapist in his private office—is considered ineffective and impractical for the needs of the common run of humanity. Many parallels are drawn by psychiatrists between community psychiatry in the civilian community and in the military community.[24] In each case, the psychiatrist is expected to maintain or contain individuals within the community and to work with various medical and nonmedical agencies in order to implement this goal. This process is similar to "command consultation," which includes obtaining information about a problem from such crucial informants as chaplains, commanders, the Judge Advocate Corps, or the Inspector General. In this way more knowledge about a problem may be acquired than a psychiatrist would find from an interview with a patient. Military experience supports the view that the person labeled as patient may not be the "real" source of trouble.[25] The psychiatrist can make his assessment and then attempt to change the individual and/or his environment so as to alleviate the reported difficulties. In community psychiatry under civilian conditions, many of these same principles and practices are followed, although control of information sources and consultation within the general community is not so readily available to the civilian psychiatrist in a school, community clinic, or welfare program, as it is to the military psychiatrist officer. How does military psychiatry match general understandings and expectations of the civilian psychiatrist in other respects?

Psychiatric Power in the Armed Forces

Differences between the private and the military practice of psychiatry are heightened by the explicit, clearly understood extent of both the formal

of the potential dangers of psychiatry in public schools, see Thomas S. Szasz, "Psychiatry in Public Schools," *Teachers College Record*, 66 (October, 1964), 57-63.

23. For a discussion of some of the ramifications of this position see R. Leifer "Community Psychiatry and Social Power," *Social Problems*, 14 (Summer, 1966), 16-22.

24. G. Caplan, "Types of Mental Health Consultation," presented at the February 5, 1962, Session, *Current Trends in Psychology in the Army Medical Service* (Washington, D. C.: Walter Reed Army Institute of Research, 1962), pp. 1315-1430.

25. See H. Rosen and H. Kiene, "The Paranoic Officer and the Officer Paranee," *American Journal of Psychiatry*, 102 (March, 1947), 614-621.

and informal power of the psychiatrist over his referral. The implicit control of the private psychiatrist over his patient through a variety of "lifemanship" tactics has been described in a variety of contexts.[26] But the power of the military psychiatrist is considerably magnified by the nature of the bureaucratic context in which he practices. First, psychiatrists like other physicians, are given advanced rank. Lawyers, psychologists, accountants, social workers, graduates of officer training programs all enter the service as junior officers; medical officers enter with superior rank up to and including the field grades depending on prior medical and military experience. And this position of organizational preeminence is even more considerable when compared to the rank of most patients. Active-duty patients are primarily enlisted men and noncommissioned officers. It is only this group which is low enough in military status to be able to afford the possible stigma of a psychiatric record.

Officers are in a different but equally difficult position. Visits to the psychiatrist do not look well on their records, especially if they are eager for advancement. Despite the view held by psychiatrists that visits to their office should not be stigmatizing, it is generally the case that persons of rank equal or superior to that of the psychiatrist will not appear for treatment or examination except under unusual circumstances.[27] Such circumstances are usually beyond their control, as when officers are in difficulties over illegal or other seriously deviant behavior or if they are ordered to report to the psychiatrist by their senior officers. Under these circumstances, as when the psychiatrist interviews anyone accused or suspected of something heinous, the formal organizational system delegates much discretionary power to the psychiatrist. He may informally indicate to the patient he is examining that it would be wise to say nothing and to have nothing incriminating on the record. The psychiatrist may decide to see the patient in therapy without this fact coming to the attention of superiors. Or he may recommend a civilian psychiatrist. Taking a different tack, he may collect and sift through a variety of additional types of information about the case through "command consultation" techniques. This information may then suggest formal and informal methods of changing or directing or even canceling the investigations which have begun.

The knowledge of the range and extent of these discretionary powers delegated to the psychiatrist by the military add considerably to the distance between patient and psychiatrist in this setting. A naïve expression of

26. See especially J. Haley, *Strategies of Psychotherapy* (New York: Grune & Stratton, 1963). There are also literary satires which show the real or potential underlying power of the psychiatrist in his relation to the patient: J. Machado do Assis, *The Psychiatrist and Other Stories* (Berkeley: University of California Press, 1963); E. Baker, *A Fine Madness* (New York: G. P. Putnam's Sons, 1964); and L. Ross, *Vertical and Horizontal* (New York: Simon and Schuster, 1963).

27. L. J. Grold and W. G. Hill, "Failure to Keep Appointments with the Army Psychiatrist: An Indicator of Conflict," *American Journal of Psychiatry*, 121 (October, 1964), 340-343.

this distance can be seen in the constant appeals made to psychiatrists by both officers and men (and the dependents of both groups) to avert or request a change of assignment. Petitioners will argue that mental illness or other severe mental disturbance may result from the current unhappy situation. Patients know that the psychiatrist can be a powerful advocate if he will champion their cause. Psychiatrists in the military indirectly acknowledge their power—or the beliefs that others hold about it—in their complaints about "manipulators" who make a variety of attempts or "gestures" to use the psychiatrist for their own ends.

The Special Problems of Military Psychiatry

Military psychiatry is not simply a title for a special arena in which the conventional practice of psychiatry takes place. Rather it is a particular kind of practice responding to the pressures and exigencies of the organization it serves. In consequence, it has developed a rationale and a series of special techniques or approaches to the problem it faces. In contrast to much of traditional psychiatric theory, military psychiatry emphasized "denial" in its resolute minimization of the seriousness of symptoms and its optimistic reassurances to the faltering soldier that "you can make it." A firm attention to the practical questions of adjustment to present circumstances belies the classical importance of introspection and self-awareness. Tolerance of temporary breakdown in functioning in order to explore the unconscious and eventually produce greater understanding is not possible when the demands of the environment cannot permit a temporary breakdown of participants. By making a virtue of necessity, military psychiatry theory "rediscovers" some of the tenets of behaviorist psychologies and moral treatment philosophies.

It could also be argued that military psychiatry has "discovered" or supplemented some of the sociological theory formulated by Edwin Lemert on the significance of labeling for the fixing of secondary deviation.[28] The urgency of the general requirement to maintain the fighting strength has led to a demonstration of how denial of symptomatology can be effective. But the denial of the label of mental illness in a closed institution like the military may be as coercive or difficult for the individual to survive as labeling of mental illness may be in other settings. Furthermore, the denial of the label in military settings may not be as effective as it seems. The psychiatric evaluation of no mental disease or defect may firmly close the gates to ready escape from the military, but it may be quite beyond the psychiatrist's power to offer instead of escape some clean or whole identity to the malingerer, troublemaker, or misfit. Commanders, legal authorities, and other military officers may be able to enforce their label of an individ-

28. E. M. Lemert, *Social Pathology* (New York: McGraw-Hill, 1951), p. 75 and footnote.

ual as a deviant independently of the psychiatrist. When the psychiatrist is also convinced that the patient is some kind of misfit (though of a kind not psychiatrically identifiable in the military context), symptom denial becomes merely an interactional tactic, a device for managing the encounter rather than an act of positive reassurance or therapy.

Military Psychiatry and the Management of Social Problems

The foregoing discussion suggests some of the problems which may be created by the theory and practice of organizational psychiatry. When the psychiatrist sees himself treating the organization rather than some direct client, there is a real danger that his skill and authority will become additional pressures available to the bureaucracy for use upon any refractory participants. The nature of psychiatric interpretations, given the rather encompassing quality of psychiatric theory, makes them peculiarly amenable (or vulnerable) to organizational specification. For example, a very short examination may suffice to evaluate an individual's mental status. In civilian commitment procedures, the court-appointed psychiatrists show an overwhelming disposition (an opinion against commitment occurs in about two percent of the cases) to find the examined ill on the basis of interviews which take less than ten minutes on the average.[29] The same pressure for rapid evaluations exists in the military setting. But here the tendency is particularly strong to find sanity rather than mental illness. Routine examinations for the administrative discharge are estimated as very brief (usually less than thirty minutes); and it is estimated that a psychiatric diagnosis of illness arises in about two in a thousand consultations.[30]

My picture of the requirements for the practice of psychiatry in the military setting is not likely to be attractive to most private practitioners. Most drafted psychiatrists who serve under two-year obligations are quite outspoken in their disinclination to continue such a career.[31] The general complaint can be summed up as "Everyone knows you can't do psychiatry in the Army." Of course, those who are identified with or committed to some type of career in military psychiatry do not agree. They see important resemblances between their work and the developing field of community psychiatry. But whatever the evaluation, what both groups observe is that

29. See T. J. Scheff, *Being Mentally Ill* (Chicago: Aldine, 1966), pp. 143-152; D. Miller and M. Schwartz, "County Lunacy Commission Hearings," *Social Problems*, 14 (Summer, 1966), 26-36.

30. E. L. Maillet, *A Study of the Readiness of Troop Commanders to Use the Services of the Army Mental Hygiene Consultation Service* (Unpublished D.S.W. dissertation, Catholic University of America, 1966), p. 168.

31. For a relatively moderate statement of their objections, see J. T. Ungerleider, "The Army, The Soldier, and The Psychiatrist," *American Journal of Psychiatry*, 114 (March, 1963), 875-877.

military psychiatry is very different from the classical psychiatry made famous by Freud and his followers and accepted by a large public. Since they are obviously not meeting the traditional expectations of the psychiatrist's role, what are military psychiatrists doing?

It is intended in this paper to suggest that employment in institutions may lead to devastating adjustments in the theory and practice of psychiatry. These adjustments have led to a situation in which goals and self-images of a subgroup differ greatly from their parent specialty. But these differences are not formally recognized. Lowered visibility and reduced contact with civilian psychiatrists obscure the differences and potential irritations related to lack of conformity with the conventions of the parent specialty. In this way the subspecialty is relatively free to develop new practices and theoretical rationales for them without coming-into conflict with colleagues holding very different ideas about the proper practice of psychiatry. Acceptance of these innovations is also made possible by the strong validation given to this subspecialty by the training it shares with all psychiatrists and by acceptance through accreditation. The American Psychiatric Association recognizes the military psychiatric residency training programs and accepts time spent in the practice of military psychiatry (however that may be) as acceptable in the fulfillment of board eligibility (the right to apply for board certification under the specialty examination system generally used in all medical specialty fields.).

But, it could be argued that the main professional support for the military subspecialty activity arises from the tacit acceptance of a division of labor. The necessity for such practice is not questioned: someone has to do it. But the practice is not prestigious and the practitioners are somewhat isolated.[32] This group derives whatever cohesion and stability it may possess not from enthusiastic support of the larger professional community but from within itself, from the processes of interaction and adaptation binding its members. It is the group of military psychiatrists themselves, with their supporters and helpers, which develops and strengthens the purposes, techniques, and value system of the subspecialty.

32. See E. C. Hughes, "Good Men and Dirty Work," *Social Problems,* 10 (Summer, 1962), 3-11, for an excellent discussion of this problem.

11

DAVID N. SOLOMON

Ethnic and Class Differences Among Hospitals as Contingencies in Medical Careers

Every occupation is in one of its aspects a role in some system of interaction.

An occupation, in essence, is not some particular set of activities; it is the part of an individual in any ongoing system of activities. The system be large or small, simple or complex. The ties between the persons in different positions may be close or so distant as not to be social; they may be formal or informal, frequent or rare. The essential is that the occupation is the place ordinarily filled by one person in an organization or complex of efforts and activities.[1]

Hughes and several of his students have directed attention to important aspects of such systems by their use of the term "career contingencies."[2] While not satisfactorily defined in the literature, various contexts indicate that the

Reprinted from *The American Journal of Sociology*, 66, No. 5 (1961), pp. 463-471, ©1961 by the University of Chicago, by permission of the author and the University of Chicago Press.

1. Everett Cherrington Hughes, "The Study of Occupations," in Robert K. Merton, Leonard Broom, and Leonard S. Cottrell, Jr., eds., *Sociology Today: Problems and Prospects* (New York: Basic Books, 1959), p. 445.

2. So far as I know, Professor Everett C. Hughes of the University of Chicago originated the concept. His students have applied it to various occupations: see, e.g., Howard S. Becker, "Some Contingencies of the Professional Dance Musician's Career," *Human Organization*, 12 (Spring, 1953), 22-26; and Harvey L. Smith, "Contingencies of Professional Differentiation," *American Journal of Sociology*, 63 January, 1958), 410-414.

Edward Gross attempts a formal definition: Career contingencies are "the major kinds of events or phenomena which can produce these patterns [orderly sequences of events connoted by the term career] and determine their probability of occurrence" (*Work and Society* [New York: Thomas Y. Crowell, 1958], p. 196). See also David N. Solomon, "Career Contingencies of Chicago Physicians" (unpublished Ph.D. dissertation, University of Chicago, 1952), p. 1: "Correlative with every occupation is a social system which constitutes the 'decisive' or 'external conditions' within which the fates of practitioners unfold. The development of a career appears as a series of steps as the individual finds his way through the system. At any one of these points, the outcome, or ultimate position of the individual is in doubt, since it is contingent upon the presence or absence of various circumstances, on the occurrence of failure to occur of certain events, both within and outside the occupation itself. These circumstances or events are the career contingencies of the particular occupational groups."

concept refers to conditions of the social system surrounding an occupation which are decisive for the success of the practitioners.[3] Success in an occupation is contingent on solving the problems, resolving the dilemmas, and passing the hurdles or obstacles which arise from the system of social interaction in which the occupational role is set.[4] Career contingencies are the features of this social system which decisively determine the life chances of those who have chosen the occupation as a career.

In many occupations the ethnic and class distinctions of the community are reflected in the system of interaction of which the occupation is a part. There is some evidence of this in the case of medical practice.[5] Moreover, the different types of medical career appear to be differently distributed through the ethnic and class structures of the medical social system.[6] In examining the career contingencies of physicians, it is therefore important to describe the social worlds of medicine in terms of ethnic or vertical lines of segregation and class or horizontal lines of stratification.

This was done in the study reported here by classifying Chicago hospitals into a set of categories which were initially *ad hoc* types based on a good deal of impressionistic knowledge of the various hospitals. The substantial differences exhibited by the resulting types of Chicago hospitals are interpreted as indicating that the system of interaction which surrounds medical practice in Chicago is not homogeneous but, rather, one which, like the community at large, exhibits ethnic and class lines of cleavage and consists of a set of social worlds, to a degree separate and discrete. Medical school and in-hospital training function as devices which sort or allocate incumbents into the various segments of the system, each of which provides a somewhat different social context for practice and is, therefore, characterized by a different variety of practice. The main purpose of this paper is the description of these ethnic and class structures, which may constitute the most important contingencies of medical careers.

On the basis of impressions gained through interviews and other less formal observation of medical practice, Chicago hospitals were classified into types

3. Max Weber discusses the "external conditions" which are "decisive" for two occupations. His context makes it plain that "external conditions" refers to the social system (see "Science as a Vocation" and "Politics as a Vocation," in *From Max Weber*, trans. H. H. Gerth and C. Wright Mills [New York: Oxford University Press, 1946], pp. 111 ff.).

4. E.g., Howard S. Becker states: "In general the major problem of the service occupations tends to be the maintenance of freedom from controls by laymen for whom one works. . . . The repercussions of this problem may be expected to exert a decisive [sic] effect on the nature of careers within such occupations" *op. cit.*, p.22).

5. E.g., Oswald Hall concluded: "The various hospitals of the community studied form a status hierarchy. The Yankee Protestant hospitals have the most adequate facilities, those organized by the Catholics follow, while those organized by the Jewish group or by medical sects are the least adequate. The prestige of the hospitals is ranked accordingly" ("The Stages of a Medical Career," *American Journal of Sociology*, 53 [March, 1948], 329-330).

6. Oswald Hall, "Types of Medical Careers," *American Journal of Sociology*, 55

which differ in the characteristics of their sponsors, affiliation with medical schools, the extent to which facilities are formally approved, and certain characteristics of doctors—ethnic origins, degree of specialization, and office location. The relevant data were obtained from three sources: the *American Hospital Directory*,[7] a sample of 854 doctors;[8] and fifty interviews, mostly with doctors, but some with laymen having knowledge of the profession.[9]

Types of Hospitals

Fifty-four hospitals, each represented in the sample by only a few doctors, were classified into four types. "Elite Protestant hospitals" are the four believed to have most prestige in the city. "Catholic hospitals" are those operated by Catholic religious orders. "Jewish hospitals" are those operated by the Jewish Charities of Chicago.[10] Finally, "other hospitals," a residual category, consists of all the remaining hospitals.[11]

SPONSORS

Three types of sponsor are found in Chicago hospitals. First, there are philanthropic patrons who give and solicit voluntary contributions, devote time and energy to the work of the hospital, and play a significant role in

(November, 1940), 243-253. See also Stanley Lieberson, "Ethnic Groups and the Practice of Medicine," *American Sociological Review,* 23 (October, 1958), 542-549. For a complete account of Hall's work, to which I am greatly indebted, see his "The Informal Organization of Medical Practice in an American City" (unpublished Ph.D. dissertation, University of Chicago, 1944).

7. *American Hospital Directory* (Chicago: American Hospital Association, 1948).

8. About sixty-two hundred names of physicians are listed, along with information about each, in the *Chicago Medical Blue Book, 1948-1949* (Chicago: McDonough & Co., 1949). About five hundred and fifty additional names were found in the *Chicago Classified Telephone Directory,* March, 1948. All these were numbered serially and over fourteen hundred selected, using Tippett's random numbers. To restrict the scope of the study, all except white males in private practice (that is, having offices) within the administrative limits of the city of Chicago were eliminated, leaving 854 for detailed consideration. Each name was also checked for additional information in the *American Medical Directory* (Chicago: American Medical Association, 1942), the *Directory of Medical Specialists* (Chicago: A. N. Marquis Co., 1942, 1946, 1949), and in the directories of the various specialty associations.

9. Forty names were selected at random from the sample, and, in addition, ten interviews were arranged with doctors or laymen indicated by other physicians or by my colleagues as likely to be willing informants. The interviews are not representative of the sample. The intention in the interviews was to stimulate informal conversation by stating generally the interest of the study in "the problems of modern medical practice," and from time to time the conversation was directed to topics of special interest 'or those on which the informant appeared to have special knowledge. The interviews were not standardized on the basis of a schedule, and no notes were taken, the content being recorded from memory within a few hours.

10. This does not imply that these are the only hospitals which are Jewish in character, which is in fact not the case, but only that these are the ones that are formally Jewish.

11. Public hospitals, whether municipal, county, state, or federal, are not centers of private practice and consequently were not considered, except as training institutions for interns and residents.

the determination and implementation of policy. Second, as is the case with Catholic hospitals, some hospitals are owned by religious orders and operated by their representatives. Finally, the sponsor may be an individual, a partnership, or a corporation which owns, operates, and controls the hospital. These owners are almost always doctors.

Every institution to some extent shares the character of its sponsors. The philanthropic patron is a person with prestige, and hospitals with this type of sponsorship enjoy more prestige than do others.[12] There are, of course, different classes of philanthropist, and thus hospitals might be further differentiated in terms of the relative status of their patrons. The ethnic identification or religion of the patrons is also an indication of the character of the institution. Finally, since "doctors' hospitals" are likely to be regarded, at least by other doctors, as commercial enterprises, they are generally of low prestige.

Elite Protestant hospitals are, with one exception, sponsored by Protestant denominations usually accorded high prestige and associated with Anglo-Saxon elements of the community. The exception, although not so listed in the *American Hospital Directory,* is in effect associated with one of the others as a facility for private patients.[13] All are supervised by lay boards and partly supported by voluntary contributions.

Other hospitals, belonging to the residual category, have several kinds of sponsor. With the possible exception of six sponsored by Protestant denominational or sectarian groups, apparently of German or North European ethnic origin,[14] and perhaps in a few others, they do not have philanthropic patrons, nor are they supported by voluntary contributions. Twenty-two are listed as nonprofit corporations, four simply as corporations. Four were listed in an earlier directory as proprietary.[15] Interviews indicate that, at least in some cases, the nonprofit designation is a euphemism covering more or less profit-oriented ownership:

> Who runs these hospitals that you're working at?
> Private individuals. They're all owned by private individuals. Oh, they have a

12. "One of the criteria of upper-class membership is evidence of 'good works' as seen in terms of philanthropy" (Oswald Hall, "Sociological Research in the Field of Medicine: Progress and Prospects," *American Sociological Review,* 16 [October, 1951], 641). See also Norman Miller, "The Jewish Leadership at Lakeport," in Alvin W. Gouldner, ed., *Studies in Leadership* (New York: Harper & Bros., 1950), Aileen D. Ross, "Organized Philanthropy in an Urban Community," *Canadian Journal of Economics and Political Science,* 18 (November, 1952), 474-486; and also her "Philanthropic Activity and the Business Career," *Social Forces,* 32 (March, 1954), 274-280.

13. The sponsors are Presbytery of Chicago, Protestant Episcopal Church, and Methodist Episcopal Church.

14. Information from the *American Hospital Directory.* The three sponsoring groups listed are Illinois Conference of the Evangelical Lutheran Church, Norwegian Lutheran Church of America, and Swedish Evangelical Mission Covenant of America. Three church-operated hospitals whose sponsors are not named are Bethany Home and Hospital of the Methodist Church, Evangelical Hospital of Chicago, and Walther Memorial Hospital, the last said by informants to be supported by a German Lutheran Group.

15. *Ibid.* 1945 edition.

dummy board so they don't have to pay income tax. That's how they get to be non-profit organizations.

Is B a community hospital, or non-profit organization, or what?
It's a community hospital. I don't know about the non-profit. They've made a lot out of it in the past few years. Of course, it wasn't so good before, but in the last few years they've made plenty. Dr. Y. owns about 90 per cent of it. He runs the hospital. We don't have any public donations or anything like that.

I understand you have a hospital of your own?
Yes, we bought that hospital three years ago. We couldn't get enough beds at *XY* and *P*, although we still carry on there. We have fifteen or twenty admissions a day for major surgery. It's a seventy-bed hospital and it's always full, but we have no waiting list. If a patient comes in we have a bed today or tomorrow, or whenever we want. It's a charitable organization—nobody makes any profit out of it, but we lay down the policy, and we keep twenty beds for other doctors. We've made it a community hospital.
You mean the other doctors have courtesy privileges?
Yes, but we have a regular staff there. We have a board but we [the] owners lay down the policy.[16]

Catholic hospitals are, by definition, those sponsored and operated by religious orders, but some also include lay philanthropic-patrons. This feature, along with others, probably differentiates them among themselves as to prestige. Perhaps the religious orders as well as the patrons might be ranked on a prestige scale. Certainly, both vary in ethnic character, as do their doctors and patients, and there are Catholic hospitals which are regarded as mainly Irish, Polish, Italian, Lithuanian, and German.

The two Jewish hospitals, operated by the Jewish Charities of Chicago, have philanthropic lay boards and thus differ from five hospitals which are Jewish in character but privately owned and therefore classified as "other hospitals." There is probably also a difference in rank between the two hospitals, but data on the status of patrons, doctors, and patients which would have established this were not obtained.[17]

AFFILIATION WITH MEDICAL SCHOOLS

Appointments to teaching posts in medical school are honorific,[18] similarly, to be a "teaching hospital" affiliated with a medical school is a mark of distinction for a hospital. Table 1 shows that all elite Protestant hospitals and both Jewish hospitals,[19] but only two of the thirty-two other hospitals

16. From interviews 39, 26, and 10, respectively.
17. Interview 35: "*XY* is the highest, but *P*'s very close. They're almost the same now. *XY* is really going along on the basis of its seniority and prestige." Interview 40: "*P*'s a very fine hospital. Just as good as *XY*. I guess we [*XY*] have—well, higher class isn't a very good word—our patients have more money. They're mostly from Highland Park and places like that."
18. Talcott Parsons, "The Professions and Social Structure," *Essays in Sociological Theory Pure and Applied* (Glencoe, Ill.: The Free Press, 1949), p. 195.
19. One of the Jewish hospitals is affiliated with a school which was recently accredited.

and only nine of sixteen Catholic hospitals, are affiliated with one or another of the medical schools in the Chicago area. (All nine Catholic hospitals are affiliated with a Catholic medical school.)

FORMAL APPROVAL

The *American Hospital Directory* indicates which hospitals are approved on the criteria shown in Table 11.1. Approval may mean only that a hospital has attained the minimum standards, but lack of approval is of greater significance.

Jewish and elite Protestant hospitals are approved in every respect. Other hospitals, a heterogeneous lot, fall along a continuum from complete approval (six hospitals) to none at all (five hospitals). They are best described in four subcategories, differentiated most clearly by approval or lack of approval of internships and residencies. The "A" subgroup have approval on all criteria, the "C" and Jewish subgroups have few approvals, while the "B" subgroup is intermediate, almost all being approved for internships, but few for residencies. Similarly, Catholic "A" hospitals are approved in all respects, while Catholic "B" hospitals have no approved residencies and fewer approvals on the other criteria.

Table 11.1 Chicago hospitals: Criteria for approval, number of hospitals, and average number of beds

Criterion for Approval	Elite Protestant hospitals	Other hospitals			other		Catholic hospitals			Jewish[a] hospitals
		A	B	C	Jewish[b]	total	A	B	total	
Affiliation with a medical school	4	2	—	—	—	2	6	3	9	2[c]
Approved nurses training school	4	6	7	2	2	17	9	2	11	2
AMA approval of internships	4	9[d]	8	1	2	20	9	6	15	2
AMA approval of residencies	4	10	2	0	1	13	9	0	9	2
Approval by ACS	4	10	9	1	4	24	9	6	15	2
CMA approval of internships[e]	4	—	—	—	—	—	—	—	—	2
Not approved	—	—	—	4	1	5	—	1	1	—
Number of hospitals	4	10	9	8	5	32	9	7	16	2
Average Number of beds	446	206	153	84	111	146	255	169	216	440

[a] Hospitals operated by the Jewish Charities of Chicago.
[b] Hospitals represented in the sample only by Jewish doctors.
[c] One is affiliated with a school only recently accredited.
[d] The one not approved is a children's hospital and thus lacks facilities for general internship.
[e] Canadian Medical Association approval indicated Jewish and elite Protestant hospitals are of international interest.

NUMBER OF BEDS

Although size may not be a valid indicator of prestige,[20] it does reflect capital investment, which is relevant. (The average number of beds per hospital for each of the groups and subgroups is shown in the bottom row of

20. Public institutions, for example, have the largest bed capacity in the city but are of low prestige, except for certain types of training.

Table 11.1). All elite Protestant hospitals, except the one for private patients only, have more than four hundred beds. The larger Jewish hospital has about six hundred and fifty beds, the smaller over two hundred. Jewish and elite Protestant hospitals are thus the largest in the city. Among other and Catholic hospitals, the subgroups with the largest number of approvals have the largest number of beds per hospital, while those with fewest approvals are the smallest.

Doctors

ETHNIC ORIGIN

Reliable lists were available which identified doctors of Jewish, Polish, Italian, and Czechoslovakian orgins. The remainder are presumably of British or North European origin. Despite the inability to differentiate the large unidentified group, the distributions are suggestive (Table 11.2).

Elite Protestant hospitals have relatively few Jewish doctors and none of the other identified groups. Jewish hospital doctors are, with two exceptions, Jewish. While other hospitals have a high proportion of Jewish doctors, more than half of these are in the five hospitals represented in the sample only by Jews. Catholic hospitals have the highest proportion of Polish, Italian, and Czechoslovakian doctors and relatively few Jews.

Table 11.2 Percentage distribution of doctors by type of hospital and ethnic identification

	Hospital affiliation					
Ethnic identification	elite Protestant	other	Catholic	Jewish	none	total
Unidentified	93.8	60.4	60.2	0.9	60.6	55.2
Jewish	6.2	37.1	14.8	98.2	21.1	33.3
Polish, Italian, Czechoslovakian	—	2.5	25.0	0.9	18.3	11.5
Total	100.0	100.0	100.0	100.0	100.0	100.0
Number in sample	64	202	88	112	388	854

SPECIALIZATION

Although the medical specialties differ in prestige and members of any specialty differ among themselves, specialty practice is in general both more remunerative and more rewarding in prestige than is general practice.[21] Moreover, certified specialists have greater prestige.

21. E.g., "The good practices of the city are the specialty practices. The statistics on income differentials between specialists and nonspecialists and the data on trends toward specialization are equally convincing on this point. The specialists are highly conscious of their superior status and refer to the general practitioners by unflattering terms such as 'signposts' and 'information booths' " (Hall, "The Stages of a Medical Career," p. 332). See also M. Leven, *The Incomes of Physicians* ("Publications of the Committee on the Costs of Medical Care," No. 24 [Chicago: University of Chicago Press,

Table 11.3 shows that a very high proportion of doctors in elite Protestant hospitals are full-time or certified specialists, most of them certified. Other and Catholic hospitals do not differ greatly in the proportions of their doctors who are specialists, but they have smaller proportions of certified specialists than do Jewish hospitals.

Table 11.3 Percentage distribution of doctors by type of hospital and degree of specializations

Degree of specialization	Hospital affiliation					
	elite Protestant	*other*	*Catholic*	*Jewish*	*none*	*total*
No specialty	6.3	32.7	42.0	46.4	74.2	52.3
Partial[a]	6.3	28.2	21.6	3.6	16.0	17.1
Full-time[a]	23.4	16.8	13.6	13.4	8.8	12.9
Certified[b]	64.0	22.3	22.8	36.6	1.0	17.7
Total	100.0	100.0	100.0	100.0	100.0	100.0
Number in sample	64	202	88	112	388	854

$$x^2 = 290 \qquad d.f. = 12 \qquad p < .001$$

a. *American Medical Directory, 1942*, p. 7 "This information . . . is based on personal data furnished by the physician."
b. "Certified" by one of the specialty associations or boards.

OFFICE LOCATION

The location of a service near the center of a city suggests a clientele that is at least citywide.[22] Decentralized establishments, on the other hand, serve a local clientele. Moreover, medical specialists concentrate near the center of a city in what is, for this and perhaps other reasons, an area of practices enjoying great prestige.

In the present sample almost two-thirds of the city's specialists have offices in the central business district ("the Loop") while, conversely, two-thirds of the doctors with offices in the Loop are specialists. While the types of hospital with the most specialists also have the highest proportions of doctors with Loop offices (Table 11.4), when specialization is controlled there remain marked differences in the proportions with Loop offices.

1932]); and Milton Friedman and Simon Kuznets, *Income from Independent Professions* (New York: National Bureau of Economic Research, 1945).
    22. "In the same period [1914-29] the area [Chicago Loop] lost 33.8 percent of its general practitioners and gained 68.5 percent in part-time specialists. But for physicians who devoted their full time to the practice of a single specialty, the gain was 118.4 percent. In other words, the Loop has become less a local and more a regional medical marketplace, for such an increase in *specialized* medical services could be explained only by reason of the extension of the size of the area from which patients would come with their demand for medical services" (Earl S. Johnson, "The Function of the Central Business District in the Metropolitan Community," in Paul K. Hatt and Albert J. Reiss, Jr., eds., *Reader in Urban Sociology* [Glencoe, Ill.: The Free Press, 1951], p. 488).

Almost all specialists in the elite Protestant hospitals and a very high proportion of specialists in Jewish hospitals are located in the Loop. In contrast, only about half the specialists in other and Catholic hospitals have Loop offices. In the case of general practitioners, other and Catholic hospitals have relatively low proportions in the Loop and Jewish hospitals a relatively high proportion—in fact, almost as high as that of specialists in other and Catholic hospitals.

Table 11.4. Percentage distribution of doctors by type of hospital, degree of specialization, and location

location office	Hospital affiliation					
	elite Protestant	other	Catholic	Jewish	none	total
Specialists						
Loop	94.6	53.2	46.9	87.5	23.7	64.4
Other	5.4	46.8	53.1	12.5	76.3	35.6
Total	100.0	100.0	100.0	100.0	100.0	100.0
Number in sample	56	79	32	56	38	261
	$x^2=70$		d.f.$=4$	$p<.001$		
General practitioners						
Loop	—a	8.9	14.3	41.1	14.6	16.9
Other	—a	91.1	85.7	58.9	85.4	83.1
Total	—a	100.0	100.0	100.0	100.0	100.0
Number in sample	8	123	56	56	350	593
	$x^2=31$		d.f.$=3$	$p<.001$		
Total						
Loop	93.8	26.2	26.1	64.3	15.5	31.4
Other	6.2	73.8	73.9	35.7	84.5	68.6
Total	100.0	100.0	100.0	100.0	100.0	100.0
Number in sample	64	202	88	112	388	854
	$x^2=223$		d.f.$=4$	$p<.001$		

a. Too few to compute percentages.

The Social System of Medicine in Chicago

The social system of medicine in Chicago—and, no doubt, in other large urban areas—is not a unified homogeneous whole but, rather, one which reflects the ethnic and class segmentation and stratification of the city. The medical community, like the community as a whole, consists of a set of social worlds which are to a degree separate and discrete.

Additional data which can be only briefly mentioned here lend support and significance to this interpretation of the differences between types of hospitals and the doctors associated with them. For example, the graduates of the various medical schools are by no means distributed randomly through the different types of hospitals; rather, each type appears to have, to some degree, its own peculiar preferences for graduates of particular schools, although doctors in the "other hospitals" are heterogeneous in this respect as well. Similarly, each type of hospital has a marked preference for doctors who have trained as interns or residents in the same type. There are thus "typical chains in which each institution aids the newcomer along to the next level"[23] and which function as devices which sort or allocate incumbents to various sectors of the system.

The interviews also indicate differences between elite Protestant and other hospitals, which together include the various strata of the Protestant system. There appear to be marked differences in what is involved in gaining access to hospital facilities, in obtaining patients, and in the nature of colleague relationships and the resulting standards of medical practice.

Elite Protestant hospitals are closed to all but members of their regular staffs. Graduating from the "right" medical school, training in the "right" type of hospital, and obtaining the sponsorship of senior colleagues in the hospital staff—all are involved in becoming a staff member, which with exceptions must occur when practice is initiated. The young specialist then seeks to build reputation among his colleagues, and if he is successful they supply him with patients through referrals. He is therefore dependent on his colleagues for patients and in other ways as well, and consequently the standards of practice are those of the colleague group with its formal and informal social organization. Since these hospitals are also the teaching hospitals, medical practice in them is associated with both education and research, and the level of competence and professional skill is maintained at a high level as a result of the colleague group's ability to control its members. Although we have no evidence of it, it is probable that their fees and income are highest.

Other hospitals, on the other hand, vary from those which are almost as closed as are elite Protestant hospitals to some which are open on a very casual basis indeed. Access to these hospitals depends on the newcomer's ability to refer (supply) patients to specialists who own the hospitals or, what amounts to the same thing, to control admissions. The young doctor must therefore build his reputation directly among patients or other nonmedical people—telephone-answering services, insurance companies, and the like—who may help him build practice, and patients become a *quid pro quo* in exchange for necessary access to hospital facilities. The nature of the relationship among colleagues is therefore quite different from what it is

23. Hall, "The Stages of a Medical Career," p. 330.

among doctors in elite Protestant hospitals, and, for the most part, doctors in other hospitals are not really colleagues at all but, rather, competitors who from time to time share a mutual interest. Under these conditions the relationship of each doctor is with a number of other individual doctors, and there is no formally or informally organized body of colleagues which takes an interest in or has power to set standards of practice. The normative orientation is restricted to matters that are essential to their interaction and does not cover quality of practice or ethics, although, of course, the individual parties to the exchange may, and in some hospitals frequently do, insist on high standards purely as a matter of individual conscience and scruple. Although, again, we have no evidence of it, fees and incomes in these hospitals are probably a good deal lower than in elite Protestant hospitals.[24]

These two types of practice which are said to characterize the different types of hospitals in the Protestant system of medicine in Chicago are, of course, the two poles of a continuum. These are not ideal types. We have among our respondents cases which exemplify the two polar types as well as others which lie somewhere along the continuum. These are empirical types, and the practices of doctors in elite Protestant hospitals lie, in general, toward the one pole while those of doctors in other hospitals lie toward the other pole; there is a zone somewhere to the right of center where there is probably a good deal of overlapping. We have evidence that similar statements could be made if Catholic and Jewish hospitals were placed on their own continua.

The different ethnic and class worlds of the medical social system are thus depicted as areas in which different varieties of medical practice flourish and in which the external conditions of practice are markedly different. The day-to-day interaction in a career can be thought of as an orbit in some system or subsystem. Careers differ in the character and boundaries of the subsystems in which they have their orbits.[25] For medical careers, one of the obviously significant contingencies, or perhaps *the* obviously significant contingency, is which of these subsystems is to be the arena in which the career will be pursued. From the point of view of any particular practitioner, the kind of career he is to have and the degree of success he is likely to achieve depend on how he fits into the scheme of segmentation and stratification.

24. For a more detailed account and complete documentation see Solomon, *op. cit.*
25. The orbit analogy is attributed to Everett C. Hughes.

12

ROSE LAUB COSER

Authority and Decision-Making in a Hospital: A Comparative Analysis

This paper presents a case analysis of the relationship between role behavior and social structure in two hospital wards. The analysis is based on daily observations made over a three-month period in the medical and surgical wards of a 360-bed research and teaching hospital on the Atlantic seaboard. Informal interviews, as well as a limited number of standardized interviews (10 each with house doctors and nurses), were used for the formulation of cues suggested by participant observation. Since only one hospital was studied, the comparisons to be made here—between the social structure of the medical team and that of the surgical team, and between the behavior of nurses on the two wards—should not be generalized beyond the case observed without further research. They are presented however with the aim of formulating hypotheses about the effect on role behavior of different types of authority structure in the hospital setting.

The surgical and the medical wards of this hospital were situated on two sides of the same floor, one floor each for men and women. An observer walking from one ward to the other, either on the male or on the female floor, would notice at first a superficial difference: joking as well as swearing, laughing as well as grumbling could be heard at the surgical nurses' station where some house doctors and some nurses gathered periodically. In contrast, on the medical ward the atmosphere can best be described as being more "polite." Joking and swearing were the exception; informal talk between doctors and nurses, if it occurred at all, was rare. Mainly medical students, who were not part of the formal ward organization, talked informally with nurses. On the surgical side, however, banter between doctors and nurses was a regular occurrence, and there one could also overhear from time to time a discussion between a nurse and some house doctor about a patient. Little if any of this occurred in the medical ward.

Reprinted from the *American Sociological Review*, 23 (1958), pp. 56-63, by permission of the author and the American Sociological Association.

The behavior of the head nurse differed significantly on these two wards. While the medical nurse went through prescribed channels in her dealings with doctors, addressing herself to the interne whose orders she was expected to fill, the surgical nurse would talk to any doctor who was available, regardless of rank. She would more specifically ask that some decisions be made rather than trying to express her views through hints, which was the nurses' custom in the medical ward.

Moreover, in the surgical ward nurses participated much more fully in rounds than in the medical ward. Descriptions of rounds by medical and and surgical nurses differed significantly. We heard in the medical ward, for example, from one of the nurses:

> If nurses go on rounds they hold the charts, they pass them to the interne, the interne to the chief resident, and then it comes back down the line and the nurse puts the chart back. All that the nurse is there for, according to them, is to hold the charts.

Another medical nurse explained:

> I get very little out of rounds. As nurses we're supposed to get something, and give something, but it never works. We're at the end of the line wheeling the charts, then I'm given orders to get something, I have to run out, when I come in again, there's something else they want me to do. . . .

In contrast, the head nurse in one of the surgical wards had this to say:

> During rounds, the nurse gains insight into the condition of the patient, finds out changes in terms of medication and treatment. She can inform the doctor what treatment the patient is on and can suggest to the doctor that the dressing procedure can be changed; she can suggest vitamins by mouth instead of by injection; she can suggest taking them off anti-biotics and point out necessary medication. . . .Occasionally the doctors would bypass the nurse, so before they forget to tell me anything I would ask; also you find out yourself when you're on rounds and that is very important.

This nurse seemed to take initiative, although she appeared to be shy and withdrawn, unlike the head nurses on the medical wards who happened to have a more outgoing personality.

In attempting to account for the different types of nurse-doctor relationship in the two wards, one could examine such factors as personality, character, and level of aspiration of the individuals. We propose, however, to discuss the phenomenon on the level of our observations, namely in terms of the network of social relations in the wards.

Social Structure of the Wards

Although the relationships in the surgical ward seemed to be easy-going, the social distance between the visiting doctor and the house doctors, and between the chief resident and those under him, was more marked among the surgeons. The contradiction between joviality and social distance was well

expressed by a surgical interne: "It is not a very strict and formal atmosphere on our ward," he said, and then added: "Of course, the chief resident
has everything; he's the despot, he decides who operates, so he takes the
cases that he is interested in. The visiting doctor, of course, may propose to
take a case over—he can overrule the chief resident."

To resolve this apparent contradiction, we must compare the formal structure of authority with the *de facto* lines of decision-making. We will see
that in the surgical ward the formal line of authority does not coincide
with the actual line of decision-making; the process of decision-making,
rather than the formal line of authority, apparently has an impact on the
role of the nurse.

As Figures 12.1 and 12.2 show, the chief of service is responsible for the

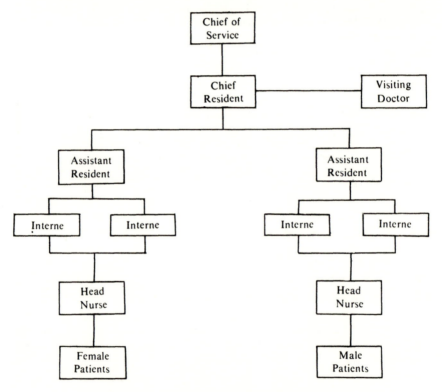

Figure 12.1. Structure of the Medical Ward:
Formal Line of Authority and Decision-Making

ward. He does not make any decisions for individual patients, however,
but delegates his authority for the care of patients to the chief resident. The
latter is responsible to the chief of service. In turn, the chief resident delegates the care of patients to the internes, each of whom is in charge
of specific patients under the chief resident's continuous supervision. The

internes pass on orders to the head nurse for the patients assigned to them. The assistant resident acts as supervisor and "consultant" to the internes.

The formal authority structure is essentially the same in both medical and surgical wards, with a simple organizational difference: there is no separation of tasks among the doctors for the male and female wards on the surgical side, as Figure 12.2 indicates. There, internes and residents walked up and down the steps to take care of their patients who were segregated by sex on two floors.

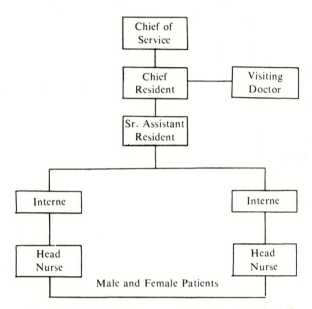

Figure 12.2. Social Structure of the Surgical Ward:
Formal Line of Authority and Decision-Making

But the way in which the house doctors made use of the authority attached to their rank differed significantly in the two wards. In the medical ward, there was consistent delegation of authority down the line. The chief resident was heard saying on rounds to one or the other of the internes, "You make the final decision, he's your patient." Such remarks were not part of the pattern on the surgical ward, where the chief resident made the decisions. The medical house officers also based their decisions, to a large extent, on consensus, with the chief resident presiding and leading the discussion while the surgical house doctors received orders from the chief resident.[1] The following incident was typical of the authority relations in the surgical ward:

1. We have adopted from Alfred H. Stanton and Morris S. Schwartz (*The Mental Hospital*, New York: Basic Books, 1954) the distinction between decisions arrived at through consensus and decisions that are made arbitrarily. (p. 258) "When a consensus is reached or assumed, the participants always feel it is completely unforced. There is no element of submissiveness, of defeat in argument. . . If there is any specific

An interne and an assistant resident were conversing about an incident that had transpired that morning, when the daughter of an elderly patient had created a scene at the nurses' station about the fact that she had been notified as late as the previous evening at eleven o'clock of her father's operation the next morning. When she came to see her father before the operation, he had already been taken to the operating room and the daughter was extremely upset about not being able to see him. The interne and the assistant resident felt that in the future something should be done to forestall similar reactions from patients' relatives; they thought that the chief resident was too busy to notify relatives in due time and that therefore they would take it upon themselves to notify a patient's relatives if the chief resident would give them sufficient advance notice. They decided to take up the problem with the chief resident at the next occasion, and did so that very afternoon. The chief resident's answer was curt: "I always notify the family on time," he said with an annoyed facial expression, and walked away. He did not wish to delegate authority in the matter, trivial though it may seem.

The chief resident's "despotism," to which the previously quoted interne referred, is part of the surgical ward's culture. Although his decision-making by fiat may seem, at first glance, to be a "bad habit," or due to a lack of knowledge about the advantages of delegation of authority and of agreement by consensus, it has its roots in the specific activity system of the surgical team which differs significantly from that of the medical team.[2] We must bear in mind that responsibility for an operation, if performed by a house officer, lies with the chief resident or with the attending surgeon. They perform the important operations. As Stanton and Schwartz have pointed out, decision by consensus is time-consuming.[3] An emergency situation, in the operating room as elsewhere, is characterized precisely by the fact that a task must be performed in the minimum possible time. Whether in military operations or surgical operations, there can be no doubt about who makes decisions, that they must be made quickly and carried out unquestioningly and instantly.

The situation is quite different for the medical team. There the problems are those of diagnosis and of different possible avenues of treatment. Such problems require deliberation, and decisions are often tentative; the results of adopted therapeutic procedures are carefully observed and pro-

---

awareness at all it is one of discovery, of clarity, or of understanding." (p. 196) On the other hand, "we define an arbitrary decision as one made by a person higher in the power hierarchy governing a person lower in it, without regard to the agreement of the latter. Most frequently, of course, it is made to override disagreement and without consulting the subordinate. . . ." (pp. 270-271).

2. For a general comparison between surgical and medical floors, see Temple Burling, Edith M. Lentz, and Robert N. Wilson, *The Give and Take in Hospitals* (New York: G. P. Putnam's Sons, 1956), chap. 16. For a dramatic description of work in the operating room, see Robert N. Wilson, "Teamwork in the Operating Room," *Human Organization,* 12 (Winter, 1954), 9-14.

3. *Op. cit.,* pp. 268, 271.

cedures may have to be modified in the process. All this demands careful consultation and deliberation, which are better accomplished through team-work than through the unquestioned authority of a single person.

In his role as teacher of medical students, moreover, the person in author-ity teaches different lessons on the two wards: in the medical ward students and house officers are taught to think and reflect, while in the surgical ward the emphasis is on action and punctual performance. If this seems too sharp a distinction, and if it is objected that surgeons should learn to think also and medical doctors should learn to act as well, it must be borne in mind that the latter ideal situation is not always approximated, especially since the physicians themselves seem to have this image of the difference between medical and surgical men. The doctors on the medical ward, asked why they chose their field of specialization rather than surgery, said, for example: "Medicine is more of an intellectual challenge"; "I enjoy the kind of mental operation you go through"; "[Surgeons] want to act and they want results, sometimes they make a mess of it." The physicians on the surgical ward displayed a similar view of the differences between medicine and surgery and differed only concerning the value they gave the same traits. When asked why they chose to be surgeons, they said that they "like working with hands," that they "prefer something that is reasonably decisive," and that "[a medical] man probably doesn't want to work with his hands."

Thus the differences in task orientation and differences in self-images would seem to account in part for the main distinction between the two wards. This distinction can be summarized as follows: On the medical ward there is a scalar delegation of authority in a large area of decision-making,[4] and the important decisions are generally made through consensus under the guidance of the visiting doctor or the chief resident. On the surgical ward there is little delegation of authority as far as decision-making is concerned and decisions about operations and important aspects of treatment of pa-tients are made by fiat. Figures 12.3 and 12.4 illustrate this difference.

The Nurse-Doctor Relationship

Under these circumstances surgical assistant residents and internes are more or less on the same level under the authority of the chief resident or the visiting doctor; this makes for a common bond between assistant residents and internes and the strengthening of internal solidarity. The rela-tive absence of actual prestige-grading, notwithstanding the formal rank differences, as they were observed among those who were practically excluded from the decision-making process, tended to eliminate some of the spirit of competition among the junior members. Moreover, with only little author-

4. The term "scalar" is here used as defined by Chester I. Barnard in "Functions and Pathology of Status Systems in Formal Organizations" in W. F. Whyte, ed., *In-dustry and Society* (New York: McGraw Hill, 1946) pp. 46-83.

ity delegated to them, they could not be consistently superior in position
to the nurse. This "negative democratization," as Karl Mannheim has called
it,[5] encourages a colleague type of relationship between the nurses and
doctors rather than a service relationship. Hence the banter and joking,
which helped further to cancel out status differences,[6] and the relative
frequency of interaction to which we referred above.

Since authority was scarcely delegated, all house officers passed on orders to the nurse, who in turn communicated with all of them. Writing
orders in the order book was not the task of internes only. This was confirmed by one of the internes who said: "Anyone on surgery writes in the
order book," and the head nurse on one of the floors corroborated this
situation when asked who gave her orders: "The internes, the residents
also give orders, all give orders; we get orders all over the place and then
you have to make your own compromise; you got to figure out what is
most important."

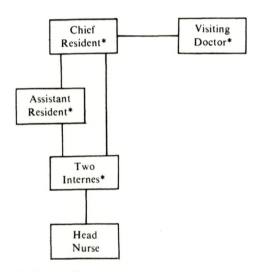

*Participate in decision-making.

*Figure 12.3. Social Structure of the Medical Ward:
Informal Line of Authority and Decision-Making*

Such a relation with the doctors puts the nurse in a strategic position. In
using her own judgment about the importance of orders, she makes decisions
about the care of patients, deciding to delay one action rather than another.
This gives her a certain amount of power.

5. Karl Mannheim, *Man and Society in an Age of Reconstruction,* (New York: Harcourt, Brace, 1951), esp. pp. 85 ff.

6. On this function of banter in status systems, see Tom Burns, "Friends, Enemies,
and Polite Fiction," *American Sociological Review,* 18 (December, 1953), 654-662.

The position of the nurse in the surgical ward brings to mind Jules Henry's analysis of the social structure of a mental hospital.[7] Henry discusses two types of social organization: the "pine-tree" type, in which authority is delegated downward step by step, as in the medical ward discussed above (see Figure 12.3); and the "oak-tree" type, in which orders come down to the same person through several channels, as in the surgical ward described here (see Figure 12.4). The latter type, Henry says, is a source of stresses and strains because the head nurse must follow orders coming from different directions that may or may not be compatible. This is probably true, to some extent, in the surgical ward described here, but it is accompanied by the fact that such a position gives the nurse more power and more active part in therapy.

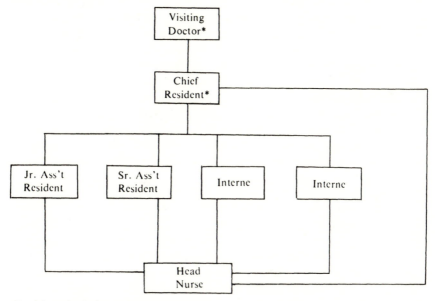

*Participate in decision-making.

*Figure 12.4. Social Structure of the Surgical Ward:
Informal Line of Authority and Decision-Making*

The head nurse on the surgical floor, often facing the necessity of compromise, must know a great deal about the conditions of patients; she is constrained to contact patients frequently and to establish a closer relationship with them. This is all the more necessary since during a large part of the day, while surgery is being performed, the surgical staff is confined to the operating room with the exception of one interne on duty in the ward. The nurse must therefore be "on her toes," checking with the duty interne only

7. Jules Henry, "The Formal Social Structure of a Psychiatric Hospital," *Psychiatry*, 17 (May, 1954) 139-152.

if absolutely necessary, since he has his hands full. Her knowledge of the
patients is thus greater than that of the nurses on the medical floor. A medical head nurse, although she tried to impress the observer with her own importance, admitted: "The nurse knows more about patients than the doctor
on surgical. On the medical floor it's about even. . . ." The doctors, in turn,
knowing that the nurse on the surgical floor has more contact with patients
than they themselves, rely on her for information and reminders, in this
way increasing her influence and decision-making role.

The doctor's expectations of the nurse differ according to ward. Asked
to define a good nurse, the doctors on the surgical ward said that she should
have foresight, intelligence, or that she must be a good assistant to the doctors, or that she should read. Some even noted that the same criteria apply
to her as to a doctor. In contrast, the physicians on the medical ward emphasized her ability to "carry out orders" and "to do her routine work well."
Only one of the medical internes declared: "Intellectual curiosity is rare but
nice if you see it," thus implying that he wouldn't really expect it. Although
our interviews with doctors are too few in number to draw any definite conclusions about expectations that medical doctors and surgeons have of nurses,
the differences in their comments support our observations made elsewhere
about some degree of autonomy and initiative among surgical nurses.

Moreover, where the rank hierarchy below the top decision-makers is not
very strict and the delegation of authority not well-defined, informal relations are built across status lines. House doctors in the surgical ward
sometimes abdicated their authority if they could rely on the nurse.[8] According to a surgical nurse, "The doctors want to be called in an emergency
only, if they know you and they feel you know what you're doing. . . .They
let us *do* things first and then call the doctor, as long as we would keep
him informed." A third-year student nurse in the surgical ward had this
to say: "In this hospital we're not allowed to draw blood or give I.V.
I do it occasionally but nobody knows. I do it just to help [the doctors]
if there are no medical student around...." Needless to say, such informal
arrangements enhance the nurse's prestige and enlarge her realm of power.

The surgical head nurse even made decisions about reference of patients
to the social service. One of the head nurses, when asked whether she participated in the social service rounds, replied: "We should have been in on
them, but I had close contact with the social worker, and I would ask her
what I wanted to know. . . . Anyhow the patients would come to me for reference to the social worker." According to the formal rules, patients are
referred to social service by the medical staff, but here, as in previous previous examples, the nurse by-passed official regulations and maintained considerable control over patients.

8. The concept of abdication of authority is here used in the sense defined by Stanton and Schwartz: "By abdication, we mean the situation in which a person who is
supposed to make a decision according to the formal organization does not make it

Nurses on the surgical ward felt less tied to rules and regulations than nurses on the medical floor. This is illustrated by their reactions to the following story upon which they were asked to comment:

Interviewer: "I would like to tell you a story that happened in another hospital. An interne was called to the floor during the night to a patient who had a heart attack. He asked the nurse on the floor to get him a tank. She told him to ask an orderly. But there was no orderly around, and she still refused to get it for him. Do you think she had a right to refuse, or do you think he had the right to expect her to get it for him?"

All nurses agreed that the nurse is not supposed to leave the floor if there is no other nurse around. However, while the answers of four of the five medical nurses were unqualified (e.g., "I would never have gotten the tank, the doctor definitely should have gotten it," or "I wouldn't think of leaving the floor for a minute when I'm alone, this is unheard of"), all five surgical nurses made important qualifications (e.g., "she should have called the supervisor," or "she could have said, you keep your ears and eyes open while I get it," or "she could say, if you keep an eye open in the meantime, I'll run and get it"). In spite of the small number of respondents these figures lend support to our observations and other interview material according to which the surgical nurse is more accustomed than the medical nurse to "find a way out," to use her initiative, and is more ready to circumvent rules and regulations.

Nurses are often accused of being "ritualistic," of attaching more importance to routine and rules than to the ends for which they are designed to serve. While the nurses on the medical floor were accused fairly often by the internes of "merely clinging to rules" and "not willing or not able to think," the head nurses on the surgical floor were never the targets of such criticisms. Indeed, the surgical nurses seemed to be capable of innovation and were often relied upon by doctors to use their own judgment and to initiate action, as we have shown.[9]

By relating the attitudes of the surgical nurses to the social structure of the ward, we have tried to confirm Merton's formulation in "Social Structure and Anomie," i.e., that "some social structures exert a definite pressure upon certain persons in the society to engage in nonconformist rather than conformist conduct."[10] There is reason to believe that in the wards that we observed, "ritualism" or "innovation" is largely a function of the specific social structure rather than merely a "professional" or "character" trait. Nurses are often in a position in which the insistence on rules serves as a

even though circumstances require that it be made." *op. cit.*, p. 274.

9. The type of therapy in the surgical ward also makes the surgical nurse's work seem more important than that of the medical nurse. As Burling, Lentz, and Wilson have pointed out, on surgical wards "the nurse's skills are tested daily and both her feeling and her prestige rise as she becomes more adept." *op. cit.*, p. 245.

10. Robert K. Merton, *Social Theory and Social Structure* (Glencoe, Ill.: The Free Press, 1957), pp. 131-160.

means to assert themselves and to display some degree of power. If their professional pride as well as their power and influence are enhanced by breaking through the routine, however, they seem to be ready to use informal means or to act as innovators to reach their goals.

If the relation of the nurse's position—and that of other occupational types, perhaps—to the structure of authority and decision-making is subject to the kinds of influence described in this case, problems of morale might well be considered in the light of their structural context.

13

ELIOT FREIDSON

BUFORD RHEA

Processes of Control
in a Company of Equals

Recently there has been an increasing amount of attention paid to professionals and scientists working in formal organizations.[1] Much of the discussion revolves around the issue of control—namely, whether or not conventional bureaucratic methods are appropriate or practical for controlling the
work of scientists and professionals. The consensus seems to be that those
workers require a kind of autonomy that is antithetical to Weber's model of
rational-legal bureaucracy, indeed, that the value of their work is actually
reduced when done "by the book" or otherwise subjected to the detailed
directives of an administrative hierarchy. The proper way for such men to
work is as members of a self-regulating "company of equals."

What exactly is a company of equals? Following Parsons, Barber has
described the pattern as:

> a social group in which each permanent member . . . is roughly equal in authori-
> ty, self-directing and self-disciplined, pursuing the goal [of his work] under the
> guidance of the . . . morality he has learned from his colleagues and which he
> shares with them. The sources of purpose and authority are in his own con-
> science and in his respect for the moral judgments of his peers. If his own con-

Reprinted from *Social Problems*, 2, No. 2 (1963), pp. 119-131, by permission of
the authors and The Society for the Study of Social Problems.

This investigation was supported in part by a Public Health Service research grant,
GM-07882.

1. See, for example, Talcott Parsons, "Introduction," in Max Weber, *The Theory
of Social and Economic Organization* (New York: Oxford University Press, 1947),
pp. 58-60; Walter I. Wardwell, "Social Integration, Bureaucratization, and Professions," *Social Forces*, 34 (1955), 356-359; Joseph Ben-David, "The Professional
Role of the Physician in Bureaucratized Medicine," *Human Relations*, 11 (1958),
225-274; David Solomon, "Professional Persons in Bureaucratic Organizations,"
Symposium on Preventive and Social Psychiatry (Washington: Walter Reed Army
Institute of Research, 1957), pp. 253-266; Mary E. W. Goss, "Influence and Authority Among Physicians in an Out-Patient Clinic," *American Sociological Review*, 26
(1961), 39-50; William Kornhauser, *Scientists in Industry: Conflict and Accommo-
dation* (Berkeley: University of California Press, 1962).

185

science is not strong enough, the disapproval of others will control him or will lead to his exclusion from the brotherhood.[2]

Patently, this is a very unorthodox way of organizing complex and responsible work, and it is described too briefly. It is rather difficult to accept the assignment of such heavy weight to individual conscience and self-direction. Colleague pressures do constitute an external source of control in the definition, but how, if a deviant is permanent and equal in authority to others, can pressure by others influence him?

Furthermore, there is the problem of the relation of the company of equals to administrative arrangements. As Barber indicates, the company of equals is an ideal rather than an empirical phenomenon. Discussing the university, he indicates that hierarchical organization and formal control by "the administration" must necessarily be added to the company of equals pattern in order that departments be coordinated and the outside environment dealt with.[3] But by and large, this, along with the dirty work of "housekeeping," seems to be all the necessity conceded to bureaucratic administration in professional or scientific settings: the critical task of controlling work can be left in the hands of the workers.

Most writers regard the infringement of bureaucratic devices on professional work as a problem, in some sense threatening.[4] However, since so little is known of how the company of equals actually works, it is by no means self-evident that bureaucratic devices are in fact so dangerous to professional work. Perhaps bureaucratic infringement is a consequence of the inadequacies of professional methods of controlling work. So we might ask, is the company of equals really self-regulating, and if so, how? Are its methods of control adequate to its goals? What are its characteristic difficulties? With one important exception,[5] little empirical material has as yet been published which can suggest how these questions might be answered. In this paper we will describe the processes of control in one "company of equals," hoping thereby to indicate some of the analytical problems raised by the idea. For reasons of both space and strategy, we will restrict ourselves to a description of internal processes, arbitrarily excluding reference to the external environment which figures in any organization.

The Clinic

We have been engaged in an intensive study of a clinic[6] staffed with highly qualified physicians and owned by a nonprofit agency. The prime workers,

---

2. Bernard Barber, *Science and the Social Order* (New York: Collier Books, 1962), p. 195.

3. *Ibid.*, pp. 197-198.

4. E.g., Kornhauser, *op. cit.*

5. Goss, *op. cit.*

6. The organization calls itself a "medical group." On the varieties of medical practice and the problems of conceptualization, see Eliot Freidson, "The Organiza-

the physicians, are not merely technical specialists, as are also secretaries and plumbers, but unquestionably "professionals" in the sense that for example, Wilensky's union experts[7] and Blau's civil servants[8] are not, but would like to be. In very few if any other occupations are the sense of individual responsibility and autonomy, and an objective position of prestige and strength so well developed for the support of a company of equals pattern.

Furthermore, the organization is staffed by exceptionally qualified physicians, all of whom are either board-certified or eligible, by virtue of their training, to take board examinations. In this sense they are "more professional" than the average run of doctors. And while it is a fairly large clinic; about 50 doctors, equipped with a fully developed administrative staff, numerous clerks and paramedical personnel, and all doctors are on salary rather than being partners, it is considerably less bureaucratic than, for example, a college (though considerably more than most clinics).

Over the past eighteen months we have examined the files of the organization, both confidential and routine, official and unofficial, we have attended all of its meetings, including those of the executive body, we have interviewed all of the doctors, most of them three or four times, we have interviewed a sample of 30 doctors who were once employed by the clinic, and of course we have interviewed the administrators. The result has been a large accumulation of data ranging from verbatim interview transcripts to notes on luncheon gossip and including sociometric ratings, minutes of meetings, and extracts from records. The present report is based on such data.

Hierarchy

Like the university, the clinic follows the principle of hierarchy, albeit unusually simply. The Medical Director is responsible for the conduct of the organization in general, including that of the physicians, and the Administrator is responsible for everyday operations, particularly but not exclusively for the conduct of the paramedical and clerical staff. The latter is organized into offices and departments, with clear lines of authority, but while the physicians are divided into various medical specialty departments, there is little division into vertical ranks. There are titular chiefs of some departments, but it is not all clear what their duties and prerogatives are, not even to them. Aside from this, there is no system of graded ranks analogous to those found at universities, and while seniority is an important source of influence, it is not a locus of hierarchical authority.

tion of Medical Practice," in H. Freeman, S. Levine and L. Reeder, eds., *Handbook of Medical Sociology* (Englewood Cliffs, N.J.: Prentice-Hall, 1963).

7. See Harold L. Wilensky, *Intellectuals in Labor Unions* (Glencoe, Ill.: The Free Press, 1956).

8. See Peter M. Blau, *The Dynamics of Bureaucracy* (Chicago: University of Chicago Press, 1955).

Clearly, the concrete elements of Barber's definition are present in the clinic. The workers have had the long period of training characteristic of professionals, they have tenure and so may be regarded as "permanent," and formal subordination and superordination among colleagues are almost nonexistent. We feel justified, then, in designating the colleague group as a company of equals, bearing in mind that, as elsewhere, administrative authority does temper colleague behavior. We will spend the remainder of this paper analyzing the role of both the administration and the colleague group in the control of work.

Rules

In most models of bureaucracy subordinates are said to be so placed by virtue of the obedience they must render to superiors and their obligation to conform to various rules and regulations. This is also partially the case for the clinic.

In the first place, the physician has "contractual" obligations, such as the number of hours he must spend in his office seeing patients, which are spelled out in some detail and which he accepts as conditions of his employment. All physicians recognize (even if unwillingly) the legitimacy of these administratively determined, "punishment-centered" regulations.[9] In addition to them, there are intramural rules whose purpose it is to ensure the coordination of effort required when a number of physicians must practice together—for example, whether it is the obstetrician or the generalist[10] who is to be responsible for providing initial emergency medical care for spontaneous abortions. These rules may be worked out by the physicians themselves, may be suggested by the administration, or may be agreed upon in joint administration-physician discussion, but in all cases they are seen as mutually agreeable expedients to solve unavoidable and obvious problems. These are clearly "representative rules." Finally, there are some rules which should but in fact do not affect the physicians —"mock rules" in Gouldner's phraseology. Some of these rules come from external sources, and if they conflict with medical or organizational efficiency and there is small chance of detection, both administration and collegium may tacitly agree to ignore them.

The variety of rules thus far parallel those found by Gouldner in the gypsum plant he studied, and are doubtless common to most formal organizations. However, we must note that none of the rules bearing on the purely technical core of medical practice—examination, diagnosis, prescription, and treatment—may be classified as punishment-centered in Gouldner's sense.

9. We refer to the analysis in Alvin Gouldner, *Patterns of Industrial Bureaucracy* (Glencoe, Ill.: The Free Press, 1954). It will be clear somewhat later in the paper, however, that "punishment-centered" rules are not so unambiguously present in our clinic as they are in the gypsum plant.

10. In this clinic there are no general practitioners. Pediatricians and internists provide everyday family services, referring to consultants what they cannot manage. We refer to the pediatricians and internists here as "generalists."

The few concrete rules which do specify elements of that core are either representative or mock in character. By and large, the most important rule bearing on the purely technical core of medical practice is more a policy statement than a regulation—it asserts that the highest possible medical standards will be maintained regardless of cost. Like many another organization in which unusually skilled work is performed, the clinic does not specify in detail the actual technical procedures to be used, but it does attempt to specify that procedures generally approved by the professional community should be used. This places determination of what is proper first of all in the hands of the workers themselves, and second, no less importantly, in the hands of any representative of the extra-clinic professional community who may be called in to evaluate the work being performed inside. This "rule" effectively prevents the development of the conflict in *technical* affairs between bureaucratic office and the expert of which Parsons made so much in his discussion of the two.[11] What conflict we observed in technical affairs was between professional opinions—for example, between that of the clinic doctors, and of professional consultants from outside the clinic.

Mention of technical affairs brings up the need to distinguish the areas of work over which control may be exercised. The technical core of medical practice is one major area. The other is the degree to which effort is organized. It is in the latter area, having no necessary relationship to technical expertness, that conflict is more likely to occur between administration and physician and among physicians. For example, the organizational need for calculability and coordination in the provision of services leads to administrative pressures on the doctor for punctuality; organizational responsibility for the patient leads to the creation of administrative channels for patient complaints. Neither the need for punctuality nor that for responsibility for the patient is questioned by most physicians. But being accountable to the organization for one's time and for one's difficulties with patients is seen to be undignified, being treated like a factory worker or a clerk. Conflict between administration and collegium, and even between colleagues in such areas as these is persistent in the clinic, and is based on quite different rules and norms than is the conflict that may occur about technical procedures.

Administrative Collection of Supervisory Information

Obviously, rules would be meaningless if one never knew when they were broken. How can conformity to the rules we outlined be ascertained by the administration when the physician does so much of his work in the privacy of his office?

First, certain gross aspects of a physician's organization of effort are noted in routine ways. Receptionists are supposed to notify the administration in the event that a physician changes his hours, does not allow her to make an appointment for an open time-period, or is habitually late.

11. Parsons, *op. cit.*, p. 60.

Similarly, when a physician rushes through his patients to finish early, or books patients earlier than he can actually see them to make sure they are "stacked up" and ready for him whenever he is ready, these and like behaviors are visible to all who would take the trouble to look. Judicious tapping of the paramedical grapevine, plus inspection of appointment books, constitute fairly regular   devices for checking on the organization of physicians' efforts. But this is the *only* regular and continuous administrative check on performance, and it yields information primarily about punctuality and speed of work, nothing about technical performance.

The patient is directly in contact with the physician during his work, and the clinic is organized to provide regular channels for patient complaints to the administration. But the patients' opinions are something few physicians will accept as valid indication of technical performance, and while some complaints do stimulate investigation, instances are fairly rare and provide only random bits of evidence.

Interestingly enough, an accurate source of information about all physicians exists, but it is used only after it is suspected that something might be wrong. The medical record for each patient is, in its wealth of detailed information, a bureaucratic delight. But although the information is continuously recorded (in part because of the legal liabilities of the work) it is not scrutinized by anyone on a routine basis. The medical chart is a working tool rather than a supervisory device, becoming a supervisory device only when interest in the case has been triggered off by some event suggesting the necessity of investigation—a patient complaint, a lawsuit, an accidental observation, and the like. It is thus only latently supervisory, used after the fact to reconstruct past performance in damning or exonerating detail.

Colleague Collection of Supervisory Information

The question is how, without routine review of the charts, information about a doctor's technical performance can be gathered at all. While the patient's complaint does provide the administration with clues to the spirit of performance, it is in the long run the collegium which must provide information on actual performance before action may be taken. Indeed, consonant with the idea of a company of equals, it is assumed in the clinic that it is the collegium which performs everyday supervision. Such supervision could be collective, i.e., a function of the company of equals as a whole, if each man's work were observable by all others or, if only observable by some, observations were uniformly communicated to the others. Neither circumstance exists either in the realm of the organization of effort or the realm of technical performance.[12]

12. Note that the following comments refer to the direct or indirect observability of work, not inferences about a man's work from his shop talk. Our comments are based on a segment of our study in which we had all the physicians in the clinic "rate" each other. Some rating criteria—such as house call habits, punctuality and

Information about a man's organization of effort is observable to the collegium on such a fragmented, selective basis that it is probably impossible for any individual to have a rounded and informed view of any other. For example, in the case of generalists, Doctor X on the emergency service in the evening is in a position to observe that he is receiving requests for housecalls from patients who were refused housecalls during the day by their own doctor, Y. But it is considerably less likely that Doctor X could ever observe that Doctor Y comes in late for his office hours, and leaves early. It is even less likely that he could observe that Doctor Y refers his patients out to consultants on the slightest pretext. In turn, while a consultant is in a very good position to learn of Y's referral habits, and possibly his mode of ordering laboratory tests, he is unlikely to know anything about Y's mode of managing his time and avoiding housecalls.

Similar selectivity and fragmentation exists in the observability of *technical* performance. Aside from gossip, or the opportunity to guess how competent a man is from the way he discusses his cases over coffee, opportunity to observe the work of colleagues varies a great deal. Part of the variation of opportunity is due to the organization of the clinic, and part to the medical division of labor.

Within such specialties as surgery which involve on-the-job teamwork in a theater, both work and its results are in the nature of the case observable and the characteristics of colleagues come to be known rather quickly to all those within the specialty itself. Within other specialties, where work is done more privately and individually, observation is more problematic. In them, a man's quality comes to be known more slowly, and more indirectly. Among generalists, some opportunity to see the work of the other is provided by the system of regularly rotating night and weekend emergency coverage, so each time a man is on duty he has the opportunity to see a few of his colleague's patients and perhaps their medical records. Over a period of time this may provide a fair sampling of a colleague's handiwork so that, all else equal, oldtimers are likely to know a good deal about each other, while new men will be little known to and know little about others. A factor in addition to time is of course popularity: unpopular doctors lose patients to popular doctors, and patients carry both records and tales.

Ordinarily, however, more patients are shared *between* specialties than within them, so that a frequently consulted specialist, especially if he is the only representative of the specialty, may be able to make a very comprehensive assessment of the internists who refer to him, whereas internists who consult each other only infrequently and even then quite selectively, may have less observational knowledge of each other than of the

---

referral habits—required the opportunity to observe the doctor's performance. Others —such as rating his medical competence—were specifically evaluational and did not actually require an opportunity to see the doctor at work. Detailed findings will be reported in another paper.

men they refer to. Certain departmental affinities bias the flow of information: pediatrics refers more to orthopedics (for turned feet) and otolaryngology (tonsils) than to urology and gynecology; urology and gynecology deal with contiguous tissue and so have occasion to see each other's patients; orthopedics and physiatry use different approaches to many of the same complaints. Some of these affinities are blocked by the clinic requirement that the generalist must be the one to refer patients; for if the specialist must return the patient to the generalist when he picks up a symptom relevant to another specialty, he is thereby denied contact with the man whose field it is. Obviously, that requirement gives the generalist the most widespread contact with all specialties.

Transmission of Supervisory Information

It should be clear that neither the administration nor the collegium observes both the doctor's organization of effort and the technical quality of that effort. Furthermore, what is observed is segmentary and rather specialized, each class of data insulated from the others: the administration collects information about office hours that is not very accessible to the collegium; the consultant collects information about the generalist that is not readily observable to other generalists; generalists collect information about each other that is not very observable to the consultants. Obviously, the colleague group cannot behave as a collectivity or company as long as these bits of information are scattered discretely through its ranks. They must all share the same information. This can occur when a man practices such persistent and thoroughgoing deviance that in one way or another it will become apparent to every individual in the company; it is more likely to occur when those bits of information are communicated each to the other and shared.

By and large, while sharing of observations does occur, it is slow and limited. While colleagues do gossip about each other, they are generally not inclined to communicate their observations bit by bit, as they collect them. There is no continuous revelation of observations which spreads information among peers. Rather, each individual usually stores up his own observations, saying little or nothing about them until he can no longer contain his indignation or until he discovers from others' hints that they too have had the same experience with the same individual. If his observations are few, and he has no strong opinion about them, he may never communicate them to others. Given the accidental character of many disclosures, and given the necessity for them to accumulate before they are shared, a considerable period of time can elapse before any widespread opinion about a man emerges.[13] And obviously, the time will vary with the strategic visibility of the specialty.

13. We ran across instances in which people who were practicing in the clinic for

In unusual cases, a sufficiently large number of observations has been stored in the memories of a sufficient number of physicians to allow a coalescence of opinion. Arriving at a certain critical mass of discontent with an individual seems to be necessary before most physicians will begin complaining about him to each other and the administration. One physician may make a rather neutral, but probing remark to a second about a third, whereupon the second may have his story to contribute, and so forth. This collective definition, though, is formed only among groups of physicians who have the opportunity to discuss such matters, and as a result there may be identifiable pockets of quite different opinion about the same man within the clinic. Opinions coalesce by specialties as well as by cliques: internists, for example, who are in close contact with obstetricians for both obstetrical and gynecological problems, may have a totally different impression of men in that department than do the pediatricians, to whom obstetricians are merely transmitters of healthy children.

Punishment

Albeit slowly and selectively, some information about deviance does come to light. How is it handled? When physicians are asked what they would do about an offending colleague, the usual response is, "Nothing." Asked what they would do if the offense were repeated, however, they answer, "I'd talk to him." "Talking-to" is in fact the most ubiquitous sanction in the clinic, and is used by both colleagues and administration as virtually the only means of punishment. From the examples we have collected, talking-to seems to involve various blends of instruction, friendly persuasion of error, shaming, and threating with retaliation.

The incidence of talking-to varies with social distance. A colleague is more likely to talk-to someone in his own department than someone outside, and a peer or junior more than a senior man. He is likely to say nothing at all to an individual outside his department, or his senior, and when he gets mad enough he will complain instead to his peers or even the administration. Talkings-to are also graded according to severity. The mildest (and by far most common) talking-to is a simple man-to-man affair. If the offender does not mend his ways the offended man may enlist the aid of other talkers, either the administrator or one or more colleagues. Eventually, if misbehavior persists and there is strong feeling about it, the offender may be talked-to by the Medical Director, or a formal committee of colleagues.

Talking-to is of course a very common informal sanction among peers in all work-groups, and is also used by superiors everywhere to warn of further sanctions. What is interesting about talking-to in the clinic is that

up to three years were unknown to some of the more remote specialists. We ran across other instances in which grave doubts about a man were felt by others in his department and were not even suspected by anyone else outside, so far as we could determine.

it is the only institutionalized punishment short of dismissal. There are no intermediate forms of direct punishment. And since formal dismissal is almost impossible, talking-to is virtually the only sanction available.

Tenure regulations require that three-quarters of the members of the clinic must vote for a doctor's dismissal before it can occur. This means that a decision by the collectivity is necessary. As we have already seen, the conditions for the formation of a collective opinion are not generally present in the system. Given the unevenness of the distribution of information in the clinic we have described, it is understandable that even a simple majority of the doctors is unlikely to be in a position to have had personal experience with an individual's deficiencies. Without personal experience with a man's deficiencies, most physicians are loath to vote for so drastic a step as expulsion on the basis of the complaints of the few colleagues or the patients who have experienced them. Only the most gross and shocking deficiency will do. The practical impossibility of dismissing a tenured doctor is thus inevitable. In fifteen years, about eighty doctors have resigned from the clinic, most of them for their own reasons, some with encouragement,[14] but none who were tenured were dismissed.

Rewards

Talking-to is thus the only practical form of direct punishment in the clinic. Aside from this, there are only rewards to motivate the physicians. Most of those rewards are bureaucratized so as to operate automatically, independent of the physician's deportment. There is, for example, a system of automatic increments, vacation with pay, bonus increments for obtaining specialty board certification, and the like. And at a certain age a man may, if he wishes, buy out of the chore of making night and weekend emergency calls. These rewards are rights of which an offender cannot be deprived. There are, however, other rewards which are particularly important because they are not bureaucratically guaranteed and because they are characteristically indirect and discretionary. Insofar as they are not mandatory, an individual can be "punished" by being "passed over" in their assignment. Some are controlled by colleagues and some by the administration.

As we have seen, the colleague group is unlikely to expel one of its members from the clinic. Other forms of direct punishment lacking, what is done about an offending colleague when talking-to does not work? By the large, the offended individuals use the technique of personal exclusion —attempting to bar a man from working with them individually or with

14. Active encouragement to resign most commonly involves making life unpleasant by frequent talkings-to and intimations of the use of devious administrative devices to "get around" formal requirements for dismissal. As in the university, tenure regulations buttressed by a conservative and ill-informed collegium create a situation that almost in the nature of the case begets covert forms of administrative harassment.

their own patients without attempting to bar him from working with or on the patients of those colleagues who have either no grievance with or no knowledge of him.[15] The offender is not referred patients, or if referral must be made, only unimportant cases are sent to him. He is not consulted about problems in his specialty or subspecialty: his advice is not sought and he is not called in to look at an interesting or peculiar case. And finally, he is not included in the system of exchanging favors that is so important in professional work: if he asked someone for a favor, he would not likely be refused, but others would not ask him for favors and so refuse him the credit that would allow him to ask with impunity for another favor in the future. All these methods of exclusion are practiced by *individuals:* they are not action of the collegium as a whole. Therefore, they do not prevent an offender from working and maintaining his work relations with the colleagues whom he has not offended. They punish him only insofar as he is sensitive to the good opinion of those individuals who exclude him.

In a somewhat different fashion does the administration employ discretionary rewards. The set of such rewards might be called a *privilege system*—special tokens, sometimes rather trivial in character, which have not been codified and bureaucratically guaranteed as rights or increments and which, taken individually, may be unique and nonrecurrent, even subject to invention by the administration. In the clinic, some of the more stable privileges involve extra money for supervising the laboratory, handling official correspondence about patient complaints, serving as special consultant, and supervising a research program. Others are more symbolic in character—for example, being invited to represent the organization to a group of distinguished visitors, being chosen to travel at clinic expense, or being allowed to take a leave of absence.

The most strategic privileges play upon the physician's image of himself. They constitute recognition of what he feels is due him at his stage of career or level of attainment. For example, among physicians the middle stage of a successful career not only involves increasing income and decreasing labor, but also being relieved of the necessity to perform the dirty work of the profession. The major form of dirty work for the generalist is the housecall, particularly at night and on weekends. Another kind of dirty work involves treating minor, uninteresting ailments and performing routine, mechanical procedures—the common cold for the generalist, refractions for the ophthalmologist, removing warts for the surgeon—otherwise called "garbage" by those who must perform them.[16] Although reduction in garbage through appointment to a consultantship, or being made chief of service, is ordinarily associated with seniority, the administration still

15. The more loosely organized system of solo practice has an even greater tendency to encourage a man to segregate himself and his patients from a poorly thought-of man without concern for other colleagues and their patients.

16. Analogous to garbage in the university is teaching introductory and other little valued courses, and even teaching as such.

has the power to exercise discretion and "pass by" one in favor of another who is cooperative or who might thereby be induced to be cooperative. Thus the grumblings about "favoritism" which surround the dispensation of all privileges by the administration.

The Normative Foundation of the System

We have seen that the elements involved in the process by which control may be exercised in this company of equals are fairly unbureaucratic in character. Access to information about work performance is not, by and large, hierarchically organized. At best it is a selective function of the division of labor; at worst a function of unsystematically random, accidental revelations to accidental observers. This state of affairs is a consequence of the fact that for most areas of performance, the administration does not exercise ordinary bureaucratic methods of gathering information, leaving the matter instead in the hands of the colleague group. And while the physicians' access to information about each others' performance is spotty, this would not be so significant if they were not also disinclined to share this information with each other. In consequence, the formation of a collective colleague opinion, and the initiation of collective colleague action are made rather difficult. Indeed, deviance is controlled almost entirely on an individual rather than collective professional basis, and by administrative exercise of discretionary rewards. Furthermore, what methods of control there are are largely normative in character.[17]

We have implied that technical performance goes generally unobserved, and, even if observed, uncommunicated, and, even if communicated, uncontrolled. This is not entirely true, for professional norms do specify the need to control incompetence and unethicality. Some of the doctors conceded that they didn't know very much about their colleagues, but they felt sure that if someone did something *really serious,* like kill a patient, they'd know about it very quickly. They felt that if a colleague were shown to be grossly and obviously incompetent or unethical there would be no question but that he would be dismissed from the clinic. And they pointed out that the really serious forms and consequences of work are brought to the hospital, where a system of professional surveillance does operate.[18] However, their idea of what is "really serious" is so extreme as to be removed from their everyday experience. What they are saying, in essence, is that butchers and moral lepers would be spotted and controlled quickly: to that extent the system works remorselessly. However, almost all forms of deviance lie somewhere between the performance of the moral leper and that of the saint. And in that middle ground the exercise of control is made more difficult by virtue

17. In this sense the clinic is a "normative organization." See Amitai Etzioni, *A Comparative Analysis of Complex Organizations* (New York: The Free Press, 1961), pp. 40-50.

18. Goss, *op. cit.*

of the perspectives and norms governing professional activity.

In medicine work is seen to have potentially dangerous consequences. Since those consequences are also relatively unpredictable and the law holds him responsible, the physician assumes some unusual risks in his work. By virtue of his willingness to assume responsibility under such circumstances, the physician claims autonomy. Also contributing to the claim as well as the grant of autonomy is the belief that there is often no single right way of tackling a problem, that the personal judgment of the man who handles the case cannot be replaced by definite, abstract rules. Colleagues who do not know the case are inclined to suspend some of their judgment of their associate's handling of it. And a sense of vulnerability stemming from this indeterminacy leads to the feeling that one shouldn't criticize an erring colleague because "it may be my turn next," or "there, but for the grace of God, go I."

This characteristic perspective on medical work thus leads to norms that encourage granting a large measure of autonomy and privacy to the physicians. It also leads to constant pressure for autonomy and privacy in the organization of effort. If one's personal judgment is that a call is an emergency, it follows that he should be free to cancel his less important appointments, keep patients waiting, even indefinitely, or push his waiting patients off on other physicians, and no one is to say nay. If one's personal judgment is that a patient in the consultation room has a trivial illness while another waiting is in a serious condition, it follows that he should be free to deal with the former perfunctorily, even brush him off if he must. In such a fashion does the way the work is organized gain a degree of freedom from scrutiny and accountability by virtue of the technical characteristics imputed to it. When one adds an extreme valuation of autonomy and dignity for their own sakes, one begins to understand the foundation supporting the system we have described.

Furthermore, the physicians expect mutual trust from their colleagues. They do not expect others to be checking up on them and they themselves try to avoid giving the impression of checking up on their colleagues. There is even a feeling of embarrassment when one accidentally observes a colleague's apparent peccadillo, and sometimes an attempt to turn the eyes away, to act as if the observation were not made. The purely accidental observation, particularly that stemming from the division of labor and in which the observer or his patient is directly involved, seems to constitute a legitimate observation that might, on occasion, be talked about with an offender, or communicated to other colleagues. Other forms of observation, with the exception of those made by a professional committee with the recognized function of review, are likely to remain either private, or resented when they are made public. One can easily see how this avoidance of "snooping" reduces the amount of information available to the company of equals, and thus increases the difficulty of corroborating and evaluating whatever few observations that happen to come to hand. And so the tendency to avoid sticking one's neck out by saying nothing to anyone is reinforced.

That professional norms rather than bureaucratic rules govern the system creates several characteristics. First of all, the system of control is not characteristically either collective or hierarchical in its operation. It is inclined to operate like the economist's free market, private individuals brought into interaction at the points where their labors meet, exercising control where their personal interests are involved. Second, the system works slowly, for a system of control can work only as rapidly as the information necessary for control can accumulate and here it does not accumulate readily. The slow pace characteristically provides a certain margin for human error that professionals are inclined to think necessary.

Third and finally, the system has a characteristic vulnerability. In the nature of the case, in order to be effective the sanctions used require that all participants be fully responsive to the norms involved. The system is quite helpless in the face of a man who does not depend upon the esteem and trust of his colleagues and who does not respond to the symbolic values of professionalism. In a very basic way the system depends upon recruiting into it properly socialized workers—workers not merely well-trained, but also responsive to the values of their colleagues. Confronted by a man who is not so incompetent or unethical as to be grossly and obviously dismissible, and who fails to show any pride as a professional, the administration and the colleague group are helpless. He cannot be flattered, shamed, or insulted and so cannot be persuaded to mend his ways or resign: all that can be done is to seal him off and try to minimize whatever damage he is believed to do.

Prerequisites for a Self-Regulating Company of Equals

Is the company of equals actually self-regulating? From the instance described, we can only answer both yes and no. There are self-regulatory mechanisms, but they are limited and contingent. Of course, our data come from but a single case, so that even if much of it rings true to our experience in universities, we cannot make any secure generalizations. However, we can use this case as a basis for tentative suggestion of the functional requisites for self-regulation in a company of equals. If nothing more, the suggestion can point to problems requiring analysis.

First of all, it should be clear that one requirement for a successfully self-regulating company of equals is a mode of recruitment which gives fair assurance that the worker has been both adequately trained and socialized into the normative system by which he can be controlled. Successful completion of a professional education is an objective measure of such technical and normative socialization, but its inadequacy seems to be implied by the characteristic tendency of professionals to rely on personal testimonials and recommendations. Such a "rational," impersonal, and specifically bureaucratic device as an examination administered to job applicants is uncommon among professionals precisely because it, like the license to practice and the professional degree, does not allow assessment of the applicant's personal qualities as a normatively socialized rather than merely technically trained professional. This deficiency is quite apart from the difficulty of measuring competence by examinations. The most effective mode of recruitment at present seems to require assessment of the applicant's "professional character" by people who have known him personally, for only by such assessment can a tolerable idea be gained of his responsiveness to the normative controls the company of equals relies on.[19]

A perfect method of recruitment does not seem to exist, but even if it did, it is unlikely to be able to take into account the way a man will change over time and in different settings. For this reason, it would seem necessary that observability of work be a second prerequisite. Only if some form of observability exists can deviant performance become known and subject to control. Obviously, more analytical attention to the concept of observability is required before it can be used precisely enough to specify the conditions for the most effective "supervision."

Third, as we have seen in our clinic, observability is not enough either. Colleagues may observe, but they may not choose to communicate their observations to others or to the offender. And they may not choose to assert control. The critical variable here, we may suggest, is a portion of the normative system of the colleague group and the self-images underlying it. Should one try to observe his colleague's performance or turn his eyes away? Should one "pass judgment"? Should one give unsolicited advice and opinions to a colleague about his behavior? These questions imply a set of values which have no necessary relation either to technical skill or to the conscientiousness with which those skills are performed. They refer to the norms dealing with one's dignity and autonomy as a professional, and with one's relation to his peers. As opposed to individual conscience, which *allows* one to be controlled by others, this set of values determines whether one will *attempt* to control others and how one will respond to other's attempts to control him.[20]

In conclusion, we may suggest that in the light of such considerations as have been discussed here, it may be possible to assess the role of the administration in the affairs of the professional more adequately than has yet been done. It is very easy to see how, under some circumstances, administrative efforts at control of work are not mere bureaucratic aggrandizement, but conscientious efforts to fill a genuine vacuum engendered by the peculiarities of the professional system of self-regulation.

19. It is in this light that one might take issue with the assessment of academic methods of recruitment in Theodore Caplow and Reece J. McGee, *The Academic Marketplace* (New York: Basic Books, 1958).

20. This might explain why there is so much bad teaching and so much good scholarship in the American university, for the former is protected from observation and control by etiquette, and the latter forced out into public scrutiny by the pressure for publication.

II

Medical Work

Managing Patients

The papers thus far have analyzed the profession of medicine with little reference to a very important aspect of practice—the client. Medicine is a consulting, not a scholarly, profession. The bulk of a consulting practitioner's work relationships involves clients, not colleagues. Clients, unlike colleagues, are not usually in the same social world as the professional; that is, they are frequently not in the same social class, ethnic group, or on the same educational level. And of course, they have not undergone the same training and socialization as the professional. Clients, therefore, do not "speak the same language" as the professional; the two do not share the same phenomenological meanings, assumptions, or concepts. Illness never means the same thing to the client and to the professional. Everett Hughes put his finger on the most obvious difference between professional and client perspectives when he said that what was routine to the professional was an emergency to the client. The client, however can ignore or handle his emergency himself if he so wishes. The professional, on the other hand, needs clients to carry out his work, to apply his knowledge, to practice his calling. He must persuade clients to accept his ministrations or be able to place them in a position where they have nothing to say about the matter.

Professional practice cannot exist without clients, but the influence of the client over the professional does not end with that simple dependence. As the papers in this section reveal, medical practice owes much of its variety and patterning to the type of client dealt with. This is not to say merely that clients of different classes, cultures, or degrees of cosmopolitanism present the practitioner with a variegated work life. The power of the client goes much deeper than that. First of all, different types of clients make different demands on the practitioner, and the way he meets these demands significantly shapes his routines of work. Secondly, different types of clients force the practitioner to do different kinds of work, not all of which carry the same prestige in his colleague-world. The everyday work life and the social identity of the professional are thus intimately related to his clientele.

The first paper in this section focuses on work routines dictated by the physical helplessness of patients who are social infants—speechless, incontinent, incapable of self-care. Although the intriguing description of the daily life of institutionalized idiots by MacAndrew and Edgerton tells what is done to the inmates, it is clear that the staff, in their intimate contact with these most physically demanding clients, do not have a clean, neat, or intellectually stimulating work life. Their work is, in Everett Hughes' words, "dirty work" only slightly glorified by a hint of professionalism. In the medical division of labor, caretaking or custodial work is usually done by paraprofessionals who, because they are low in prestige, are delegated such work, and who are low in prestige because they do such work.

There is another sociologically pertinent aspect to the work described in this paper. Although the actual content of the work is dictated by the physical helplessness of the client, the staff has complete control over the timing of eating, sleeping, washing, and dressing; the client is a unit in a production line. In many large custodial and treatment institutions, where the client is only moderately helpless physically and otherwise a fully competent adult, the staff nevertheless, for purposes of convenience and efficiency, imposes the same sort of "batch" routines. In the more common instances, the staff *imposes* physical incompetence on the client in order to maintain control over the work routine.

Another kind of control over work is attempted by higher-level professionals. The demands their clients make on them are not the physical kind made on paraprofessionals; the clients of physicians and nurses are more apt to make intellectual and psychological demands. When clients can choose, they may demand reasons for cooperating with treatment. Then, when they have accepted treatment, they may demand solicitousness and sympathy. The image of the professional is one who is concerned but detached, omniscient, and effective in his treatment. There are many situations, however, in which the intellectual and emotional demands of clients threaten the detachment and omniscience of the physician. Such situations are often encountered when treatment has not been effective and the prognosis is bad. If the physician tells the patient the truth—that he will not be cured—his professional image as a healer is tarnished. What is more, he is likely to be faced with an outpouring of emotion directed at him.

The two papers by Quint and by Davis are concerned with what professionals do when faced with this problem of psychological "dirty work." Quint, a nurse herself, details the way doctors and nurses try to avoid long conversations with patients dying of cancer and tend to limit their work to the technical side of treatment, the area over which they feel they have the most control. Davis describes another technique used by physicians to avoid the "onerous and time-consuming" task of dealing with the distraught—in this case, parents of children who will be crippled for life. Instead of telling parents the true prognosis, physicians pretend it is still uncertain and thus avoid an emotional scene they would have to take care of. In Davis's cases, the physicians sacrificed the prestige they might have gained from total omniscience in order to avoid a challenge to their detachment—or concern.

Such avoidance techniques on the part of medical personnel result in a deep-seated resentment by patients in hospitals. They frequently resent either not receiving any sympathy or understanding for their plight or not receiving any concrete information at all. Shiloh, in his study of hospitalized patients in Israel, discovered that what patients resented most about the hospital was the lack of information about their condition, treatment, and prognosis. Being kept in a state of ignorance was particularly annoying to those patients whose social status outside the hospital led them to expect, as Shiloh puts it, "to be equal partners with the hospital in the mutual goals of successful treatment and prompt discharge, and they expected the hospital to provide them with the information necessary for the consummation of these mutual goals." Such information would also have enabled them to argue with their physicians, so they were kept in ignorance —passive recipients of care, not "equal partners," as they wished. In sum, control over patients who are not intellectually helpless is managed by careful control over their access to information in order to protect the authority and aura of the professional.

As we have seen, the prestige level of an occupation is closely related to the type of work done, so it is not surprising that members of upwardly mobile occupations try to avoid doing work they consider demeaning. Not surprisingly, avoiding "dirty" clients is one way of avoiding "dirty work." In the last paper of this section, a study of professional social climbing, Walsh and Elling argue that the negative attitudes of public-health nurses toward lower-class clients is indicative of their desire to raise the prestige level of their profession by shaking off low-prestige clients. They considered lower-class clients most often "difficult" and "unpleasant" and preferred middle-class clients. Ironically, in Shiloh's study, lower-class patients were least irritated about the lack of information, while high-status patients were most likely to make a fuss, which demonstrates that all professionals are likely to have trouble managing some clients.

Earlier papers showed that the professional's autonomy over his work was hard won, as was his social prestige. These analyses of the effects of clients on professional work indicate that autonomy and prestige must be carefully nurtured every working day. As a result, many professional activities are probably best viewed as stemming from a conflict over control of the situation. The particular form this conflict takes depends on the relative social status of professional and client, and on the extent of institutionalized control the professional wields, but in a symbolic sense, *all* patients are idiots to professionals.

BIBLIOGRAPHIC SUGGESTIONS

The standard analysis of the doctor-patient relationship is Talcott Parsons, *The Social System* (Glencoe, Ill.: The Free Press, 1951), Chapter 10. Parsons focuses on the complementary obligations of patient and physician in the pursuit of their mutual goal of moving the patient out of the sick role and back to his usual social roles. An extensive treatment of the doctor-patient relationship which discusses the problems of autonomy, prestige, and conflict over control of the situation is Eliot Freidson, *Patients' Views of Medical Practice* (New York: Russell Sage Foundation, 1961), Part 3. Freidson discusses the consulting professional's problem of persuading lay clients that he is indeed an expert authority in "The Impurity of Professional Authority," *Institutions and the Person*, Howard S. Becker et al., eds. (Chicago: Aldine, 1968), pp. 25-34. The insights in Erving Goffman, *The Presentation of Self in Everyday Life* (Garden City, N.Y.: Doubleday Anchor, 1959), the well-known account of impression management in work and other settings, can usefully be applied to the social aspects of medical work.

There is an enormous literature on patients in mental hospitals which graphically details staff-imposed control, but the best place to begin reading in the area of custodial institutions is Erving Goffman, *Asylums* (Garden City, N.Y.: Doubleday Anchor, 1961). This widely cited book provides an analytic framework into which other, more descriptive studies can be placed. Some standard references on patients in mental hospitals are Alfred H. Stanton and Morris S. Schwartz, *The Mental Hospital* (New York: Basic Books, 1954); William Caudill, *The Psychiatric Hospital as a Small Society* (Cambridge: Harvard University Press, 1958); and H. Warren Dunham and S. Kirson Weinberg, *The Culture of the State Mental Hospital* (Detroit: Wayne State University Press, 1960). A study of patients in a different kind of custodial institution is Julius A. Roth and Elizabeth M. Eddy, *Rehabilitation for the Unwanted* (New York: Atherton Press, 1967), which uses many of Goffman's concepts to describe the life of patients in a long-term rehabilitation program. René C. Fox, *Experiment Perilous* (Glencoe, Ill.: The Free Press, 1959), offers an interesting contrast to the above books, in that it presents an account of the institutional life of the highly praised subjects of a prestigious medical team. Both patients and professionals were at the very top of the medical stratification system, and their prestige was demonstrated by every aspect of hospital life.

Most of the studies of short-term patients in general hospitals are straightforward description, with little attempt at sociological analysis. Ann Cartwright, *Human Relations and Hospital Care* (London: Routledge and Kegan Paul, 1964), reports on patients in British hospitals, and Elizabeth Barnes, *People in Hospital* (London: Macmillan, 1961) reports on patients in hospitals of various countries. Raymond S. Duff and August B. Hollingshead, *Sickness and Society* (New York: Harper & Row, 1968), is an extensive study of a large New England medical center which provides an excellent picture of the different types of care given patients of different social classes. Rose Laub Coser, *Life on the Ward* (East Lansing: Michigan State University Press, 1962), is one of the few studies of life in a general hospital from the patient's point of view.

Information control in hospitals has been treated at length in several perceptive books. Barney G. Glaser and Anselm L. Strauss, *Awareness of Dying* (Chicago: Aldine, 1965), thoroughly discusses who tells what to terminal patients, and the effect of information or lack of it on patients, families, and medical personnel. Jeanne C. Quint, *The Nurse and the Dying Patient* (New York: MacMillan, 1967), covers the same subject with particular reference to nurse-patient relationships. Fred Davis, *Passage Through Crisis* (Indianapolis: Bobbs-Merrill, 1963) takes up the problem of information control in incurable illness, and Julius A. Roth, *Timetables* (Indianapolis: Bobbs-Merrill, 1963), deals with the problem in the case of a partially chronic, but curable illness. In all these studies, the question of who controls the situation, the professional or the patient, is a pertinent part of the discussion. A collection of articles which deal mostly with nurse-patient interaction and which contains useful additional data on communication and the patient's point of view is James K. Skipper, Jr., and Robert C. Leonard, *Social Interaction and Patient Care* (Philadelphia: J. B. Lippincott, 1965).

14

CRAIG MACANDREW

ROBERT EDGERTON

The Everyday Life of
Institutionalized "Idiots"

It has been variously estimated that there are 100,000 idiots in the United States today. Because approximately half of these, including almost all of the adults, are in public institutions, common sense knowledge of idiots is typically both sketchy and ridden with clichés. Unfortunately, our scientific knowledge concerning idiots is not a great deal better. While there is a substantial, but spotty, body of medical information at hand, detailed understanding of the psychological functioning of idiots is notably deficient[1] and knowledge of their social behavior is virtually nonexistent.[2]

There is a sense, of course, in which we know what idiots are: operationally, they are those who score less than 20 on a standard IQ test and who are judged to be organically incapable of scoring higher. They are, then, the most profound of mental incompetents, as is indicated by the following typical professional definition:

Reprinted from *Human Organization*, 23 (1964), pp. 312-318, by permission of the authors and publisher.

The authors wish to express their gratitude to Dr. George Tarjan, Dr. Harvey F. Dingman, and the staff of Pacific State Hospital for the opportunity to conduct this inquiry. Observations were carried out from October, 1962, through April, 1963.

This research was supported in part by the National Institute of Mental Health, Grant No. 5-R11-MH469: Data Processing in Mental Deficiency, Pacific State Hospital, Pomona, California.

The term "idiot" has been replaced in the field of mental retardation by the term "profound mental retardation." This latter term is preferred because, among other things, it lacks the pejorative common-sense connotation which has become attached to its more commonly recognized predecessor. However, "profound mental retardation" is both cumbrous to use repeatedly and is not well known, we have found, to social scientists working outside the field of mental retardation. We have therefore elected to use the earlier, better known term, but without, needless to say, intending anything invidious thereby.

1. G. A. Kelly, "The Theory and Technique of Assessment," *Annual Revue of Psychology*, 9 (1958), 323-352.

2. See S. B. Sarason and T. Gladwin, "Psychological and Cultural Problems in Mental Subnormality: A Review of Research," *American Journal of Mental Deficiency*, 62 (1958), 1115-1307.

> The idiot is . . . . a person so deeply defective in mind from birth, or from an early age, as to be unable to guard himself against common physical danger.[3]

Specifically, we are instructed that:

> They have eyes but they see not; ears, but they hear not; they have no intelligence and no consciousness of pleasure or pain; in fact, their normal state is one entire negation.[4]

We are also advised that they are typically incapable of speech:

> Their utterances mostly consist of inarticulate grunts, screeches, and discordant yells.[5]

Finally, we are informed that they are characteristically physically handicapped and frequently disfigured; references to their appearance often use words such as "stunted, misshapen, hideous, bestial," and the like. In a word, what we know—or least what we think we know—about idiots is little more than a slightly elaborated set of first impressions.

Most importantly, we know practically nothing about their everyday conduct—about what they actually *do* in the course of living their lives in the institutions which are their typical abodes. In this article we attempt to provide a description of the everyday lives of institutionalized idiots as they are actually lived in one such institution. To our knowledge, the literature contains no such systematic description. In the discussion section we recommend the uniquely informing character of a detailed understanding of such profoundly retarded beings to certain of the perennial problems which are peculiar to a proper study of mankind—not the least of which is the elucidation of the very notion of "man" itself.

The Physical Setting

Pacific State Hospital is a large state institution for the mentally retarded. Its 494-acre grounds are occupied by over 3,000 patients and 1,500 staff members who respectively live and work in an elaborate, self-contained complex of lawns, parks, roads, and some 70 major buildings. Located outside the city of Pomona, California, the hospital was founded in its present location in 1927 as Pacific Colony. While this location was characterized by rural seclusion at the time of its founding, it has since become increasingly surrounded by the expanding residential and commercial areas of the Southern California megalopolis and is now less than a mile from one of the major links in the greater Los Angeles freeway system. This agglutination process is pithily evidenced in the population statistics of the area: while the population of Pomona stood at 20,000 in 1927, it will soon top 100,000 and its rate of growth shows little sign of leveling off.

3. A. F. Tredgold, *Mental Deficiency* (New York: William Wood, 1956), p. 199.
4. *Ibid.*, p. 205.
5. *Ibid.*, p. 202.

Accompanying this change in environs, at least equally dramatic changes have taken place in administrative philosophy. While the inmates of Pacific Colony once cultivated acres of farm land under a policy of primarily custodial care,[6] the custodial tradition was radically revised some ten years ago when the administrative orientation shifted to one of treatment and rehabilitation. In the process, the "colony" became a "hospital," the "cottages" became "wards," and the "inmates" became "patients."

Included in the hospital's 3,000 resident mentally defective patients are approximately 900 idiots who are domiciled in various wards throughout the institution. The present paper is concerned with one such ward, a ward reserved for the most severely retarded ambulatory adult male patients (N=82) in the hospital. Built in 1954, at a cost in excess of $210,000, Ward Y is a low, tile-roofed building separated from several other wards of similar design by stretches of lawns and shrubbery. While the ward is large and well constructed, both its design and detailing reflect the characteristic institutional stamp of unimaginative drabness and of a grossly inadequate provision for the entrance of natural light.

Patients and Staff

The 82 patients who reside in Ward Y range in age from 15 to 52; their average age is 27.1 (S.D.=8.45). As for their measured intelligence, if we remove eight patients—about whom more in a moment—who comprise a clearly demarcated minor second mode in their IQ distribution, the mean IQ of the remaining 74 patients is 15.4 (S.D.=9.05). In terms of the contemporary nomenclature, these remaining 74 patients are, without exception, either severely or profoundly retarded. The eight relatively high IQ patients have been assigned to Ward Y for diverse reasons—as helpers, because they cannot get along on the higher grade wards, etc. Most of them have come to perform a number of assigned duties on the ward. In addition to these eight "in residence" helpers, six additional mildly retarded patients are detailed to Ward Y to assist the staff during morning and afternoon hours.

The staff consists of from 11 to 13 male attendants and 3 female attendants all of whom bear the title of psychiatric technicians. Their work hours are set up on a standard three-shift basis with 7 on the day shift (6:30 A.M.—3:00 P.M.), 5 to 6 on the afternoon shift (2:45 P.M.—11:15 P.M.), and 2 to 3 on the night shift (11:00 P.M.—7:00 A.M.).

First Impressions of Ward Y

Words, however well-chosen, cannot begin adequately to convey the combined sights, sounds, and smells which initially confront and affront the out-

6. That custodial care was the clear intent of the Legislature at the time of the Colony's founding is evidenced in the summary of the bill contained in the report of

sider on his first visit. What follows is at best an approximation.

Despite the size of Ward Y, the simultaneous presence of its 82 patients evokes an immediate impression of overcrowding. Additionally, most of the patients are marked by such obvious malformations that their abnormal status appears evident at a glance. One sees heads that are too large or too small, asymmetrical faces, distorted eyes, noses and mouths, ears that are torn or cauliflowered, and bodies that present every conceivable sign of malproportion and malfunction. Most patients are barefooted, many are without shirts and an occasional patient is—at least momentarily—naked. What clothing is worn is often grossly ill-fitting. In a word, the first impression is that of a mass—a mass of undifferentiated, disabled, frequently grotesque caricatures of human beings.

Within moments, however, the mass begins to differentiate itself and individuals take form. A blond teen-ager flits about rapidly flapping his arms in a bird-like manner, emitting bird-like peeping sounds all the while. A large Buddha-like man sits motionless in a corner, staring straight ahead. A middle-aged man limps slowly in a circle grunting, mumbling, and occasionally shaking his head violently. A shirtless patient lies quietly on a bench while a small patient circles about him furiously twirling a cloth with his left hand. A blind youngster sits quietly digging his index fingers into his eyes, twitching massively and finally resolving himself into motionless rigidity. A red-haired patient kneels and peers intently down a water drain. A portly patient sits off in a corner rocking. Another patient rocks from a position on all fours. Still another patient, lying supine rolls first to one side and then to the other. Several patients walk slowly and aimlessly around, as if in a trance, showing no recognition of anyone or anything. A microcephalic darts quickly about, grinning, drooling and making unintelligible sounds. An early twentyish mongol wearing an oversized cowboy hat strides about with his hands firmly grasping the toy guns in his waistband holsters. Others smile emptily, many lie quietly, still others from time to time erupt into brief frenzies of motion or sound.

A few patients approach the newcomer to say, "Daddy," or "Wanna go home," or to give their name or to offer some paradoxical phrase such as "tapioca too, ooga, ooga." One or another patient may attempt to touch, pull, or grasp the stranger, but such attempts at interaction are usually of the most fleeting duration. Others may approach and observe from a distance before moving away. Most pay no attention to a new face.

In the background, strange and wondrous sounds originate from all sides. Few words can be distinguished (although many utterances, in their inflection,

---

the California Committee on Mental Deficiency appointed by Act of the Legislature in 1915. "Purpose of the Institution: The institution should provide adequate custodial care and training for its inmates . . . Provision should be made for the scientific study of the group of individuals thus gathered, with a view to discovering the best means of correcting the social conditions which make it necessary to maintain such institutions."

resemble English speech); rather, screams, howls, grunts, and cries predominate and reverberate in a cacophony of only sometimes human noise. At the same time, loud and rhythmic music is coming out of the loudspeaker system.

There are, finally, the odors. Although many patients are not toilet trained, there is no strong fecal odor. Neither is there a distinct smell of sweat. Yet there is a peculiar smell of something indefinable. Perhaps it is a combination of institutional food and kitchen smells, soap, disinfectant, feces, urine, and the close confinement of many human bodies.

In sum, Ward Y and its inhabitants constitute a staggering visual, auditory, and olfactory assault on the presupposedly invariant character of the natural, normal world of everyday life. Here, to a monumental degree, things are different.

The Daily Routine

The day on Ward Y begins at 6:00 A.M. when the lights go on and the relatively high-IQ helpers begin to get out of bed. By 6:15 these helpers are dressed and together with the employees they begin to rouse the more defective patients from their sleep. These patients are awakened in groups of 12, the number being determined by the number of toilets on the ward. With few exceptions, they sleep without clothing, and thus they are led, nude, into the bathroom where each is toileted. After they eliminate, helpers apply toilet-paper appropriately, wash their hands, and lead them out of the washrooms. Each is then dressed in denim trousers with an elastic waistband and a shirt. This completed, they are permitted to go into the day hall where they mill about while the next group of 12 is awakened, toileted, washed, and dressed. As this is going on, one or two employees strip those beds which have been soiled during the night and helpers follow them making up all the beds.

By 7:15 A.M. most of the toileting, washing, and dressing has been completed and the most capable helpers are given their breakfasts in the dining room. No food is prepared on the ward; it all comes from a central kitchen and is delivered to the several wards by food truck. By 7:30, the helpers have finished and the 23 least capable patients—referred to by the staff as "the babies"—are led into the dining room. Since the babies are capable neither of carrying a tray nor of feeding themselves, they are individually led to a table, seated, and literally spoon-fed by an employee or a "detail." Feeding the 23 babies consumes about 30 minutes. Thus at about 8:00, the babies have finished their breakfast and are led out of the dining room and back to the bathroom where they are again toileted and washed before being led to the play yard where their incontinence is both less disturbing to, and more easily handled by, the staff. As the babies leave, the remaining 50-odd patients, most of whom have been standing in line in the corridor just outside the dining room, are allowed to enter. Just before the door is opened, those who have not been waiting outside are herded into this corridor by an employee whose job it is to check the entire ward for strays. Upon entering, they are led single file to a cafeteria-like serving line where they pick up a tray and proceed along the counter. Both food and utensils are placed on the tray by employees or "details" as they move along. Some of these relatively more competent patients seem only dimly aware of what is happening and must be led by an employee both along the serving line and to a table. Others, however, exhibit great interest in the food, chatter excitedly, and once through the serving line walk off toward a table unaided and undirected.

As soon as all the patients have filed into the dining room, the door is locked. This measure is taken to prevent the premature exit of patients who might get into trouble if they were allowed to wander about the ward without supervision. In a very few minutes, all have been served and are seated, usually four to a table. Each has a spoon but no knife or fork. Their deportment at the table varies greatly. At some tables, the eating may proceed in a reasonably—indeed, remarkably—decorous fashion, but at other tables such is not at all the case. Whole hard-boiled eggs are eaten at a gulp, oatmeal with milk is eaten with the fingers, prunes drop to the floor, trays are over-turned, neighbors have cups of milk poured or sloshed on them, and so on. While in the course of breakfast two or three arguments typically arise which on occasion lead to fights or tantrums, and while there are always some wanderers who leave their tables and stroll about, breakfast progresses, for the most part, with a significant semblance of order and propriety. Once breakfast is completed, about thirty minutes after commencement, these patients are led out of the dining room, leaving behind them an ample residue of spilled food and drink on tables, chairs, and floor. As they file out, helpers, details, and employees clean up behind them.

Leaving the dining room, these patients, like the babies, are led once more to the bathroom, where each is again undressed and toileted. Again, toilet paper is handled only by helpers and employees for when left to their own devices, some have been known to flush entire rolls down the toilet— a sport which occasions major dislocations in the plumbing. After being toileted, each patient's hands are once again washed. Next comes tooth brushing; each patient has his own toothbrush identified by name, but only a few are capable of brushing their teeth unaided. Consequently, most patients, still undressed, wander about the bathroom waiting to have their teeth brushed by a helper or an employee. When a patient is finished, he files out of the bathroom where he is met at the door by another helper who wipes the excess toothpaste and saliva from his mouth with a cloth. This completed, he is once again dressed.

About 9:00 A.M.—some three hours after arising—all the patients are at last ready to meet the day. It is at this point that play activity, which for most patients is a euphemism for free time, begins. Just as in the case of the early activities—toileting, dressing, and feeding—the patients are again separated into competence groupings but now there is a territorial dimension to their division. The least competent patients, approximately 55 in number, go to the outside play yard (or in bad weather to the porch), while the more competent patients remain within the ward proper.

The play yard is a large asphalt-paved rectangle enclosed on two sides by the ward itself and on the other two sides by an 8½ ft.-high wire fence. Within the enclosure are several wooden benches, a tether ball, and two roofed structures which provide shade. Aside from the tether ball, which is typically not in use, the only objects provided for patients' amusement are balls of various sizes which an employee occasionally makes available. Employees and helpers sometimes attempt to induce organized activity by engaging a few of the relatively more able patients in throwing a ball back and forth. Such activity is never sustained for any length of time, however; few of the patients are interested in such activities and those who are interested can neither catch nor throw in any effective manner. Besides these natural handicaps, a few of the patients delight in capturing the ball and throwing or kicking it over the fence, whence the employee must retrieve it.

Thus, while the patients in the play yard are under constant supervision, they are in fact left almost entirely to their own singularly limited devices. At least 20 patients do nothing but sit, rock, or lie quietly. The activity of the remaining 30 or so consists of running, pacing, crying, or shouting, and this typically in a manner oblivious of their surroundings. Aside from an occasional ephemeral outburst when, for instance, two patients bump into each other or when one pushes or strikes another, there is little interaction between them. What interaction does occur is almost entirely limited to the tactual: there is occasional cuddling, stroking, huddling together, and amorphous, exploratory probing. These interactions have the quality of "pure happenings"; they are characteristically without relation either to past or future: in a word, they have the appearance of occurring outside of history. Occasionally one patient may approach another and launch into an outpouring of jibberish, gesturing frantically all the while, only to be met by a vacant stare or, contrariwise, he may stop in mid-passage as inexplicably as he began. Here, truly, one sees the *in-vivo* prototype of a "billiard-ball" theory of personality.

To the consternation of the staff, one activity which does occur with inexplicable frequency is spontaneous disrobing. A major task for the supervising employee and his two details consists in maintaining the minimal proprieties of everyday dress. While most patients are bare-footed and while shirts are more often off than on, nothing whatsoever is done about the former and, except in case of sunburn, little, if anything is done about the latter. Trousers, however, are intimately involved with considerations of decency and their absence is quite another matter indeed. Trousers must be put back onto patients who simply remove them, and they must be removed from patients who have soiled themselves. Approximately 25 patients on Ward Y are totally incontinent and another 25 are sometimes so. As has already been noted, virtually all of these are in the group sent to the play yard. There are two clothes hampers in the yard, one containing clean clothes and the other soiled clothes. As trousers are soiled, they are thrown into the one hamper and clean ones are taken from the other. Because trouser sizes are not marked, and because both patients and garments come in many sizes, one often sees some patients enshrouded by enormous pants and others constricted by tiny ones.

Inextricably combined with these matters of moral appropriateness is an imperative concern for the physical health of the patients. Enteric disease—especially bacillary dysentery and its complications—is an ever-present danger. Fecal matter is not always ignored by the incontinent idiot: it is sometimes smeared, played with, thrown, and even eaten. It is for these reasons, too, that incontinence is counted as a matter requiring urgent staff attention. Nor is every patient aware that all water is not fit to drink; some patients have been known to drink water out of the toilet bowls and from the shower room floors. There is, too, the constant danger that despite the plentiful administration of tranquilizers, certain of the patients might at any moment do grave physical damage to themselves or others. Such outbursts are as a rule without apparent cause; a patient may bite, scratch, or gouge either himself or another patient. These occurrences are sufficiently frequent that periods of calm may correctly be seen as preceding the storms that will inevitably follow. There is, finally, the danger of accidental injury. Seizures occur unpredictably and handicapped patients such as these not infrequently slip and fall. The possibility of accidental injury is so great for some patients that the staff seldom permits them to enter the play yard because they feel a fall on its rough asphalt surface would be more likely to cause injury than would a similar fall on the polished cement floors of the ward.

Among the 25 or 30 patients who remain inside, the problems of incontinence and nudity are much less pressing. The demands for supervision are lessened by confining all patients to the dayroom and TV room, access between which is open at all times. Such confinement is accomplished by the simple policy of locking all other doors. Within the confines of these two rooms, then, the patients typically sit, sleep, watch TV, or pace about aimlessly; only rarely do they interact with one another. Their interaction with staff, too, is limited to brief encounters which more frequently than not consist of staff directives to refrain from doing one thing or another—to stay out of the office, to leave so-and-so alone, to stop masturbating, to stop hitting one's head against the wall, etc. Much time is spent in staring intently at one or another staff member as he goes about his duties. In general, the scene one confronts in the dayroom is not greatly different from that of the play yard.

From a pool of 20 select patients, rotating groups of six or seven are daily given special training in the occupational therapy room. This training consists of such activities as coloring in coloring books, playing with plastic toys, listening to music, and practicing some elementary manipulative skills. Aside from this, those who remain inside the ward are, like their counterparts in the play yard, left for the most part to their own devices.

Throughout this period of play activity most of the staff is engaged in a variety of routine tasks. One employee, as we noted, supervises the play yard; another spends all or most of the day in the ward clinic dispensing medication and treating minor injuries or illnesses; another must supervise details and helpers in cleaning the dining room, bathroom, and the ward in general; one employee is required to be responsible for the patients who are in the occupational therapy room; another must each day take those patients who are scheduled for clinic appointments to the hospital. Finally, the ward charge must be on hand to meet the ward physician when he calls, must make out a number of written reports, and must oversee all activity on the ward.

At 11:00 A.M. play activity stops, and preparations for lunch begin. All patients are again toileted and washed, with the babies being undressed in order both to make toileting proceed more effectively and to insure against the stuffing of clothing into the toilets. The daily luncheon preparation occupies both patients and staff for the better part of an hour. Lunch itself begins around noon and follows the same pattern as breakfast: helpers first, babies next, then the rest of the patients. Following the meal, each patient is again toileted and washed. The entire luncheon operation lasts from 11:00 A.M. to about 1:30 P.M.

At 1:30 play activity is resumed. It follows the morning pattern in all major details and lasts until 4:00 P.M. On a nice day, 50 or more patients are usually taken to an open grassy area ("the park") about a quarter of a mile distant from the ward where they are allowed to roam about. Little advantage is taken of this opportunity, however; the patients generally remain clustered together around the supervising staff members. Aside from this trip away from the ward, the afternoon activities parallel those of the morning.

At 4:00 P.M. toileting and washing begins again in preparation for the evening meal which lasts from 5:00 to 6:00, once more along the same pattern. The evening meal too is followed by a brief toileting and washing which is generally concluded by 6:30. This, in turn, is followed by the third play activity period of the day, which lasts until about 7:30. This time the porch replaces the play yard and the TV room tends to draw a larger audience than during the day. During this period, patients are frequently assembled and marched around the day hall for several minutes (ostensibly in order to work off unspent energy in preparation for bedtime).

The hour between 7:30 P.M. and 8:30 P.M. is devoted to bedtime preparation. After being toileted, each patient is directed under the shower where

employees apply soap here and there, supervise the rinsing, and then towel
the patients dry. They are next inspected for cuts, bruises, rashes and the
like, and following this they are at last sent off to bed. As noted earlier, almost all patients sleep without clothing. While the beds are labeled with the
patient's names, none of the patients, of course, can read. Although some
know their own bed, many do not and must be led there by staff. The beds
of patients who characteristically get up during the night, of those given to
nocturnal noise making, and of those subject to frequent convulsive seizures
are placed close to the office in order that night-shift employees can observe
them more closely and respond to them when necessary with minimal disturbance to the remaining patients.

While an occasional patient is simply unable to sleep, in which case he
is typically dressed and brought into the day room where he sits silently
until morning, the most striking feature of the night is the ease with which
it passes.

Periodically Recurring Events

There are other events in the lives of the idiots which, while they are no
less constitutive of the routine of their institutional life, do not occur daily.
In this category we include: the weekly bath, the fortnightly pinworm inspection, the monthly weighing, the monthly haircut, and the aperiodic visits of relatives.

One night a week all patients are given baths. The procedure is as follows: the drain in the large shower room is plugged, the room is flooded
and soap is liberally added to the water. Small groups of patients enter, sit
on the floor and soak themselves. Two male employees then strip to their
shorts, wade into the now pond-like shower room and scrub the patients.
This completed, the patients are led under the showers to be rinsed and then
are taken out of the shower room where they are dried. Following this,
they are given their daily cut, bruise, and rash inspection and their finger-
nails and toenails are clipped as needed, while the next group of patients
is being led in to soak.

Once every two weeks, all patients are inspected for pinworms. About
midnight, after all have settled down, two employees enter the dormitory
and turn the patients one by one onto their stomachs. The buttocks are then
spread and with the aid of a flashlight the presence or absence of pinworms
is determined. This seemingly bizarre practice is so routinized that little
disturbance is created; in fact, many of the patients do not even awaken.

Once each month all patients are weighed. A large scale is set up in the
day room and the patients are disrobed and lined up for weighing. If a
patient cannot or will not stand quietly on the scale, an employee must
hold him still until a reading is obtained. Not only is this weighing a part
of standard records-keeping, but the discovery of any marked changes in

weight causes serious staff concern and typically leads to requests that patients evidencing these weight changes be examined medically.

A hospital barber spends one day a month on Ward Y and cuts as many patients' hair as he has time for. Those whom the barber misses—at least 20 and often more than this—must be given haircuts by one or another employee. For reasons of efficiency, ease of care, and prevention of disease, patients are given crew-cuts (the only patients exempted are those whose parents object to this kind of haircut). Patients are also shaved at least once a week. Shaving takes place in the ward barber shop, and is ordinarily performed by a helper who uses an electric razor. Some patients, however, are frightened by the buzzing noise of the electric razor and must be shaved with a safety razor; in these cases, an employee does the shaving.

Patients on Ward Y received a total of 812 visits during the last year—an average of 15.6 visits per week. Although there is an occasional open house or family party, visits usually consist of one or both parents of a patient spending a part of the day with their son in the ward's reception room, on the hospital grounds, or off the grounds entirely. When patients are scheduled to receive visitors—and administrative efforts are made to schedule these visits in advance—they are bathed, shaved, and dressed in company clothes immediately prior to the appointed visit.

The round of life here described is notably bleak and impersonal in its objective characteristics. However, the attitude of the staff does much to balance this. Ward employees do, in fact, evince an entirely sincere interest in the patients and regularly display both kindness and sympathy toward them. Nor is either staff or administration content with merely guiding their charge through an endless succession of similar appearing days. For example, on Saturday nights one staff member often shows travelogues, cartoons, and home movies on the ward. These films are projected onto the wall of the day hall and are viewed by all patients. Also, on most Saturday afternoons there is a party. Girls for these occasions are provided by Ward Q, which houses equally retarded ambulatory female patients. One week the party is on Ward Y, the next week it is held on the female ward. Only the toilet trained and better behaved patients participate; the others remain on the porch or in the play yard, indifferent to the festivities. Party-going patients are dressed in their best clothing, the ward is decorated, refreshments are served, phonograph records are played, and dancing is attempted with at least an occasional semblance of partial success. It should also be noted that the hospital provides a variety of recreational activities in which varying numbers of patients from Ward Y sometimes participate. Thus, the more competent patients are frequently taken to the hospital canteen, and sometimes to the swimming pool, or to listen to music. Once every month or so, some are taken off the hospital grounds to public parks, the beaches, restaurants, amusement parks, zoos, fairs, sport events, and the like. Needless to say, however, the participation of the least competent patients in these off-ward activities is of necessity strictly limited.

This said, it remains that these special events, while instantial of the good intentions of both staff and administration, stand in stark contrast to the mundane ward routine which *is* the patients' everyday life.

Discussion

At least one child out of every 1,000 born in the United States will be an idiot—a person totally incapable throughout life of caring for his own needs. Many of these will be completely infirm and will live a vegetative existence confined either to a hospital crib or to a wheelchair. Even those who are ambulatory, like the patients on Ward Y, will require institutional care of a most comprehensive nature. The preceding account of the institutional lives of the patients on Ward Y should have given some indication of the nature of the problems an institution faces in providing such care.

The cost of this care—roughly $300,000 per year for the 82 patients on Ward Y—is considerable. Not only is institutional care for the profoundly retarded costly, it is both practically and morally problematic for it is subject to the vicissitudes of parental pressures, of state budgets, of administrative and legislative dicta, and of conflicting professional interests and circumstances. While students of social organization have directed much attention to institutions for the mentally ill, interest in institutions for the mentally retarded has been virtually nonexistent.

This singular neglect is the more curious when one considers the paradigmatic relevance of the mentally retarded to so many of social sciences' perennial issues. We invite, for instance, the consideration of the profoundly retarded as instructive examples of human beings whose capacity for culture is dramatically impaired. So construed, they stand on the threshold between man and not-man, and thus permit simultaneous inquiry into both the nature of man and the nature of culture-bearing animals.

Idiots' capacity for language is minimal (although it is greater than that of any of the non-human primates). This lack of language skills is, of course, related to their impoverished cultural and social behavior, but even the most rudimentary explication of the nature of this relationship awaits consideration. While they respond to some symbols, they create symbols only rarely if at all, they sustain little culture, develop few rules of their own, evidence relatively little exploratory curiosity, and their interaction with one another is both minimal and peculiarly ahistorical. In at least certain respects, then, they are *less* human than some infra-human species. In short, the relationship between language, social interaction, and rule-oriented behavior is available here *in vivo* in a manner different from that found either among normal humans or normal nonhumans.

We recommend, too, that in the interaction between patients and staff it is possible to obtain a unique perspective on such concerns as responsibility, trust, competence, reciprocity, and the like—all of which have been from the beginning and remain quintessential to a proper study of mankind. Here such matters find a natural laboratory, for staff is necessarily concerned both with creating and sustaining the human character of its charge against a background of continually recurring evidence to the contrary.

In summary, the whole area of mental retardation is, for the social scientist, a research backwater; and profound mental retardation is totally ignored. The foregoing description of the everyday lives of institutionalized idiots is intended to provide an introduction to these profoundly incompetent beings. Our own research has already taken us into analyses of both the practical and theoretical problems posed by such as these. By describing what has previously not been recorded and by recommending its theoretical relevance, we would hope to interest others in similar inquiry.

15

JEANNE C. QUINT

Institutionalized Practices
of Information Control

As the curiosity of the boy prompted him to tap lightly on the hornet's nest, with a noisy, unexpected, and dreadful result, so interest in certain human problems can precipitate not only loud buzzing noises but also a few painful and unanticipated stings. My curiosity about the problems encountered by persons who undergo surgical disfigurement led to a study of adjustment following mastectomy and, in turn, to a more general problem: The fearsome meaning which the word cancer carries in our society and the effect of this cultural definition on human behavior—on what happens to the person who finds himself, quite suddenly, a victim of an unwanted and dread disease. Propaganda of the Cancer Society notwithstanding, cancer carries a death-sentence connotation which is shared by members of the health professions as well as society in general. If nothing else, this study demonstrates that living with this new identity, facing the possibility of a painful and difficult way of dying, is not an easy task and is often a lonely one because laymen and professional people alike withdraw from interactions which stimulate personal identification with the problem. To judge from the findings of this study, to have cancer in our society is to bear a stigma. That is, the person with cancer has an undesired attribute which often leads to isolation from others in the environment.[1]

Reprinted from *Psychiatry*, 28 (1965), pp. 119-132, by special permission of the author and the William Alanson White Psychiatric Foundation, Inc., copyright holder.

This paper derives, in part, from a study supported by National Institute of Mental Health Grant No. M-5495, and sponsored by the School of Nursing and the Dept. of Surgery, School of Medicine, University of California, Los Angeles. The author acknowledges with appreciation the help and support of Barney G. Glaser, Anselm L. Strauss, Stewart E. Perry, Otto E. Guttentag, Wiley F. Barker, and William P. Longmire.

1. The progressive isolation, specifically with respect to talking about cancer and the possibility of death, encountered by women during the year following mastectomy has been detailed in Jeanne C. Quint, "Mastectomy—Symbol of Cure or Warning Sign?" *GP*, 29 (1964), 119-124.

This paper describes some institutionalized practices and individual tactics used by physicians and nurses in their dealings with cancer patients and then considers the cultural and subcultural origins of these behavior patterns. Not only are generalized attitudes toward cancer reflected in these behaviors, but also certain values of the medical and nursing subcultures as well; and generalized sets of actions for all patients are commonly observed in spite of the frequently repeated remark, "Every patient must be treated as an individual." These tactical maneuvers seem to be ways of controlling social interaction between people with differing amounts of access to privileged information which has significant personal meaning for one or both interactants. Finally, since many of these practices may actually function as barriers to effective patient care by interfering with the cancer patient's efforts to deal more openly with his problem, they are of practical concern, and so there are some clear action implications. Before considering these matters in detail, however, I want to give some general information about the mastectomy study and to describe briefly the methods used for data collection and analysis.

Study and Design Methods

The central problem of the study was to understand the social consequences of a treatment procedure which produced two serious changes in the persons observed. More specifically, mastectomy was considered a significant experience because it initiated a transformation along two basic dimensions of human identity: That of being a woman, and the more fundamental one of human existence. I anticipated that the first year following mastectomy, the transition year, would be difficult, and the woman's perspective was of principal concern. However, a related second aim was to understand how family members perceived this event and dealt with it in their everyday lives. A third area of interest was precipitated when ongoing data analysis showed that encounters with medical and nursing personnel were important for two reasons: First, some of these encounters were described by the women participants as critically important incidents; and second, the kind and sequence of encounters they reported were highly variable and resulted in wide differences in what they knew about what was happening to them and why. Thus, it was deemed necessary to obtain more concrete knowledge about the social structure of the medical center in which the mastectomies were performed and to understand how intraorganizational relationships affected what happened to these women.

The problem was formulated for field research with a fluid design and of an exploratory nature. The data were collected through interview and through participant observation by the two nurses who cared for the 21 subjects during their hospitalization. These same two field workers, another nurse and I, conducted the five posthospitalization interviews with each patient.[2] To

2. A more explicit discussion of the early planning phase is given in "Delineation of Qualitative Aspects of Nursing Care," *Nursing Rsc.*, 11 (1962), 204-206.

provide direction for these five home visits, interview guides were developed, but it was anticipated that each of us would vary approaches and tactics to meet the requirements of particular situations. The interviews were focused on the general areas of reaction to the incision and methods used for coping with problems of personal appearance, social activities and relationships with others, unexpected events, and future orientation. Near the end of the year, one interview was conducted with a family member, if the woman gave her consent, and these interviews focused on these three areas: The impact of the experience on the woman, the impact on the family, and the future orientation of both.

Near the end of the first year of the study an intensive three-month period was devoted to making observations in the hospital and outpatient department in order to understand more clearly the social structure and interrelationships of the groups and departments most centrally involved in treating these women both during hospitalization and afterwards. In addition, in order to have some familiarity with the surgeon's perspective on the problems faced by women after mastectomy, interviews were conducted with 14 physicians, all of whom were in private practice either part time or full time. (The two part-time participants held academic appointments in medical schools; the others had clinical appointments.) None of these physicians were providing treatment to the subjects participating in the study.

Data-gathering activities covered a period of 18 months. Interest categories were not predetermined but emerged as the data were assessed for frequencies, unusual events, and patterning of responses. For example, it became apparent early that concern about cancer recurrence and death occurs frequently, and this finding influenced both the sources and the kinds of data which were used subsequently. Once all the data were at hand, it was possible to begin a systematic inspection of them, to identify significant categories, and to specify relationships between the categories. For instance, healing time was found to have important personal and social consequences. Delay in healing forced postponement of use of a breast prosthesis and usually kept the woman socially isolated for a longer interval. Moreover, such delay precipitated thoughts about cancer recurrence and frequently stimulated efforts to secure statements of reassurance which were not always forthcoming from the physicians who were asked. The data showed that concern about cancer recurrence cut across differences in socioeconomic backgrounds; but there is some indication that the management of many aspects of day-to-day living was related to social-class differences, and the data are now being examined from this perspective.

One final point: The subject matter being investigated was emotionally disturbing to the entire project staff, but particularly so to the nurse-fieldworkers who could not escape personal involvement.[3] Although precautions of

3. See Jeanne C. Quint, "The First Year After Mastectomy: The Patients and the Nurse Researchers," in *Designs for Nurse-Patient Interaction*, Convention Clin. Sessions, American Nurses' Association, 9 (1964), pp. 5-12.

many kinds were used to promote detachment, ultimately personal involvement in an emotionally disturbing human experience became a datum. Data analysis has taken a new turn now that time has passed; the notes can be perused more readily from the viewpoint of observer and reporter rather than that of active participant in a human engagement.

Cultural Attitudes Toward Cancer
as Reflected in Doctor and Nurse Behavior

In analyzing the experience of the subjects in this study, it soon became clear that what they were told about their cancer and the surgical procedure was couched in generalities rather than specifics; and often they were not well informed about the relative success of the surgery and the extent of cancer involvement found. Moreover, physicians and nurses made it very difficult for them to ask direct questions about the matter or even to let them say that they were concerned about it, and the barriers to verbal communication were noticeably higher the more extensive the cancer involvement. I began to speculate that the association of cancer with death was operating to influence the behavior of both surgeons and nurses when they engaged in interactions with these patients.

In spite of some individual variations in patient-management procedures, the surgeons with whom we talked used many of the same practices. The postoperative announcement in the hospital was commonly given as a statement of chance, such as: "We found no extension under the arms and there's a 90 percent chance you'll be alive in five years." When positive axillary nodes were found, the odds were less favorable but were usually stretched in the positive direction in the report made to the patient, though family members were usually given a frank statement on the immediate situation and the prognosis. Another commonly used practice was to allow the patient to assume the initiative in asking for details. Thus, if a patient inquired specifically, the surgeon might tell her of the existence of positive nodes, though he might not voluntarily offer this information. Although some surgeons reported that they gave precise details about the number of positive nodes found, others responded with a nonspecific statement. One physician observed:

> I simply tell all of the patients that we have had to remove the breast and up into the axillary region, that we took everything that we saw was involved and that we feel we have gotten the disease.

Extensive inquiry or prolonged conversation about the matter was often prevented by the use of the comment, "If this had been my wife, this is what I would have wanted."

Replies of house staff interviewed revealed their common use of certain avoidance tactics when dealing with cancer patients. The word "cancer" was infrequently used in conversations with patients, whereas the word "tumor" was commonly heard in these exchanges. When a cancer could not be completely removed, it was common practice to tell the patient "we cut it out," but explanatory details were not given unless they were specifically requested. Also, the house staff gave time priorities to patients who offered them challenging opportunities, and patients with extensive cancer involvement did not fall into this classification—if one can judge from the time allotted to them on hospital rounds.

Posthospitalization office visits were usually focused on treatment, and again it was common practice to let the patients take the lead in conversational choices. According to what we were told, few women ask direct questions about the extent of cancer invasion or talk about their fear of recurrence, and none of the surgeons with whom we discussed the matter asked their patients whether this was a source of worry. One physician made this observation, however:

> It's not so much that they talk about it, and perhaps this is the reason I feel it's so important to continue to see them frequently . . . .it's more that you can *feel* their fear, and they're all afraid of this.

Only one of the surgeons with whom we discussed this problem made a practice of giving the patient and the family members the same information, and he (in his words) "lays it on the line" with them but maintains an optimistic attitude "whenever there is anything to be optimistic about." He tells the family members that he is giving the patient the same information, and he meets the protests of "I don't want her to know" by saying, "I'm sorry, but I cannot do that. I feel that it is essential that she know the facts." His principal reason for this practice is to prevent the problems which arise when there is a discrepancy in information given to the patient, and, according to him, the problem of a discrepancy increases whenever more than one physician is involved in a case. He commented further that he does not know how this is resolved within the family, but ultimately the family members almost always tell him that they feel he was correct in the honest and direct approach he used with the patient. When asked to comment about the difficulties that confront a doctor in telling a patient the extent of his cancer, this physician said:

> It's only a problem for the doctor if he makes it a problem. In the hospital, I watched this go on with patients, and believe me it doesn't work. This is at least one reason why I have decided to try to be honest and straightforward with the patients, as seems feasible at all, at the time; and I must say with much more gratifying results.

Some of the women who delayed too long in seeking treatment told of their experiences with physicians. During her first office visit one woman reported that the doctor said: "Do you want me to be good to you? You have only six months to live. You have terminal cancer." Another woman, after many fearful months of indecision, went to a clinic for her first examination and was given a similar blunt announcement by a resident physician who then stood outside the dressing-room door with another physician discussing the survival chances for someone who had waited so long before seeking medical help. A woman who did not wish to consent to hypophesectomy was told by the physician: "You're writing your own suicide note by not having it done now." One can speculate that these actions reflect a deep-seated fear of death from cancer on the part of the physician just as much as do the more commonly used avoidance tactics. Perhaps the fear is intensified because the physician recognizes that treatment at this stage has little chance of offering a cure, and the patient who further delays treatment places him in a helpless position.

Conversations with nurses, as well as observations made in the hospital, showed that the nursing staff too used many avoidance strategies in their dealings with cancer patients, and these were of two kinds: First, there were gestures and actions which made it difficult for a patient to initiate conversation about her fears; and second, there were conversational tactics used to interrupt patient discourse that threatened to get out of hand by focusing directly on either the diagnosis or the prognosis. Both techniques were effective in limiting a patient's opportunities to talk about her illness or to raise questions about what was happening to her.

In general, the nursing staff had contact with patients in the performance of specific assignments—rarely primarily for socialization purposes. The exceptions to this were patients whom the staff obviously liked as persons, and often the nurses spent extra time with preferred patients.[4] It was evident that the preferred patients were the ones who handled their illnesses in a way which was not disturbing to the staff and which did not create difficult problems for them. For example, the various nurses with whom we talked did not enjoy assignment to patients who continuously cried or felt sorry for themselves. In their approaches to patients, the nurses moved rapidly and performed their tasks efficiently. Patients described them in this way: "They look so busy." In addition, the ward pactice of rotating patient assignments made it difficult for patients to establish relationships with particular nurses but also served to protect the staff from becoming well acquainted with the human problems of the patients they were serving.

Much of the time the nurses were able to avoid conversational difficulties with patients by using tactics which directed the discussion into safe channels. Thus, the nurse could focus attention on the procedure being done, or could teach the patient about such matters as arm exercises, or could make small talk; but she seldom encouraged open talk about the illness itself or about cancer. Sometimes, of course, a nurse did encounter a patient who asked directly: "Do I have cancer?," or "Am I going to die?" In response to this type of question the nurses reported using a variety of tactics to avoid giving a direct answer, such as referring the patient to the

4. The finding that nurses spend more time with patients whom they like has also been reported by Francoise R. Morimoto in "Favoritism in Personnel-Patient Interaction," *Nursing Rsc.*, 4 (1955), 109-112.

physician, changing the subject, lapsing into silence, or making such statements as "We all have to go some time." In only one instance did the
data reveal a nurse openly confronting a patient with knowledge of her cancer before knowing what the doctor had told her, and this was done by a
private-duty nurse who, in response to the patient's question about radical
mastectomy, answered directly, "Yes, it was." It is perhaps relevant
to note that the nurse who answered the patient's question in this manner
was well acquainted with the problems which follow mastectomy since her
sister had undergone the surgery several years earlier.

The nurses with whom we talked reported that mastectomy patients did
not talk openly to them about their worries or fears, but some nurses
thought that the possibility of recurrence of cancer was a common concern.
One nurse stated:

> I think this is what would worry *me*. I don't know about the patients. They've
> never really expressed this.

She continued by saying that she thought a person could accept a mastectomy more readily if she could know that this was to be the end of the surgery, with the remark: "I think the fear would be greater, knowing what
can happen."

Our observations indicated that the nurses did not routinely ask the physicians for specific information about the possibility of metastases, and one
can surmise that this technique served a protective function in two ways:
First, by shielding the nurse from feelings of sadness, and second, by making it easier for the nurses to respond to patients' questions by saying, "I
don't know. You'll have to ask your doctor." That some patients with
cancer nevertheless do upset the nurses was indicated by another nurse who
made this comment:

> It's more bothersome to the staff, though, if the patient can't face the fact that
> she's got cancer. A couple of patients we had returned recently with metastases
> of the brain, and that's a little disturbing.

She went on to say that such cases gave one a hopeless feeling. As her comments suggest, when cancer patients are very upset or are terminal, the
nurses are less able to protect themselves from the reality that "this could
happen to me, too."

We learned from the patients that the nurses they encountered in doctors'
offices or in the clinic seldom engaged in prolonged conversation with them,
but when they did, the conversation was focused either on a treatment procedure or on information about breast prostheses. The only nurses who sanctioned their talking about cancer were the two fieldworkers functioning not
as nurses but as interviewers for the purposes of this study; and we did not
find it easy to have these conversations. In fact, the experience of the fieldworkers is additional evidence that permitting patients with cancer to talk
openly about their concerns is not an easy task for the listener but requires
time and support from others if one is to be relatively comfortable in dis-

cussing a topic which carries underlying fear for both participants. Midway in the course of this study I reported to a consultant:

> It's when I am with these women who are really getting the full impact of what it's like to have cancer that it really gets me down. I not only feel *for* them, I begin to feel *with* them, to the point that I have physical symptoms. Isn't it it a way of saying I'm scared too?

Because we permitted these women to talk about important personal and stressful experiences, whereas others would not tolerate such behavior, we became significant human beings in their lives, but the experience brought important consequences for us as well. Not only were we vulnerable as women, identifying with a frightening event which could happen to any woman, but also we had to struggle without identities as nurses who are supposed to be impersonal and uninvolved with patients. We were caught in feelings of compassion and sadness and human concern, and we frequently suffered the anguish of *wanting to do something*.

Some situations we found particularly depressing and disconcerting. For example, one woman had been told by the surgeon, "In three months or so you'll never know this happened to you"; yet the wound was still unhealed at the end of a year. Morose at the time of her last interview, she commented:

> It's disconcerting. When that drain under my arm opened up and started to drain every day, I talked to them about it. All they said was, "Just let it drain." Well, in the meantime it's closed up again. But it still is disturbing to me. *Why, why should it* suddenly break open?

On one occasion, six months after surgery, a clinic patient called us—in great anguish because one doctor had told her that X-ray was imperative, whereas another doctor had released her. She reported:

> I went to work for three days, and my arm got so red and swollen that I got fired. Since I have been to that outpatient department, I have seen about twelve different doctors. How do they know what was removed? They've got me into a nervous wreck up there. It costs me a fortune to get there. Do they think that I would go if there wasn't something wrong with me? They don't realize what pressure they are putting me under. I went up there because I was vomiting for three days, and I was worried.

As women, we found ourselves distressed by many of the frustrations and difficulties described by these women during the year we were in contact with them. In addition, we were exposed to the stresses and strains which they and their families experienced during this period of adjustment to a major change in their lives.

Women whose incisions were delayed in healing or who developed secondary complications became edgy when their physical signs and symptoms failed to abate. One woman who found herself losing strength and unable to continue with her usual activities reported ten months after surgery:

> It has a tendency to make me highly nervous. My sister told me a week ago; she said, "I refuse to do anything more for you because there's nothing that

will please you." And *I'm not* that way. I've just been in so much misery. A person that's going through this needs all the encouragement in the world, and it's the worst thing in the world that a person will turn on anybody when they've got this disease.

Seven months after surgery another woman reported that her nerves were very edgy and that her husband irritated her unbearably. She said:

I have a terrible hatred. I can't tell you why but I do, and I'm crying a lot. He can just *look* at me, and I'll bawl. I don't know what it is—my nerves, letdown. Everything irritates me. *Everything! He* irritates me. The people in the market irritate me. I just want to do something to shut them up, to *leave me alone.*

In a separate interview her husband stated:

She was drinking before, but she's drinking heavier now. I know how she would feel, especially being a woman, but she's got to do something about it because a man just can't live with someone like this and expect to be sane in six months. He won't be. He won't be.

Within two weeks following this interview they were separated. In another family, a husband and wife discussed more openly problems which arose, but he made this observation to the fieldworker: "Sometimes I don't know what to say to reassure her."

While the central issue these women faced was the possibility of death from cancer, most of them faced it relatively alone because their families and friends, as well as the doctors and nurses, blocked them from discussing this. As one husband said:

I figure it's over with, and both of us want to forget it. So there's no use in bringing it up.

For many of these women, the fieldworkers provided the only outlet for talking about their real worries, and we learned something of what it is like to live with cancer. That this experience carries deep meaning comes through in a poignant comment from one woman:

This not knowing is just terrible. You know, you have this feeling of not knowing whether your time is up.

Sometimes our feelings of outrage and helplessness interfered with our effectiveness as fieldworkers, and we found outselves trying to put pressure on the physician to "do something," yet our efforts in some instances provoked frank antagonism. The doctor was particularly vulnerable when the patient's prognosis was poor, and he could offer little help; yet it was under the same circumstances that we found ourselves captured in our own tensions and interceding in an inappropriate manner. On one occasion, for example, a physician frankly ridiculed the project and, over coffee with one of the secretaries, referred to it caustically as a "terminal cancer study." He said that he avoided the nurse fieldworker whenever he saw her coming because she asked such stupid questions. In one instance she had asked him if he knew that Mrs. X had stomach trouble, and he commented to the secretary, "Well, what do you expect? She's got cancer."

The difficulties which open talk with cancer patients can precipitate for nurses are illustrated by some problems we faced in conversations with these women. Because they identified us as nurses and trusted us as persons, they felt free (more so than with the physicians) to ask questions about their progress and prognosis, and these situations were difficult for us to manage. To have someone ask, "How am I, really?" is an uncomfortable experience when one knows that the patient's condition is deteriorating, and we had no choice but to refer her to her physician for an answer. Although we entered the patients' homes as fieldworkers, not as practicing nurses, we could not evade our feelings as nurses and the helplessness and hopelessness which some encounters carried for us. That we sometimes communicated other information was pointed out by one woman who observed:

> You know something you're not telling me, but you don't want to tell me, and I'll have to ask someone else.

That cancer and its association with death is anxiety-provoking to those in the health professions in general is further revealed by the difficulties we encountered in finding colleagues who would listen when we needed to talk, both about the difficulties we encountered and the feelings which these experiences engendered. We found few persons who could provide support for us, and we shared a form of conversational isolation similar to that of the women participants. The reporting of the findings has provided additional evidence that these data carry tremendous emotional impact, and I have found that social scientists as well as those in the health professions are sometimes upset by these accounts.

Some Findings From Other Studies

In a study of the psychological problems of adjustment to cancer of the breast, Renneker and Cutler stated that about half of the 50 women whose interviews they reported on were living in a world in which people around them avoided using the word cancer. They offer these observations:

> The word cancer was freely used by the interviewer throughout the sessions. The responses elicited were dramatic: A few women were so relieved to hear someone say cancer that, like children with a new word, they said it again and again. All appeared to accept it with relief.[5]

They also found that when the surgeon avoided using the word cancer, a woman took this as evidence that her diagnosis was equivalent to a death sentence. When the surgeon did not speak of the cancer spontaneously, she interpreted his silence to mean that she was going to die—that he wanted neither to say this nor to lie about it.

5. Richard Renneker and Max Cutler, "Psychological Problems of Adjustment to Cancer of the Breast," *Journal American Medical Association*, 148 (1952), 836.

In another study, which attempted to determine what physicians in one community told patients with cancer, the investigators found that 31 percent either always or usually told their patients they had cancer, whereas 69 percent either usually did not tell them or never told them. Of greater interest, perhaps, are the differences which appear when the responses are analyzed by specialty groups. Whereas 94 percent of the dermatologists always told their patients, only 12 percent of the radiologists did so, with other specialty groups ranging between these two extremes. The authors of this study note that those who rarely tell patients are the physicians who tend to see more patients in the later stages of the disease or who are responsible for terminal care. They suggest that physicians treating internal cancers are influenced by the factor that they see the prognosis as unfavorable.[6]

Kelly and Friesen in an outpatient department opinion poll found that 89 percent of cancer patients wanted to know they had cancer, 82 percent of noncancer patients would want to know if they had cancer; and 98 percent of patients being followed in a cancer detection center wanted to be told if they had cancer.[7] The authors indicate that the higher proportion found in the latter group is probably to be expected since cancer detection is their object in undergoing regular examinations. It is interesting to note also that of the same group of cancer patients who responded 89 percent in favor of knowing, only 73 percent thought that people in general should be told, perhaps reflecting the notion that people in general are less capable of handling bad news than they. The cancer patients were also asked whether they agreed or disagreed with this statement: "Doctors and patients' relatives are occasionally inclined to believe that they are protecting patients from worry by not telling them they have cancer." The patients almost overwhelmingly disagreed. In the opinion of these authors, patients want to be informed if they have cancer far more often than the average physician would anticipate.

Cultural Values, Social Interaction, and Cancer Disclosure

Most of the practices of information control described in this paper achieve two general goals. First, the patient himself must usually take the offensive in getting information about the extent of his cancer involvement. Second, he is prevented much of the time from openly expressing concern about whether or not he is going to die from cancer, how, and when. In the terms used by Glaser and Strauss, under most circumstances those in the health professions use many tactics to maintain a closed awareness context around

6. William J. Fitts and I. S. Ravdin, "What Philadelphia Physicians Tell Patients with Cancer," *Journal American Medical Association,* 153 (1953), 901-904.
7. William D. Kelly and Stanley R. Friesen, "Do Cancer Patients Want To Be Told?" *Surgery,* 27 (1950), 822-826.

the cancer patient—that is, to keep him uninformed of his true identity.[8] Although these authors stress the developmental aspects of interaction, including the strategies used by those seeking information, in this paper attention is given only to the maneuvers used by those with privileged information about a patient's diagnosis and prognosis either to control the amount of information which is given to him or to exert control over his actions. Expressed in another way, I am here concerned with the strategies used by those who hold positions of power with respect to the other interactant.

The problem is compounded, however, because the information in question carries significant meaning for both participants. Fear of death from cancer might even be viewed as a universal phenomenon since few, if any, persons select it as a preferred way of dying.[9] In essence, cancer carries unpleasant associations for both participants, but it has an additional significance for members of the health professions. Sometimes cancer cannot be cured and, under these conditions, doctors and nurses can no longer cling to the image of themselves as savers of lives but rather must face the reality of professional failure. It is not surprising that many institutionalized practices have developed to protect professionals not only from unpleasant and emotionally disturbing scenes with these patients but also to cushion involvement with their own identity feelings, both personal and professional, when these are threatened.

Thus, many tactics are used to control the amount of information given to the cancer patient and thereby to foster the idea that he will recover, even though this may not always be the case. Such actions are supported by medical and nursing rationales which stress the importance of maintaining hope in the face of uncertainty, but they also reflect a primary value of this society—the wish to deny the reality of death.[10] Many of the avoidance tactics used by health professionals are no different from those used by laymen to manage distressing situations, whereas others clearly make use of the doctor's or nurse's privileged position and are supported by organizational practices and team efforts.

In the first place, hospitals are organized so as to maximize the difficulties for any patient seeking medical information, but the cancer patient has the distinct disadvantage of having an illness which no one really wants to discuss with him. To that end, the use of rotating assignments and group rounds assists the staff in avoiding prolonged contact with the same patients, particularly those who might ask troublesome questions, and the

8. The relationship between awareness of another's identity and social interaction under different structural conditions is discussed by Barney G. Glaser and Anselm L. Strauss in "Awareness Contexts and Social Interaction," *American Sociological Review*, 29 (1964), 669-679.

9. See Daniel Cappon, "Attitudes of and Toward the Dying," *Canadian Medical Association Journal*, 87 (1962), 693-700.

10. Robert Fulton and Gilbert Geis, "Death and Social Values," *Indian Journal Social Research*, 2 (1962), 30.

word gets around rather fast about "difficult patients." Moreover, a team organization which lacks clear-cut delegation of responsibility provides a convenient tool for staff members who wish to pass the buck. An atmosphere of busy activity with primacy given to life-saving actions provides another useful out, and such a work context makes it easy for staff members both to control the amount of time allotted to a patient and also to justify it. In other words, both consciously and unconsciously, the staff make use of strategies which effectively limit patients' opportunities to negotiate for information. If one views the hospital as a locale where personnel and patients are enmeshed in a complex negotiative process to accomplish, in part at least, their individual purposes, as Strauss and his co-workers suggest, the cancer patient is additionally handicapped by a diagnosis which physicians and nurses find both personally and professionally threatening.[11]

Time management is one matter; impression management in face-to-face interaction is quite another, since people express themselves or convey information by both verbal and gestural means, and the messages conveyed may or may not be congruent. When physicians and nurses attempt to communicate by word and deed a particular identity to the cancer patient, they try to coordinate both aspects of sign activity along the same avenue or in the same direction, perhaps not always successfully.

Physicians and nurses have somewhat different problems to manage in these interactions since physicians are the legitimate definers of the patient's diagnostic identity, whereas nurses are expected to support physicians in their decisions to withhold or to give particular kinds of information. In effect, nurses are supported in their individual and group maneuvers by a professional rationale which affirms that only the physician can disclose a patient's diagnosis to him. Nurses are remarkably adept at blocking patient inquiry about delicate matters by both verbal and nonverbal means, and an efficient professional demeanor checks many patients. Nurses are also successful much of the time in maintaining control of conversation in one of three ways: Either they focus on the treatment and on getting well, or they avoid direct questions, or they talk about matters far removed from the hospital or the office. In the first instance, they use an occupationally determined strategy; in the others, they employ conversational devices brought from middle-class society in general. This professional rationale also serves an important self-protective function since the nurse can legitimately avoid seeking out information which is not essential for succesful performance of her job and which, in fact, might make the job more difficult to accomplish were she better informed.

Where the nurse runs into difficulty is with the patient who does not stay in proper character but confronts her directly with questions or subjects which

11. Anselm L. Strauss, Leonard Schatzman, Danuta Ehrlich, Rue Bucher, and Melvin Sabshin, "The Hospital and Its Negotiated Order," in *The Hospital in Modern Society*, Eliot Freidson, ed. (New York: The Free Press, 1963), pp. 147-169.

are professionally embarassing or personally disturbing, and when this occurs, she falls back on different strategies. That is, she resorts to techniques which cut short any conversation threatening to discredit her identity. With a few exceptions, the strategies employed are not unique to nurses but rather are commonly used in many settings to block conversation which threatens to make one or both participants uneasy or upset. Under the circumstances being discussed, however, nurses are faced with threats to two identitites: As nurses, and also as human beings who know deep inside that death lies ahead for all men. Thus it is that avoidance maneuvers protect the self-image of the nurse as a saver of lives but also prevent strong feelings and fears about death from being brought to the surface.

The physician's problem in face-to-face interaction is not so much how to avoid the topic altogether as it is how to give the patient sufficient information to insure cooperation in treatment and at the same time avoid unnecessary and prolonged scenes. In distinguishing between clinical uncertainty and functional uncertainty, Davis suggests two modes of communication that reveal a discrepancy between what the doctor knows and what he tells the patient: First, dissimulation—the rendering of a prognosis which the physician knows to be unsubstantiated clinically, and second, evasion—the failure to communicate a clinically substantiated prognosis.[12] He notes further that the physician may perpetuate uncertainty in his communication with the family even after he is no longer in doubt about the patient's condition, in order to manage the treatment situation without the added problem of handling emotional reactions which a frank discussion of the prognosis might provoke. He observes that the hospital-anchored physician, more than the community-based practitioner, is supported in these endeavors by a "bustling, time-conscious work milieu."[13]

The use of evasion by physicians is directly related to a negative prognosis, but even those who more openly give concrete information to cancer patients are prone to use evasion in a subtle way. For example, the use of statistical chance to project a patient's future to the patient is an equivocation if family members are given a different account of the situation. The practice of giving incomplete and sometimes misleading information is supported by medical rationales which assert that the physician cannot deny hope to the patient, and the doctor who accepts this viewpoint can use various strategies to control the face-to-face interaction with his patients. For instance, he can focus complete attention on recovery, provide nonspecific answers to medical questions, avoid use of the word "cancer" and other potentially dangerous phrases, limit the time available for consultation, and refrain from discussing questions about the future. In addition, he can use his position to cut short conversation which threatens to become distressing or difficult to manage. By using any of these strategies, the physician can

12. Fred Davis, "Uncertainty in Medical Prognosis: Clinical and Functional," in this volume.
13. *Ibid*, p. 245.

protect his identity in two ways. He can more easily maintain the image, both to himself and to the patient, that he has the power to cure human ailments; and, also important, he can protect himself from involvement in the human problems of the other person. Thus it is that the physician, like the nurse, tends to block conversation which threatens to undermine his personal and professional values. Indeed, the use of the "shock announcement" with cancer patients who have delayed in seeking help is yet another way for the physician to cope with a situation which threatens these values.

The invisible stigma of the cancer patient presents a threat to physicians and nurses because of the patient's claim to normalcy is either ambiguous and uncertain, or depressingly clear. In any event, the cancer patient—perhaps more than any other—reminds those in the health professions that their powers to cure are limited and also reminds them that dying, the last experience of the human predicament, may not come in kindly ways. Those physicians and nurses who can more openly discuss both diagnosis and prognosis with cancer patients have somehow come to terms with the reality of death. However, in a society which treats death like a noxious disease, it is not surprising that many people in the health professions who carry the task of protecting people from death have well-developed strategies for maintaining poise and control in situations which threaten these basic identities.[14]

Some Action Implications

As has been implied in this description, the institutionalized practices of information control have both clinical and psychological costs for cancer patients. With this perspective in mind, I want now to suggest the need for some changes in medical and nursing education and practice. When patients and family members are presented with contradictory information, as was found to be the usual pattern in our study, the problem for the patients became one of coping with an uncertainty sometimes heightened by a sensitivity to the fact that others were withholding information from them. Renneker and Cutler suggest that concealment can lead to unfortunate consequences by promoting distrust in the physician and subsequent withdrawal from cooperation in postoperative treatment procedures.[15] Perhaps physicians and nurses who take the position that "we must never take away the patient's hope" by telling the truth are responding to their own feelings of helplessness and hopelessness. In addition, the education of both groups has focused attention on the saving of lives and has offered little training in the art of helping patients to live with an untreatable illness.[16]

14. The relationship between identity and cultural definitions of death is emphasized by Robert Fulton in "Death and the Self," *Journal Religion and Health*, 3 (1964), 359-368.

15. See footnote 5.

16. The relationship of death to life, rather than to disease, has been given relatively little attention in schools of medicine and nursing. See Otto E. Guttentag, "The

A physician has suggested that when the doctor makes decisions *for* the patient rather than in consultation with him as another human being, he is treating that patient like a machine rather than a man.[17] When those in the health professions and the family join together in a pact of secrecy, they are removing from the patient the right to participate in making decisions about his future and are denying him the opportunity to decide how he wants to live with his fatal illness.

The physician holds a critically important and extremely difficult position in regard to this matter, since it is he who carries the legal and moral responsibility for telling the patient his diagnosis and for explaining the therapeutic regimes which he can offer.[18] As has been indicated, many physicians have difficulty in giving cancer patients a realistic appraisal of the situation; yet many patients would prefer hearing bad news rather than worrying about the unknown. The practice of giving the patient and his family members different versions of his true condition may actually impose great psychological strain on him, for he becomes very sensitive to conversational silences and to withdrawal of contact by other people. Perhaps, also, cancer patients can better mobilize their psychological resources when they are better informed about their condition.

To judge from the findings of this study, what patients are told—or not told—by physicians may be as much a part of the treatment as the surgery itself, yet this aspect of the practice of medicine has received minimal attention in medical teaching. In fact, the image of the physician as a saver of lives is accentuated by medical education, and it is with this perspective that students learn to classify patients. Thus, patients who cannot be cured are found to rate low. In addition, medical school effectively insulates students from many problems which they will meet in practice—such as how to talk to a patient with an inoperable tumor.[19] Even programs developed to incorporate the psychological aspects of medicine emphasize medical interviewing as an information-getting process, with little mention made of the when, how, and what of information-giving.[20] Oken found that medical school training had little to do with determining physicians' policies about what to tell cancer patients. He concluded that physicians made these decisions principally on the basis of personal conviction, heavily weighted

Meaning of Death in Medical Theory," *Stanford Medical Bulletin,* 17 (1959), 165-170; also Jeanne C. Quint and Anselm L. Strauss in "Nursing Students, Assignments and Dying Patients," *Nursing Outlook,* 12 (1964), 24-27.

17, Otto E. Guttentag, "On Defining Medicine," *Christian Scholar,* 46 (1963) 205-206.

18. Alan R. Moritz and C. Joseph Stetler, *Handbook of Legal Medicine* (St. Louis: Mosby, 1964), pp. 153-154.

19. Howard S. Becker, Blanche Geer, Everett C. Hughes, and Anselm L. Strauss, *Boys in White* (Chicago: University of Chicago Press, 1961), pp. 316-318.

20. George L. Engel, William L. Green, Jr., Franz Reichsman, Arthur Schmale, and Norman Ashenburg, "A Graduate and Undergraduate Teaching Program on the Psychological Aspects of Medicine," *Journal Medical Education,* 32 (1957), 859-870.

with emotional justification, rather than on critical observation. Moreover, the physicians in his survey viewed cancer with the same pessimism as did the general public.[21]

As I perceive this, the problem facing physicians is not simply a question of whether or not to tell the patient he has cancer. It has more to do with conveying appropriate information at the right time and in such a way that the patient does not feel lost or confused or abandoned. To make this kind of determination, the physician needs to make use of behavioral clues as well as physical signs and symptoms in deciding what action to take at a particular time, and he needs to be aware that his actions contribute to the patient's reactions and subsequent actions. It is one thing for the doctor to bluntly announce, "Well, things look pretty bad," and walk out of the room; it is quite another for him to sit down with the patient and present an unfavorable situation with objectivity and compassion. As one woman told us, "I think the doctor's more concerned about the tumors than he is about anything else." There is a serious responsibility which often confronts the physician in these matters: The patient's right to accept or reject a recommended treatment which cannot be guaranteed to help him or to save his life. Ayd states the physician's responsibility as follows:

> He has the duty to make it clear to the patient that there are available extraordinary means which may save his life and the physician is obligated to use them if the patient wants him to do so. At the same time a doctor must recognize that he does not have the right to urge a dangerous remedy or a new procedure without just cause.[22]

Expressing this in another way, one might ask: Does the patient, rather than his family, have the right to decide how he wants to live with his disease?

If physicians are to change their practices in talking with cancer patients about their illness, I suggest that training for this should begin in medical school. This is a formidable task because it involves helping medical students recognize how their fears and attitudes about cancer affect their interactions with these patients, and such training is time-consuming and difficult. Moreover, its success may well depend on the availability of the physician-teachers who are themselves at ease in talking with patients, and with students, about difficult and distressing matters. The medical school is in a position to contribute in yet another way by encouraging research on human responses and adaptations to living with cancer—and other diseases carrying a fatal connotation—for only by systematic study of the personal and social consequences of disease can treatment of the person have a fully scientific base.

21. Donald Oken, "What to Tell Cancer Patients," *Journal American Medical Association*, 175 (1961), 1120-1128.
22. Frank J. Ayd, "The Hopeless Case," *Journal American Medical Association*, 181 (1962), 1101.

Nursing has always been concerned with the care and comfort of the patient, and I submit that the professional nurse can play an important part in helping both the patient and the physician cope with the difficult problems which a cancer diagnosis brings. Let me make it clear that it is not the nurse's function to assume the physician's responsibility of telling the patient the diagnosis, but she can help the patient face reality by letting him talk about his cancer when he is ready to do so, and she can be an important communication link between the patient and the physician. Nurses in doctor's offices and in clinics are in a crucial position to offer this kind of service, as are those engaged in private duty or serving in public health agencies which provide home care services, but they can do so only if they recognize such action as an important nursing function and can comfortably offer it. Second, to be effective in helping the patient, the nurse should neither wait for the physician to tell her what to do nor should she wait for the patient to ask for help. She should take the initiative in talking to both, in interpreting misunderstandings which arise, and in keeping herself informed so that the patient is protected from information discrepancies. Further, she needs to be sensitive to the importance of timing and should be able to recognize the behavioral clues which indicate when a change in tactics is required. Perhaps most of all, she should have a philosophy of nursing care based on the patient's right to participate in critical decisions affecting him and his future. Finally, there may be instances when the physician needs moral support in facing his difficult task, and the nurse may find herself in a position to offer this kind of assistance to him.

Not all nurses can provide such a service to cancer patients, nor should they be expected to do so, and the difficulties involved should not be underestimated. When a patient with cancer begins to talk about it, he may be angry or sad, and the nurse is faced with handling her own feelings. Many physicians may not be able to accept this kind of assistance from the nurse, and she may face anger or criticism from them for her efforts. Others may not recognize the valuable contribution a sensitive nurse can make to a patient's well-being and will resist making use of her talents. Perhaps the professional nurse who is willing to assume this kind of responsibility for patient care needs to become skilled in talking with physicians as well as with patients, so that doctors become better informed of the value of this important service. Indeed, professional schools of nursing may want to place greater emphasis on this aspect of nursing practice in their educational programs. Moreover, these schools need to recognize both the kind of training required and the amount of time such training takes for student nurses to develop their abilities to talk more openly with cancer patients about topics which provoke feelings of helplessness.

To bring about such changes in nursing practice is a difficult matter. Indeed, the problem is truly a question of changing attitudes which are based on deeply entrenched cultural and subcultural values and which underpin, at least in part, the basic nurse identity. The question of altering physician practices is even more complex and serious since the physician in our society, even more than the nurse, is expected to ward off death; yet the basic problem faced by cancer patients will continue unless physicians in cooperation with other professional personnel in the health field are ready to face its reality. Probably little change can be expected so long as the social and psychological aspects of patient care remain essentially nonaccountable and less important than the highly technical life-saving procedures which modern medicine continues to emphasize. For example, hospital personnel are not held accountable for interpersonal aspects of care given to dying patients in the same way that they are responsible for carrying out certain technical procedures.[23] Moreover, avoidance of personal responsibility by practitioners continues to be reinforced by institutionalized medical practices which quite effectively shield physicians and nurses from involvement with individual patients and assist them in maintaining a world in which the reality of death can be denied or at least temporarily ignored.[24]

At the beginning of this paper, I suggested that to have cancer is to bear a stigma which can lead to social isolation. In discussing the expectations and behavior of normal persons toward a person carrying a discrediting stigma, Goffman made this observation:

> The stigmatized individual is asked to act so as to imply neither that his burden is heavy nor that bearing it has made him different from us; at the same time he must keep himself at that remove from us which ensures our painlessly being able to confirm this belief about him. Put differently, he is advised to reciprocate naturally with an acceptance of himself and us, an acceptance of him that we have not quite extended to him in the first place.[25]

The patient with cancer has a heavy burden, and his burden strikes fear in all of us so that we find it easier to minimize our personal identification with him. However, when some of us in the health professions join laymen in isolating the person with cancer, we may be adding to the burden rather than lightening it.

23. See Anselm L. Strauss, Barney G. Glaser, and Jeanne C. Quint, "The Non-Accountability of Terminal Care," *Hospitals,* 38 (1964), 73-77.

24. A contrast between the "image" of rehabilitation and the reality of rehabilitation is sharply drawn by Elizabeth M. Eddy in "Rites of Passage in a Total Institution," *Human Organization*, 23 (1964), 67-75.

25. Erving Goffman, *Stigma: Notes on the Management of Spoiled Identity* (Englewood Cliffs, N.J.: Prentice-Hall, 1963), p. 122.

16

FRED DAVIS

Uncertainty in Medical Prognosis, Clinical and Functional

Medical sociology is indebted to Talcott Parsons for having called attention to the important influence of uncertainty on the relationship between doctor and patient in the treatment of illness and disease.[1] This is described as a primary source of strain in the physician's role, not only because clinically it so often obscures and vitiates definitive diagnoses and prognoses, but also because in an optimistic and solution-demanding culture such as ours it poses serious and delicate problems in the communicating of the unknown and the problematic to the patient and his family. In line with this view, Renée Fox has recently made an insightful analysis of the curriculum of a medical school, showing how, both from a formal and an informal standpoint, one of its functions is to socialize the student to cope more successfully with uncertainty.[2]

Granting the self-evident plausibility of the hypothesis, sociological studies of medical practice thus far have neglected to assess empirically its scope and significance in the actual treatment of specific illnesses or diseases[3]. As a ready-made explanation of a disturbing element in the rela-

Reprinted from the *American Journal of Sociology*, 66 (1960), pp. 41-47, by permission of the author and the University of Chicago Press.

Revised version of a paper read at the annual meeting of the American Sociological Society, Chicago, September, 1959. I wish to thank Anselm Strauss, Julius A. Roth, and Stephen A. Richardson for their valuable criticisms. Acknowledgment is also due my former colleagues, Harvey A. Robinson, Joseph S. Bierman, Toba Tahl, Arthur Silverstein, and Martin Gorten, of the Polio Project, Psychiatric Institute, University of Maryland Medical School, with whom I collaborated in research. The project was aided by a grant from the National Foundation.

1. Talcott Parsons, *The Social System* (Glencoe, Ill.: The Free Press, 1951), pp. 466-469.

2. Renee Fox, "Training for Uncertainty," in R. K. Merton, G. Reader, and P. L. Kendall, eds., *The Student Physician* (Cambridge, Mass.: Harvard University Press, 1957), pp. 207-241.

3. Partial exception must be made for the work of Julius A. Roth. See *Time Tables* (Indianapolis: Bobbs-Merrill, 1963).

tionship between doctor and patient, the concept—uncertainty—stands in danger of being applied in a catch-all fashion whenever, for example, the sociologist notes that communication from doctor to patient is characterized by duplicity, evasion, or other forms of strain. That other factors, having relatively little to do with uncertainty, can also systematically generate strain in the relationship may unfortunately be ignored because of the disposition to subsume phenomena under pre-existent categories.

The present paper examines the scope and significance of uncertainty as evidenced in the treatment of a particular disease. Specifically, it seeks to distinguish between *real* uncertainty as a clinical and scientific phenomenon and the uses to which uncertainty—real or pretended, *functional* uncertainty— lends itself in the management of patients and their families by hospital physicians and other treatment personnel. By extrapolation this distinction suggests a fourfold typology of patterns of communication from doctor to patient, analysis of which highlights important sources of strain other than uncertainty.

The disease in question is paralytic poliomyelitis, and the subjects are fourteen Baltimore families, in each of which a young child had contracted the disease. These were studied longitudinally over a two-year period by an interdisciplinary team of social scientists and research physicians whose broad interest was in assessing the total impact of the experience on child and family. Except for one family that dropped out midway in the study, in each case the child with polio and his parents were interviewed at inter- vals from the time of the child's admission to a pediatrics ward in the acute stage of the disease to approximately a year and a half following his dis- charge from a convalescent hospital.

From the very first interview with the parents, held within a week or so following the child's admission in the hospital, to the fourteenth and final interview with them some two years later, the research was aimed at de- termining at every stage what the parents knew and understood about polio in general and their child's condition in particular and through whom and how they came to acquire such knowledge and understanding as they had on these matters. In addition to being interviewed in home and office, the parents were also observed from time to time in the hospital on visiting days—this being their only regular opportunity to discuss their child's condi- tion with the physician-in-charge as he made his round of the ward. It might be noted here that, with few exceptions, the parents soon came to re- gard these encounters as especially frustrating and of little value in getting information on questions which were troubling them. Although the situation on visiting day did not permit the observers to come away with word-for- word records of what went on, their perfunctory character was sufficiently evident to substantiate the descriptions later given by the parents in inter- view. As one mother remarked:

Well, they "the doctors" don't tell you anything, hardly. They don't seem to want to. I mean, you start asking questions and they say, "Well, I only have about three minutes to talk to you." And the things that you ask, they don't seem to want to answer you. So I don't ask them anything any more.

Finally, to round out coverage of the network of communication involving the parents, interviews were held with the hospital physicians, physiotherapists, and other ancillary personnel responsible for the child's treatment and care. Here a major goal was to learn what their diagnosis and prognosis were of the child's condition and on what medical considerations these were based.

By bringing together the interview and observational data gathered from these several sources, it was possible to compare and contrast, at successive stages of the disease and its treatment, what the parents knew and understood of the child's condition with what the doctors knew and understood. One must assume that the doctor's knowledge of the disease and its physical effects is more accurate, comprehensive, and profound than that of the parents. The problem, then, could be stated: How much information was communicated to the parents? How was it communicated? And what consequences did this communication have on the parents' expectations of the child's illness and prospects for recovery?[4] And, since in paralytic poliomyelitis (as in many other diseases and illnesses) uncertainty does affect the making of diagnoses and prognoses, an attempt was made to assess the scope, significance, and duration of uncertainty for the doctor. This then provided some basis for inferring the extent to which the parents' knowledge and expectations, or lack thereof, could also be attributed ultimately to uncertainty.

For purposes of simplicity, the discussion that follows is restricted to uncertainty only as it impinges on the prognosis of residual disability expected as a result of the poliomyelitic attack. This subsumes questions of such relatively great moment to child and parent as: Would he be permanently handicapped? Would he require the aid of braces and other supportive appliances? Would his handicap be so severe as to prevent him from engaging in a wide range of normal motor activities or be barely detectable?

Now the pathological course of paralytic poliomyelitis is such that, during the first weeks following onset, it is difficult in most cases for even the most skilled diagnostician to make anything like a definite prognosis of probable residual impairment and functional disability. During the acute phase of the disease and for a period thereafter, the examining physician has no practical way of directly measuring or indirectly inferring the amount of permanent damage or destruction sustained by the horn cells of the spinal cord as a result of the viral attack. (It is basically the condition of these cells,

4. See Fred Davis, "Definitions of Time and Recovery in Paralytic Polio Convalescence," *American Journal of Sociology*, 61 (May, 1956), 582-587.

and not that of the muscles neurologically activated by them, that accounts for the paralysis.) Roughly, a one- to three-month period for spontaneous recovery of the damaged spinal cells—a highly unpredictable matter in itself —must first be allowed for before the effects of the disease are sufficiently stabilized to permit a clinically well-founded prognosis.

During the initial period of the child's hospitalization, therefore, the physician is hardly ever able to tell the parents anything definite about the child's prospects of regaining lost muscular function. In view of the very real uncertainty, to attempt to do so would indeed be hazardous. To the parents' insistent questions, "How will he come out of it?" "Will he have to wear a brace?" "Will his walk be normal?" and so on, the invariable response of treatment personnel was that they did not know and that only time would tell. Thus during these first weeks the parents came to adopt a longer time perspective and more qualified outlook than they had to begin with.[5]

By about the sixth week to the third month following onset of the disease, however, the orthopedist and physiotherapist are in position to make reasonably sound prognoses of the amount and type of residual handicap. This is done on the basis of periodic muscle examinations from which the amount and rate of return of affected muscular capacity is plotted. The guiding contingencies for prognosis are:

> Muscles that have shown early and rapidly developing return of strength will probably make a full recovery. Those which have but moderate or little strength at the end of this period will probably never make complete recovery. Muscles which are completely paralyzed at the end of this period will probably always remain so. In other words, at the end of this period the spinal motor cells have or have not recovered their physiologic activity and no further change in them may be expected.[6]

By this time, therefore, the element of clinical uncertainty regarding outcome, so conspicuously present when the child is first stricken, is greatly reduced for the physician, if not altogether eliminated.[7] Was there then a commensurate gain in the parents' understanding of the child's condition after this six-week to three-month period had passed? Did they then, as did the

5. *Ibid.*, pp. 583-585.

6. The American Orthopaedic Association, "Infantile Paralysis, or Acute Poliomyelitis: A Brief Primer of the Disease and Its Treatment,"*Journal of the American Medical Association*, 131 (August 24, 1946), 1414.

7. As in nearly all applied fields of endeavor, medicine necessarily deals in probabilities rather than absolutes. Hence some measure of uncertainty is always present, the crucial question being the matter of degree and not the mere presence. Admittedly, no hard-and-fast lines can be drawn at the point at which uncertainty acquires therapeutic significance; but, if the concept is to have any analytical value at all, it cannot be applied to all instances of illness in which it is possible to concede the existence of some degree of uncertainty, however slight. If this were done, there would not be an instance to which it did not apply.

doctors, come to view certain outcomes as highly probable and others as improbable?

On the basis of intensive and repeated interviewing of the parents over a two-year period, the answer to these questions is that, except for one case in which the muscle check pointed clearly to full recovery, the parents were neither told nor explicitly prepared by the treatment personnel to expect an outcome significantly different from that which they understandably hoped for, namely, a complete and natural recovery for the child. This does not imply that the doctors issued falsely optimistic prognoses or that, through indirection and other subtleties, they sought to encourage the parents to expect more by way of recovery than was possible. Rather, what typically transpired was that the parents were kept in the dark. The doctors' answers to their questions were couched for the most part in such hedging, evasive, or unintelligibly technical terms[8] as to cause them, from many such contacts, to expect a more favorable recovery than could be justified by the facts then known. As one treatment-staff member put it, "We try not to tell them too much. It's better if they find out for themselves in a natural sort of way."

Indeed, it was disheartening to note how, for many of the parents, "the natural way" consisted of a painfully slow and prolonged dwindling of expectations for a complete and natural recovery. This is ironical when one considers that as early as two to three months following onset the doctors and physiotherapists were able to tell members of the research team with considerable confidence that one child would require bracing for an indefinite period; that another would never walk with a normal gait; that a third would require a bone-fusion operation before he would be able to hold himself erect; and so on. By contrast, the parents of these children came to know these prognoses much later, if at all. And even then their understanding of them was in most instances partial and subject to considerable distortion.

But what is of special interest here is the way in which uncertainty, a *real* factor in the early diagnosis and treatment of the paralyzed child, came more and more to serve the purely managerial ends of the treatment personnel in their interaction with parents. Long after the doctor himself was no longer in doubt about the outcome, the perpetuation of uncertainty in doctor-to-family communication, although perhaps neither premeditated nor intended, can nonetheless best be understood in terms of its functions in the treatment system. These are several, and closely connected.

Foremost is the way in which the pretense of uncertainty as to outcome serves to reduce materially the expenditure of additional time, effort, and involvement which a frank and straightforward prognosis to the family might entail. The doctor implicitly recognizes that, were he to tell the family that the child would remain crippled or otherwise impaired to some significant

8. Cf. Bernard Kutner, "Surgeons and Their Patients," in E. Gartly Jaco, ed., *Patients, Physicians, and Illness* (Glencoe, Ill.: The Free Press, 1958), p. 390.

extent, he would easily become embroiled in much more than a simple, factual medical prognosis. Presenting so unwelcome a prospect is bound to meet with a strong—and, according to many of the treatment personnel, "unmanageable"—emotional reaction from parents; among other things, it so threatens basic life-values which they cherish for the child, such as physical attractiveness, vocational achievement, a good marriage, and, perhaps most of all, his being perceived and responded to in society as "normal, like everyone else." Moreover, to the extent to which the doctor feels some professional compunction to so inform the parents, the bustling, time-conscious work milieu of the hospital supports him in the convenient rationalization that, even were he to take the trouble, the family could not or would not understand what he had to tell them anyway.[9] Therefore, in hedging, being evasive, equivocating, and cutting short his contact with the parents, the doctor was able to avoid "scenes" with them and having to explain to and comfort them, tasks, at least in the hospital, often viewed as onerous and time-consuming.

Second, since the parents had been told repeatedly during the first weeks of the child's illness that the outcome was subject to great uncertainty, it was not difficult for them, once having accepted the idea, to maintain and even to exaggerate it, particularly in those cases in which the child's progress fell short of full recovery. For, equivocally, uncertainty can be grounds for hope as well as despair; and when, for example, after six months of convalescence the child returned home crippled, the parents could and characteristically did interpret uncertainty to mean that he still stood a good chance of making a full and natural recovery in the indefinite future. The belief in a recuperative moratorium was held long after there was any real possibility of the child's making a full recovery, and with a number of families it had the unfortunate effect of diverting them from taking full advantage of available rehabilitation procedures and therapies. In fact, with few exceptions the parents typically mistook rehabilitation for cure, and, because little was done to correct this misapprehension, they often passively consented to a regimen prescribed for the child which they might have rejected had they known that it had nothing to do with effecting a cure.[10]

Last, it must be noted that in the art (as opposed to the science and technique) of medicine, a sociologically inescapable facet of treatment—often irrespective of how much is clinically known or unknown—is frequently that of somehow getting the patient and his family to accept, "put up with," or

9. *Ibid.*, p. 391. Particularly with working-class families, of which there were ten out of fourteen in the study, the propensity of doctors (and other professionals, for that matter) to resort to this particular rationalization is accentuated accordingly. However, the barriers toward giving any parent this kind of information appeared so pervasive that the four lower-middle-class and middle-class families fared hardly any better.

10. See W. E. Moore and M. N. Tumin, "Some Social Functions of Ignorance," *American Sociological Review*, 14 (December, 1949), 787-795.

"make the best of" the socially and physically disadvantageous consequences of illness. Both patient and family are understandably reluctant to do this at first, if for no other reason than that it usually entails a dramatic revaluation in identity and self-conception. Not only in paralytic poliomyelitis but in numerous other chronic and long-term illnesses, such as cardiac disease, cancer, tuberculosis, mental illness, and diabetes, such is usually the case. Depending on a number of variables, not the least of which are those of personality, the cultural background of the family, and the treatment setting, a number of strategems beside that of rendering a full and frank diagnosis and prognosis (even when clinically known) are open to the physician who must carry the family through this difficult period.[11] Whereas the evasiveness and equivocality of hospital treatment staff described here may not have been as skilled or effective a means for accomplishing this as others which come to mind, it must in fairness be recognized that there is still little agreement within medical circles on what practice should be in these circumstances. (The perennial debate on whether a patient and his family should be told that he is dying of cancer, and when and how much they should be told, is an extreme though highly relevant case in point.) And perhaps the easiest recourse of the hospital practitioner—who, organizationally, is better barricaded and further removed from the family than, for example, the neighborhood physician—is to avoid it altogether.

Clearly, then, clinical uncertainty is not responsible for all that is not communicated to the patient and his family. Other factors, interests, and circumstances intrude in the rendering of medical prognoses, with the result that what the patient is told is uncertain and problematic may often not be so at all. And, conversely, what he is made to feel is quite certain may actually be highly uncertain. As the rough fourfold schema of Figure 16.1 suggests, there are at least two modes of communication [(2) and (3)] that reveal a discrepancy between what the doctor knows and what he tells the patient. Before turning to these, however, we shall consider two "pure," non-discrepant modes [(1) and (4)].

The first of these, "Communication" (1), refers to the common occurrence in which the physician can, in accordance with the state of medical knowledge and his own skill, make a reasonably definite prognosis of the condition requiring treatment and communicate it to the patient in terms sufficiently comprehensible to him. Though not always as uncomplicated as it sounds, this is perhaps the main kind of exchange of information between doctors and patients, particularly as regards the simple and minor ailments brought daily to the average practitioner's attention. It is also, of course, the ideal mode of communication toward which the relationship of doctor and patient universally aspires.

11. Doctors are by no means the only ones who are routinely called upon to shepherd others through difficult status transitions (See Erving Goffman, "On

	CERTAINTY	UNCERTAINTY
PROGNOSIS GIVEN PATIENT	(1) Communication	(2) Dissimulation
PROGNOSIS NOT GIVEN PATIENT	(3) Evasion	(4) Admission of Uncertainty

Figure 16.1

On the other hand, an "Admission of Uncertainty" (4), where no other prognosis is clinically justifiable, is by its nature a more difficult and unstable mode of communication, the manifestations of which will vary considerably, depending on the personal and institutional contexts of practice. Such instability derives mainly from certain mutually reinforcing interests of the two parties: the doctor, who as a matter of professional obligation seeks to narrow the range of uncertainty as far as possible, and the patient, who wishes simply and often naively to know what is wrong and how he can be made to feel better. These and other pressures that would prevent an open admission of uncertainty can more easily be resisted in the bureaucratized hospital setting—as, indeed, they initially were in the case of the families of the children with polio—than, for example, in neighborhood private practice. For, given the widespread intolerance of uncertainty in our culture, the hospital-anchored physician is better insulated from the prejudices, sensitivities, and economic sanctions of those he treats than is his neighborhood counterpart.[12] The latter, particularly if his practice comes mainly from word-of-mouth referrals by an established clientele, runs the potentially costly risk of driving patients elsewhere, that is, to a more "accomodating" competitor, if he states his uncertainty in too bald and unrelieved a manner. Differential economic and reputational risks of this kind in medical practice may be, incidentally, not wholly unrelated to the increasing contemporary tendency to assign the untreatable, chronic, or highly problematic condition to the relatively impersonal hospital setting, where whatever may occur redounds less decisively to the disadvantage (or credit) of any single responsible individual unless it be of the patient.

Owing in large part to a currently inadequate scientific grounding, certain fields of medical practice, as psychiatry, permit little more than admissions of uncertainty in a very large number of cases. Yet, even here, it is to be questioned whether the office psychiatrist can as a matter of course adopt the

Cooling the Mark out," *Psychiatry*, 15 [November, 1952], 451-463).

12. Cf. Eliot Freidson, "Client Control and Medical Practice," *American Journal of Sociology*, 65 (January, 1960), 374-382.

same unyielding, noncommittal, antiprognostic stance with his private, fee-paying patients as does the state-hospital psychiatrist with the severely mental-ly ill and their families—this despite the fact that nowadays, as with pneu-monia and the common cold, the psychopathology treated in the mental hospital affords better grounds for prognosis than do the psychoneuroses and character disorders seen in the consulting room. Nonetheless, in the case of the latter, there is usually held out—after all due qualification and reservation—a vague, implied possibility that somehow "a better adjust-ment," "a more satisfactory utilization of personality resources," etc., may be induced.

As these remarks imply, "Dissimulation" (2)—the rendering of a prognosis which the physician knows to be unsubstantiated clinically—is the more like-ly if the doctor's reputation and livelihood are derived for the most part from the favorable opinions and referrals of an independent lay clientele. Sheer professional vanity may, of course, also enter in. The subtleties, ruses, and deceptions that betoken dissimulation, from the innocuous sugar-pill placebo to unwarranted major surgery, are too many and too imaginatively varied to consider here. But it is essentially this guise of medical practice that has historically been the butt of much lively ridicule and satire, as, for example, in the fumbling presumptions of Sterne's Dr. Slop and the excruciating ministrations of Romains' Dr. Knock. More venial forms of the art are sometimes resorted to in order to delay until the physician has had a chance to observe how a condition develops or until protracted laboratory investigations are completed. Since so many of the undiagnosable illnesses and ailments that are brought to doctors would "take care of them-selves" in any case, the judicious employment of dissimulation is perhaps not so hazardous from the therapeutic standpoint as one might at first conclude. That it often affords the patient a significant measure of psycho-logical relief from anxiety is, in fact, cited by some in its defense, albeit with the qualification that it should not be used in cases where anything serious might be expected.

"Evasion" (3)—the failure to communicate a clinically substantiated prog-nosis—has already been considered at some length. As noted, this was the primary mode of communication employed by the hospital treatment staff when confronted with the queries and concerns of the parents. Little need be added here except to emphasize that the informal institutionaliza-tion of this mode is closely related to the practitioner's ability to remove himself from the many "technically secondary" (i.e., nonorganic) problems and issues that often follow in the wake of serious illness in the family. The large hospital, with its complex proliferation of specialized services and per-sonnel, is particularly conducive to it, especially if the attending physician is not the patient's own but someone assigned to him.[13]

13. See T. Burling, E. M. Lentz, and R. N. Wilson, *The Give and Take in Hospitals* (New York: G. P. Putnam's Sons, 1956), pp. 317-333. The treatment of polio is

The discussion carries no implication that physicians will, in accordance with the setting of their practice and the kinds of illnesses they treat, invariably, or even primarily, address themselves to questions of prognostic certainty and uncertainty in the manner outlined. Nor is it suggested that important shifts from one mode of communication to another do not occur at different stages of treatment of particular patients. Our aim has been rather to temper to some extent the predominantly cognitive emphasis that the issue of uncertainty has received in medical sociology, as if all that passed for uncertainty or certainty in the communication between doctor and patient were wholly a function of the current state of scientific and clinical knowledge. In demonstrating that other values and interests also influence the doctor-patient transaction, we have done little more than exemplify a familiar sociological axiom, namely, that this, too, is anchored in society, and we must perforce take account of its numerous nonrational and irrational elements.

---

highly specialized, and in none of the fourteen cases was the hospitalized child treated by a family physician. Moreover, the very considerable costs of treatment, far beyond the means of all but the wealthy, were borne in whole or very large part by the National Foundation and not by the families themselves. This served to reduce further the claims the parents felt they could make on the doctor's time and attention.

17

AILON SHILOH

Equalitarian and Hierarchal Patients: An Investigation among Hadassah Hospital Patients

The Problem

The hospital has been termed one of the most complex social organizations of any place of work in the Western culture. Social organization in this sense refers to the formal and informal network of professions and roles through which the coordinated tasks considered necessary to patient care are structured and executed. The modern university hospital considerably complicates this network in that it adds on such multiple goals as teaching and research. Such a hospital operates at once, as one scientist has put it, as something of a hotel, treatment center, laboratory, and university.[1]

Human beings deemed sufficiently malfunctioning to warrant their admittance into such a hospital are immediately plunged into this complex social organization with its multiple roles and goals.

The process of hospitalization, for such patients, is often the involuntary exposure to, and participation in, this social complex while undergoing treatment for diagnosed or discovered malfunctions.

It has occasionally been considered that the manner in which the patient comprehends this complex could have a direct bearing on his personal hospital prognosis and posthospital performance.

Reprinted from *Medical Care*, 3 (1965), pp. 87-95, by permission of the author and the publisher.

This investigation was initiated and conducted with the encouragement and stimulation of Professor Sidney L. Kark. Dr. Jack Karpas, Deputy Director-General of the Hadassah Medical Organization, provided invaluable administrative assistance. Professors Joannes Juda Groen, Nathan Rabinovici, Moshe Rachmilewitz, and Nathan Saltz, and the personnel of the internal medicine and surgery wards wherein the investigation was conducted, are thanked for their exemplary courtesy and cooperation. Financial assistance from the Israel Institute for Anthropological Research is gratefully acknowledged.
    1. R. N. Wilson, "The Social Structure of a General Hospital," *The Annals of the*

This consideration has been seriously investigated in a number of studies of chronic mental patients. By various methods, Belknap,[2] Caudill,[3] Goffman,[4] and Greenblatt,[5] for example, have demonstrated that the manner in which the patient comprehends the social organization into which he has been placed may directly affect his health progress during and after hospitalization.

So demonstrative have been these studies of patient comprehension that many authorities agree with Ozarin's trenchant conclusion: "... much of the pathological behavior of patients is a result of their hospital experience rather than a manifestation of their mental illness."[6]

The obvious conclusion, suggests Vitale,[7] is that mental chronic hospitalized behavior is profoundly determined by the institution and that, accordingly, it, as well as the patient, merits serious consideration.

While there is a growing literature on this subject (see Rosenberg[8] for a recent bibliography) only a few studies have been concerned with the broader aspects of long-term institutionalized behavior (e.g. Borman[9]).

Very few serious studies, however, notes Wilson,[10] have been concerned with the reaction of the normal short-term patient under exposure to the rapid-turnover general hospital. Their patterns of comprehensions may be frequently commented on in such hospital journals as *Modern Hospital, Hospital Management, Hospitals,* and *Hospital Progress*, but the emphasis too frequently is derived from or oriented to the hospital staff, rather than the hospital patient.

Wilson has termed such a patient *terra incognita* in that he is often the "...forgotten man of hospital research." There are, noted Wilson, still few current studies that focus directly on the patient's hospital experience.

In a review article, Esther Lucile Brown[11] considered the psychosocial needs and the degree to which the hospital structure and staff perceive and cater to these needs.

American Academy of Political and Social Science, 346 (1963), 67.

2. I. Belknap, *Human Problems of a State Mental Hospital* (New York: McGraw-Hill, 1956).

3. W. Caudill, *The Psychiatric Hospital as a Small Society* (Cambridge: Harvard University Press, 1958).

4. E. Goffman, *Asylums* (New York: Doubleday, 1961).

5. M. Greenblatt, D. J. Levinson and R. H. Williams, eds., *The Patient and the Mental Hospital* (New York: The Free Press, 1957).

6. L. D. Ozarin, "Moral Treatment and the Mental Hospital," *American Journal of Psychiatry*, 3 (1954), 371-378.

7. J. H. Vitale, "The Therapeutic Community: A Review Article," mimeographed report, no date.

8. L. Rosenberg, "The Social Behavior of Hospitalized Psychiatric Patients: A Preliminary Bibliography, mimeographed report, University of Chicago (1963).

9. L. D. Borman, "Institutions and the Institutionalized Patient," mimeographed report (1963).

10. *Op. cit.,* pp. 70-71.

11. Esther L. Brown, "Meeting Patient's Psychosocial Needs in the General Hospital," *Annals of the American Academy of Political and Social Science,* 346 (1963), 117-125.

In this article, and also in an earlier monograph,[12] Dr. Brown concluded that despite the fact that the concept of "total patient care" was extensively promoted, in reality the hospital and the hospital staff are still trained almost exclusively to treat disease and to make patients physically comfortable.

Thus, many patients, she summarized: "...perceive their hospitalization as characterized by unallayed anxiety, loneliness, boredom, or frustration."

The present study has attempted to consider only certain aspects of this overall problem and has targeted its investigation on patients' comprehension of and reaction to specific aspects of their hospitalization experience.

The Hospital Setting

The Rothschild-Hadassah University Hospital is located above the village of Ein Karem along the western border of Jerusalem. The hospital consists of twenty-eight medical and surgical departments and thirty-five institutes and laboratories, and is staffed by 1,600 doctors, nurses, and workers.[13]

Annually, some 16,000 in-patients, 200,000 out-patients and 15,000 emergency cases are treated. Students of the Schools of Medicine, Dentistry, and Nursing use the hospital as their focal learning center. In addition, a comprehensive research program of basic and clinical medicine is structured and conducted.

Patients interviewed in this study were selected from the surgery and internal medicine departments. In December 1962,[14] the nominal bed strength for the two internal medicine wards was 82; and for the two surgery wards 44. For all four wards, bed occupancy was over 90 percent and individual patient average length of stay was 14 days. Per 100 discharged patients, between 3 to 5 percent of the patients died in hospital.

Methodology

Interview techniques were tested, revised, and finalized during an introductory period on the four wards in the autumn of 1963, and the formal interviews were conducted during the winter of 1963-64.

Each interview consisted of three parts: a one-page closed questionnaire recording basic demographic data particular to each patient; followed by a series of four open-end questions addressed to each patient concerning the

12. Esther L. Brown, *Newer Dimensions of Patient Care, Part II: Improving Staff Motivation and Competence in the General Hospital* (New York: Russell Sage Foundation, 1962).

13. I am indebted to Mr. Lucien Harris for his prompt assistance in providing me with factual data concerning the hospital staff and programme.

14. *Statistical Report for the Year 1962,* Hadassah Medical Organization, Jerusalem (1963).

(1) nature, (2) cause, (3) treatment, and (4) prognosis of his hospital condition.

("What was the condition that put you into hospital?"; "What do you think caused this condition?"; "What treatment are you receiving for this condition here in hospital?"; "What do you expect this condition to be when you leave the hospital?")

The third part consisted of four sketches each representing a specific hospital scene. As each sketch was shown, in the order Figures 17.1 to 17.4, the patient was asked: "In your opinion, what does this sketch represent?"

The patient population interviewed represented a random selection of the patients hospitalized in the four wards during the period of study.

The Interviewed Patient Population

Sixty patients were interviewed, all of them Jewish and citizens of Israel. Except for six patients who were, singly, from Haifa, Bnei Braq, Beersheva, a kibbutz in the Jordan Valley, a kibbutz in the Judean Hills, and a moshav near Ashdod, they all lived in Jerusalem.

Of the total 60 patients, 30 of whom were from the internal medicine wards and 30 from the surgery wards, slightly under half were males (28:60), and almost two-thirds were between the ages of 30 to 59 (39:60).

Eighty percent of these patients were married. Of the remainder—two females under 18 and four adult males were single; and six of the patients aged 60 and over were widowed.

One-quarter of the patients were *sabras*—native-born Israelis—and another quarter of the patients were from countries of the Middle East. Except for three patients born in English-speaking countries of the West, all the remaining patients were born in Eastern European countries.

Of the 45 foreign-born patients, 20 were resident in the country prior to the independence of the state (May 1948), 12 had immigrated during the years 1948 to 1953, 10 had immigrated during the years 1953 to 1958, and 3 had immigrated since 1958.

In addition to the three members of agricultural settlements, patients' occupations ranged along an urban occupational distribution from the professional to managerial, clerical, and skilled workers, to the semiskilled and unskilled workers.

Findings

The four open-end questions addressed to the patients concerning the nature, cause, treatment, and prognosis of the condition necessitating their hospitalization revealed a distinct gap between the comprehension possessed by patients concerning their prehospitalization and hospitalization experience.

Without exception, patients were prompt to reply, articulate, and replete with details as to the nature and cause of their condition prior to hospitalization, at the very time that they were hesitant, brief, and vague in their replies as to the treatment and prognosis aspects of this condition within the hospital.

In reply to the two questions: "What was the condition that put you into hospital?" and "What do you think caused this condition?", patients were wont to launch into five- to ten-minute recitations describing the internal and external manifestations of the conditions and detailing the personal, familial, and community factors determining its present aggravation.

("Three years ago I was carrying a heavy sack of vegetables up four flights of stairs during a *chamsin* . . . "; "Two weeks ago we got a new director who took an immediate dislike to me . . . "; "After the birth of my fourth child, I began to put on weight . . . "; "For a long time I've had trouble with my stomach, but last Friday, on my way home from the synagogue, I got these sudden, sharp pains . . . "; "About a week ago, I began to turn yellow all over . . .).

Of the 60 patients, 3 attributed the cause of their condition to supernatural forces: an adult male born in Turkey but resident in Israel for over forty years attributed his weak condition to the evil eye put on him by a fellow co-worker; a Yemenite woman, resident in Israel since 1950, attributed her intestinal difficulties to "a sin" she had committed in her youth; and a recent Moroccan immigrant, suffering from high fever and aching joints, described her immigrant flat as cold, windy, and damp, and concluded "the evil spirits that live there made me ill."

Among the 27 European-born patients, there were eight references to concentration-camp experiences as the cause of their present condition.

A young Czech woman explained that on the day she arrived in Auschwitz, as a girl of 14, her mother, father, four brothers and sisters, aunt and grandmother were taken away and gassed. Now happily married and the mother of three children, she suffers from severe stomach cramps and chest pains which began, she says, on that day.

A Polish woman, suffering from dysentery, dizziness, weakness, and high blood pressure, worked in forced labor in the concentration camp and, she said, "The body must pay for it."

A Rumanian male, suffering from heart trouble, worked in an office disposing of Jewish "evidence." "Now," he concluded, "what else can I expect."

A young Czech male, who also spent his childhood in Auschwitz, and whose entire family perished there, explained his recurrent stomach pains as due to his starting "to live a normal life too late."

A Hungarian woman, who lost her husband and child in Auschwitz, attributed the cause of the swelling in her legs and the sharp pains around her heart to the fact that "All those years I kept it in me and stayed alive."

A Hungarian male, hospitalized for weight loss, sweating, dizziness, and diarrhea, explained that since Treblinka, "I have forgotten how to laugh."

Two patients suffering from rheumatism and bronchitis attributed the cause to concentration camp exposure, and one male, suffering from severe lower extremity malfunctioning, attributed it simply to "routine beatings."

TREATMENT AND PROGNOSIS

In reply to the two questions: "What treatment are you receiving for this condition here in hospital?" and "What do you expect this condition to be when you leave the hospital?" patients replied, after long pauses, hesitantly, briefly, vaguely, and often with a series of disjointed words or phrases.

Treatment consisted of "examinations," "an operation," "diet," "rest," "aspirins," "pills," "red pills," "injections," "drops," "a lot of things," "many things."

Other patients replied: "How do I know?"; "I don't know"; "You're asking me?"; "Why ask me"; "I don't know about such things"; "It's written down in my file."

A Yemenite woman complained that she wasn't receiving any treatment at all. They were only taking blood from her and she was weak and needed every drop that she had.

An Iraqui woman replied, "God knows! They're always taking blood from me. Look, my right arm is dead!"

A Moroccan laborer, scheduled to undergo an operation the next day, after long thought replied, "I don't know."

One aged Polish widower replied that he didn't know what his treatment was because "I'm a good patient. I don't ask questions." Four other patients replied in a similar vein.

A religious Polish shopkeeper explained that he was on his way to Heaven but the treatment in Hadassah restored him to life. Just what that treatment consisted of, he was not certain—"Ask the messenger of God, the physician."

Five further religious patients stated that they prayed all the time while in hospital that God would strengthen his messengers—the physicians. What their hospital treatment consisted of was of secondary importance to the fact that God was determining it.

Of the total 60 patients, only 2 stated that they did not know or care to comprehend their hospital treatment.

One middle-aged male patient replied that while in Auschwitz, where he had worked as a grave digger, he had made an agreement with Satan that as long as he worked long and hard Satan would leave him alone. "And," concluded the patient, "I'm still working long and hard."

Another patient, a Hungarian widower, stated: "The doctors here go their way and I go my way. They don't listen to me so I don't listen to them. Dr.—— of Tel-Aviv is my doctor and I am taking all his medicine even here in hospital."

The only interviewed patient who subsequently died in hospital expressed strong fears concerning his lack of comprehension of his hospital treatment.

("Tell me, what kind of an operation am I going to have? Do I really need it?")

Patients manifested a similar lack of comprehension as to the exact prognosis of the condition for which they had been hospitalized and none of them mentioned any aspect of posthospital performance as possibly essential or useful to ensure or maintain a positive prognosis.

Most frequently, after long silences, patients would reply that they expected to be "all right." Seven orthodox Jews replied with an invocation to God ("*Baruch Ha'Shem*").

Twelve patients replied that they were looking forward to going home to rest and obtain some sleep. As one of these patients states, "I'm in hospital to get cured, I'll go home to get well."

Eighteen patients were negative as to their hospitalized condition prognosis. One patient expected to go home to starve ("I'm too weak to work and there is no one to care for me. I'll just quietly starve to death"), five others stated specifically that they expected to go home to die as they could see no way of altering or improving their way of life.

Seven others, women, stated that there was so much work waiting for them at home that they soon expected to be back in hospital, and five patients replied, gloomily, that as there was no one to care for them at home, they could only stay well by remaining in hospital.

Of the three patients who had attributed the course of their hospitalized condition to supernatural force, not one was sanguine as to the hospital prognosis.

The Yemenite patient who considered her illness to have been caused by a personal sin replied that she expected to go home to die. "It doesn't matter," she kept repeating, "I return home to die."

The Turkish adult who claimed that his illness was caused by a fellow-worker wanted to know what the doctors were going to do to prevent the evil eye from attacking him again, and the Moroccan immigrant who attributed her complaints to evil spirits resident in her flat asked if she could spend the rest of the rainy season in the hospital in order to remain well.

One patient explained that she was sure she was being sent home too early, before she was fully recovered, but when she had mentioned this to the physician, he replied, she claimed, "You are well enough to return home. Hadassah is not a hotel."

"EQUALITARIAN" AND "HIERARCHAL" PATIENTS

During the course of these interviews it soon became apparent that at least two types of patients were being investigated: the "Equalitarians"— those desirous of efficiently achieving a successful treatment, a positive prognosis, and a prompt hospital discharge by joint participation with the hospital on an equal basis; and the "Hierarchals"—those desirious of achieving similar goals, though perhaps not always as efficiently and promptly, by occupying perceived subservient hospital roles.

The reaction of equalitarian patients to their manifest lack of comprehension of the treatment and prognosis aspects of their hospital condition was that of resentment.

In varying degrees of articulation they stated that while they had realized that their entry into hospital necessitated a loss of personal independence they had not realized how little responsibility for making decisions would be left to them.

Once within the walls of the hospital, on the hospital bed, they complained that they were rarely asked to participate in making crucial decisions or even made aware that such decisions had to be made.

Equalitarian patients reported that they were subjected to tests and examinations, injections and probes, often of a strange, painful, frightening, or embarrassing nature, generally in semipublic conditions, and yet, they complained, it was rarely explained to them why the tests were being conducted or what the findings were.

These patients were acutely aware of their lack of comprehension of the treatment and prognosis aspects of their hospitalized condition and their resentment would be manifest in the ambivalent manner with which they acknowledged any improvement in their physical condition.

While such patients would indicate general satisfaction with the purely technical and professional aspects of their hospital treatment, they were irritated by the impersonal, noncommunicative process with which it was conducted.

Equalitarian patients were quick to emphasize the technical achievement within the hospital, the undoubted professional proficiency of the hospital staff, and the obvious pressure under which the personnel were working, but they coupled this with irritation at the hospital role assigned to them as patients—to be docile, passive, prone recipients.

One such patient summed up a long harangue of this nature by stating, "I'm all right as long as I know what is happening to me, but here I don't know anything."

Equalitarian patients were prone to voice niggling complaints about the hospital: "There's been dust under my bed for a week"; "Why can't I have a flask of cold water always by my bedside?"; "This ward is so noisy"; "Typical plain, cold hospital food"; "I hate these pyjamas"; and emphasize how much they were looking forward to returning home.

Hierarchal patients did not view their lack of comprehension with the same gravity.

For these patients it was a relief that others assumed the responsibilities, made the decisions, initiated and consummated the programs. These patients were more content to lie in bed and be the passive recipients.

The tests and examinations impressed them with the complexity and excellence of the care they were receiving, and any attached unpleasantness was interpreted as an unfortunate necessary by-product.

Hierarchal patients were pleased with the material comforts of the hospital and grateful for the attention and treatment they were receiving.

Any supposed depersonalization was interpreted by them as the normal pattern of behavior within a hierachy where they, as patients, were on the lowest rung.

Such patients were in no particular hurry to return home. They found the hospital to be "relaxing," "warm," "clean and comfortable." They enjoyed "eating good food" and being "well-cared for."

These patients stated a reluctance to be discharged from the hospital "too quickly" and suggested that they remain in hospital until they are "really better."

What *did* worry hierarchal patients was that, in addition to being ill, they had problems—generally of a financial or familial nature—and it was about these problems that they were articulate and requested assistance.

Hierarchal patients often perceived the hospital and its apparently unlimited resources as a logical source of assistance for solving these problems and, when this assistance was generally limited to the improvement of their physical health, they too became resentful.

The fact was, it soon became clear, equalitarian and hierarchal patients manifested striking dissimilar patterns of perceived patient role and expected hospital role, and their reactions to their mutual lack of comprehension of the treatment and prognosis aspects of their hospitalized condition was merely one indication of these dissimilarities.

Another indication of these dissimilarities was picked up in the responses to the four hospital sketches (Figures 17.1 to 17.4), the third part of the interview.

Equalitarian patients consistently interpreted Figure 17.1 from their own personal negative experiences.

"A typical hospital scene. I asked the nurse to give me a clean washcloth, I like to wash frequently, and she said 'all right.' That was three days ago."

"That man has just had a serious operation and wants a nurse. That will take a long time."

"The patient is in pain and calling for the nurse. She is alone and frightened."

"That's me yesterday waiting two hours for the nurse. I just cried and cried."

"If that's at night, he is in luck—night nurses come promptly."

"That patient can't get down from her bed and is calling for the nurse—very unpleasant."

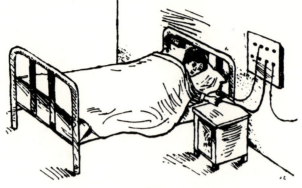

Figure 17.1

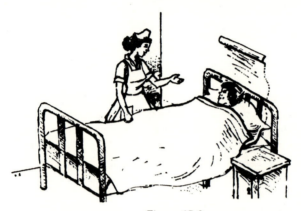

Figure 17.2

Confronted with the same sketch, hierarchal patients were more prone to emphasize their own reluctance to "bother" the nurses.

> "Patient calling for a nurse. I never do. I take care of myself."
> "Patient calling for a nurse. I've not once called for a nurse."
> "Patient calling for a nurse. Doesn't look too serious."
> "Young girl calling for a nurse. They come quickly but I rarely call them."
> "Woman calling for a nurse. She'll come in a few minutes."
> "Personally I never need to ring, and when I do I just wait."
> "I don't like to bother the nurses."

Both equalitarian and hierarchal patients, with one latter exception, replied to Figure 17.2 by voluntarily praising the nurses, emphasizing how hard they worked, how short-staffed they appeared to be, and yet how often they managed to be as friendly as the nurse in the sketch.

However, whereas hierarchal patients were wont to emphasize the pleasant manner of the nurses and how nice it made them, the patients, feel when the nurses spoke with them, equalitarian patients would go on and indicate that being nice wasn't enough; there should be more nurses to allow them to do their job properly—caring for the patients.

Hierarchal patients: "You see the nurse coming to compliment and cheer up a bed-ridden patient. I really feel better when the nurse comes to chat with me." "You see how the patient feels better when the nurse comes to chat with her." "They come around like that in the morning. Sometimes it cheers me up for the whole day."

"The nurses are so friendly and talk with me just like anyone else."

Equalitarian patients: "Well, she finally came."

"Look, her hands are empty, and until she returns with a glass of water . . . "

"When they come to me like that it is usually with medicine."

"It looks like one of the student nurses."

One hierarchal patient complained that he had been in the hospital for twenty-three days and still couldn't get a pair of night socks. "The nurses here are snobs," he concluded.)

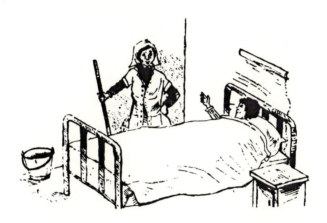

Figure 17.3

Figure 17.3 again highlighted the essential differences between the two types of patients.

Hierarchal patients repeatedly identified the cleaning woman as listening to and helping the patient. They would then go on to volunteer the name of their own cleaning women and the manner in which they chatted with them.

"Esther cleans here. She is very nice."

"I usually ask them what the weather is like outside."

"Shoshana is going to have a baby soon and will have to stop working. She's very worried."

"I speak with the cleaner when she comes by, why not? She is a nice person."

"You'd be surprised at what my cleaner knows about this ward."

"We speak French to each other. She is the only person here who talks to me."

"I'm friendly with all the workers here. It can be very helpful."

Equalitarian patients found this sketch to quite limited. In a disappointed tone they would answer: "Oh, that's a cleaning woman." "A cleaner." "Patient saying hello to the cleaner. I do, as well."

"Looks like some cleaner listening to a *noodnik* of a patient," "I think that our cleaning woman is neater than that."

In response to Figure 17.3, hierarchal patients, as against equalitarian patients, consistenly exhibited a greater identification with the cleaning woman, a stronger awareness of her personality, and a much higher degree of relationship.

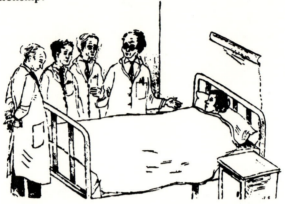

Figure 17.4

Figure 17.4 elicited an immediate and positive interest from all the patients, although, again, actual responses differed between the two types of patients.

Equalitarian patients were wont to indicate that the ward rounds of the professor and his staff were the highlight of their hospital experiences because it afforded them the opportunity to learn something of their hospitalized conditions, its treatment, and prognosis.

Equalitarian patients were quick to point out that there should be more doctors grouped around the bed ("Multiply that number by at least five.") and then went on to state that they, as the patient in the sketch, followed the proceedings with avid interest.

"Here is where I learn what is going on."
"I'm like one of the medical students."
"Afterwards I ask the nurse about any words that I don't understand."
"Believe me, it's always interesting."

Hierarchal patients also considered the ward rounds of the professor and his staff to be a very important aspect of their hospital experience; however, whereas equalitarian patients saw them as unique learning experiences, hierarchal patients were more prone to consider them as further evidence of the great care and attention being given to them.

Hierarchal patients repeatedly emphasized how comforted they felt when the professor and his staff grouped themselves round the bed and how the report and discussion indicated to the patient how much individual care he was receiving. The actual content of these proceedings was rarely as important as the actual demonstration itself.

Recapitulation

The findings of this investigation of 60 Hadassah Hospital patients and their patterns of comprehension of and reaction to specific aspects of their hospitalization experience may be summarized briefly:

(i)   Patients were prompt to reply, were articulate and replete with details as to the nature and cause of their pre-hospitalized condition at the very time that they were hesitant, brief, and vague as to the treatment and prognosis aspects of their condition within the hospital.

(ii)   Patients' reactions to this clear lack of comprehension of these aspects of their hospitalization experiences could be grouped and termed by differences in perceived patient role and expected hospital role.

(iii)   Equalitarian patients perceived their role to be that of equal partners with the hospital in the mutual goals of successful treatment and prompt discharge, and they expected the hospital to provide them with the information necessary for the consummation of these mutual goals.

(iv)   Hierarchal patients perceived their role to be that of passive, grateful recipients within a rich-in-resources hospital, and they expected the hospital to assist them in solving certain of their personal, as well as purely physical, problems.

(v)   Both equalitarian and hierarchal patients were resentful, accordingly, when the hospital did not manifest a satisfactory agreement with these perceived or expected roles.

(vi)   Further insight into the differences between equalitarian and hierarchal patients was provided by an analysis of their reactions to four hospital sketches (Figures 17.1 to 17.4).

(vii)   Equalitarian patients were wont to complain of poor staff service, although not directed at the nurses *per se,* were indifferent to the cleaning staff around them every day, and enjoyed the medical ward rounds as an opportunity to learn about their hospital condition, treatment, and prognosis.

(viii)   Hierarchal patients were reluctant to call for staff, more desirous of attending to their own needs, buoyed up by personal visits of nurses, on familiar and even intimate terms with the cleaning staff, and appreciative of the medical ward rounds as an additional demonstration of the professional care and attention they were receiving.

Discussion

It is not without justification that Wilson has called the short-term general hospital patient *terra incognita*. The fact is, despite the massive number of studies conducted within the hospital, only a few have been concerned directly with the patient as an individual human being.

Furthermore, despite the growing literature documenting critical differences in ill-health and behavior among the world populations and cultures (see, for example, Apple,[15] Jaco,[16] Koos,[17] Paul,[18] and Rubin[19]), rarely have such studies been conducted among sick persons within the confines of the general hospital.

On the theoretical level, Talcott Parsons[20] has structured the value system of the American white middle-class toward the sick, and Esther Lucile Brown,[21] in an exhaustive three-part review of general hospitals, has emphasized that patients may manifest different needs, but critical hospital studies are still lacking for their adequate substantiation and amplification.

In one approach, Ernest Dichter[22] conducted a large-scale investigation into the attitudes and motivations of 160 hospital patients and concluded, as his "most significant finding," that patients regress to a child's irrationality.

Weston LaBarre[23] spelled out the "family" that such patients construct wherein the physician becomes the "father" and the nurse becomes the "mother," and Sam Schulman[24] went on to a detailed analysis of the mother surrogate role of the nurse within such a "family."

Whatever the validity of these generalizations, they tend to consider hospital patients in the mass—as a unified, homogeneous group—at the very

15. D. Apple, ed., *Sociological Studies of Health and Sickness* (New York: McGraw-Hill, 1960).

16. E. G. Jaco, ed., *Patients, Physicians, and Illness* (Glencoe, Ill.: The Free Press, 1958).

17. E. L. Koos, *The Health of Regionville* (New York: Columbia University Press, 1954).

18 B.J. Paul, *Health, Culture, and Community* (New York: Russell Sage Foundation, 1955).

19. V. Rubin, ed., "Culture, Society, and Health," *The Annals* 84 (1960).

20. T. Parsons, "Definitions of Health and Illness in the Light of American Values and Social Structure", pp. 165-187, and, with with R. Fox, "Illness, Therapy, and the Modern Urban American Family," pp. 234-245, in Jaco, *op. cit.*

21. Esther L. Brown, *Newer Dimensions of Patient Care:* Part 1. "The Use of the Physical and Social Environment of the General Hospital for Therapeutic Purposes" (1961), Part 2. "Improving Staff Motivation and Competence in the General Hospital" (1962), Part 3. "Patients as People" (1964). (New York: Russell Sage Foundation).

22. E. Dichter, "The Hospital-Patient Relationship," *Modern Hospital* (1954, 1955).

23. W. LaBarre, "The Patient and His Families," *Casework Papers* (1958) Reprinted in *Child-Family Digest* (1959), 9-18.

24. S. Schulman, "Basic Functional Roles in Nursing: Mother, Surrogate, and Healer," pp. 528-537, in Jaco, *op. cit.*

time that numerous studies at the community level are throwing up subtle and profound cultural differences.

One of the very few hospital studies which has attempted to investigate beyond these generalizations, and therefore which is of value in discussing the present Hadassah findings, is Rose Laub Coser's study of 53 patients in a predominantly Jewish hospital in the eastern United States.[25]

After an intensive period of observation within the hospital, Dr. Coser interviewed these patients on the day of their discharge from the medical and surgical wards (Appendix).

She found two types of patient adaption to the hospital—those "hospital-oriented" and those "outside-oriented."

According to Dr. Coser, "outside-oriented" patients tended to be younger, see the hospital more in instrumental terms, and manifest the desire to be discharged quickly. These patients tended to be surgical rather than medical patients and were more productive of answers regarding their ideas of a "good doctor" and "good nurse."

"Hospital-oriented" patients, predominantly looking for gratification of primary needs, usually felt that the hospital provided them with a "home," were more prone to acquiesce in the hospital setting, felt less deprived of their normal life, and made few or no suggestions for the possible improvement of the comfort of the patients.

There is the attraction to postulate a similarity between "equalitarian" and "outside-oriented" patients, and "hierarchal" and "hospital-oriented" patients, and further studies targeted on the utilization of both methods of investigation may demonstrate this postulated similarity.

The problem of methods, of course, cannot be too casually considered. Although Poincaré is quoted as stating that the natural sciences report on findings, and the social sciences report on methods,[26] Jack Elinson,[27] in a comprehensive review of methodology in medical sociology, found the theoretical level to be characterized by a "low degree of articulation," and he cited discouraging vagaries and generalities of common terminological concepts.

The questions and sketches utilized in this study were carefully prepared so as to minimize cross-cultural differences, but they need to be tested in a wider context within the hospital, and a closer analysis of the characteristics comprising equalitarian and hierarchal type patients must be correlated to such components as age, sex, ethnic group, social class, and hospitalized ward—all of which may be of direct relevance.

25. Rose L. Coser, *Life In the Ward* (East Lansing: Michigan State University Press, 1962).

26. Quoted on p. 14 by Bernard Berelson and Gary A. Steiner, *Human Behavior: An Inventory of Scientific Findings* (New York: Harcourt, Brace, 1964).

27. J. Elinson, "Methods of Sociomedical Research," in *Handbook of Medical Sociology*, H. E. Freeman, S. Levine, and L. G. Reeder, eds. (Englewood Cliffs, N.J.: Prentice-Hall, 1963), pp. 449-471.

Simmons and Wolff [28] have reported social class behavioral differences among hospital patients that bear a familiarity to the descriptions of Coser and the present study.

Despite differences in methods, locality, and terminology, it may be that "upper class" (Simmons and Wolff), "outside-oriented" (Coser), and "equalitarian" (Shiloh) patients are comparable groups, and the same may also apply to "lower class," "hospital-oriented," and "hierarchal" patients.

It is only by direct hospital patient investigations that these patterns can be more precisely defined and more fully characterized.

The large-scale follow-up study must also deal with belief in the supernatural, particularly in the causation of body malfunctioning, and its influence on hospital treatment and prognosis.

Evidence from the present study indicates that this crucial reality for the hospital patient is unclearly appraised and inadequately treated in Western medical practice.

In a series of recent articles, Lewis and Lopreato[29] have updated Malinowski's[30] original contribution and have provided a useful, testable hypothesis for its application in the field of medicine:

("Arationality [of a magico-religious or metaphysical nature] in the prevention or treatment of an illness stand in *(a)* direct relation to perceived chance or danger inherent in the illness, and *(b)* in inverse relation to medical knowledge about that illness.")[31]

There are at least two more aspects of these findings which merit discussion. As noted, all the patients in this study were Israeli Jews.

Zborowski,[32] Croog,[33] and Mechanic,[34] in their recent studies in the United States, have reported that American Jews differ from their Christian brethren in their reaction to pain (Zborowski), sensitivity to and concern with physical symptoms (Croog), illness behavior (Mechanic).

These studies have demonstrated, according to the authors, that the Jews are sufficiently different to warrant calling them, in Mechanic's term, the "special case."

28. L. W. Simmons and H. G. Wolff, *Social Science in Medicine* (New York: Russell Sage Foundation, 1954).

29. L. S. Lewis, "Knowledge, Danger, Certainty, and the Theory of Magic," *American Journal of Sociology*, 69 (1963), 7-12; and L. S. Lewis and J. Lopreato, "Arationality, Ignorance, and Perceived Danger in Medical Practices," *American Sociological Review* 27 (1962), 508-514.

30. B. Malinowski, "Magic, Science, and Religion," in *Science, Religion, and Reality*, James Needham, ed. (New York: Macmillan, 1925).

31. Lewis and Lopreato, *op. cit*, p. 508 (italics in original).

32. M. Zborowski, "Cultural Components in Responses to Pain," pp. 256-268 in Jaco, *op. cit.*

33. S. H. Croog, "Ethnic Origins, Educational Level, and Responses to a Health Questionnaire," *Human Organization*, 20 (1961), 65-69.

34. D. Mechanic, "Religion, Religiosity, and Illness Behavior: The Special Case of the Jews," *Human Organization*, 22 (1961), 202-208.

The reasoning to be tested, of course, is to what extent such attributed behavior is a correct description and appraisal of reality. Although the Jerusalem study was not structured to consider this problem directly, findings indicate that such generalizations of "Jewish" behavior may be misleading or shallow.

The evidence from the concentration-camp patients and their tendency to manifest conditions of a nonspecific, generalized malfunctioning nature may provide critical insight into certain of the disorders and survivals among former concentration-camp victims as reported by Nathan *et al,*[35] and suggests a further application of Dvorjetsky's theory of "delayed pathology."[36]

These few considerations for the type of large-scale follow-up investigations desirable are of more than academic interest—they are of direct relevance for optimal functioning of the administrative and professional hospital staff.

Whitehorn,[37] for example, has spelled out in no uncertain terms the current paradoxical decline in public esteem for physicians, when, technically, they are showing the greatest efficiency in curing disease and postponing death.

Although it would seem logical that public esteem for physicians should run parallel with their demonstrated effectiveness in curing disease, Whitehorn has argued that it has not, and he has suggested that much of this decline may be due to the physicians largely ignoring the "personal factors in health and disease, while remaining preoccupied with impersonal factors" (p. 34).

Wilson[38] has attempted to pinpoint this changing physician role by contrasting the traditional charismatic aura surrounding the physician with the present technically skilled, team-approach role assigned to him by a growing number of sophisticated and knowledgeable patients.

In the future, perceives Wilson, the physician's role will be greatly diminished in status, authority, knowledge, and action.

Further evidence of such essential dissatisfaction with the medical profession and the hospital is prominent in such recent studies as Gerda L. Cohen's[39] dramatic account of *What's Wrong with Hospitals.* Ann Cartwright's [40] study of human relations and hospital care, which revealed, among other things, that three out of five patients were dissatisfied in some degree with the

35. T. S. Nathan, L. Eitinger, and H. D. Winnick, "A Psychiatric Study of Survivors of the Nazi Holocaust. A Study in Hospitalized Patients," *Israeli Annals Psychiatry and Related Disciplines,* 2 (1964).

36. M. Dvorjetsky, "Ulcers of the Digestive Tract in Israel," *Dapim Refuim,* 23 (1964).

37. J. C. Whitehorn, "The Doctor's Image of Man," in *Man's Image in Medicine and Anthropology,* I. Galdstone, ed., Monograph IV, Institute of Social and Historical Medicine, The New York Academy of Medicine (New York: International Universities Press, 1963), pp. 3-49.

38. R. N. Wilson, "The Physician's Changing Hospital Role," *Human Organization,* 18 (1959-1960).

39. G. L. Cohen, *What's Wrong With Hospitals?* (London: Penguin, 1964).

40. Ann Cartwright, *Human Relations and Hospital Care* (London: Routledge and Kegan Paul, 1964).

information given to them about their own condition, and Stanley H. King's[41] eloquent advocacy of the need for a "back to the patient" movement.

Appendix. Interview Guide To Patients [42].

1.   When you are sick, would you rather be at home or in hospital?
2.   What do you miss most while you're in the hospital?
3.   What is your idea of a good doctor?
4.   What is your idea of a good nurse?
5.   What is your idea of a good patient?
6.   How do you like the rounds?
7.   How do you like the wards?
8.   Are there any suggestions that you would care to make for a possible improvement of the patients' comfort?
9.   Are you ever bored or restless while you're in the hospital?
10. What will be the first thing you will do when you get home?

41.   S. H.King, *Perceptions of Illness and Medical Practice* (New York: Russell Sage Foundation, 1962).

42. Coser, *op. cit.*, p. 149.

18

JAMES LEO WALSH
RAY H. ELLING

Professionalism and the Poor – Structural Effects and Professional Behavior

While still in its infancy, the comparative study of relations between human service personnel ranked on different levels of the occupational prestige hierachy and impoverished or lower-class clients can be particularly revealing in efforts to understand the role of social stratification as it affects health and welfare activities. In turn, qualification and better understanding of the deep irony Veblen identified as "trained incapacity" can result from such studies, making it possible to design more acceptable and effective forms of human service. This infant area of inquiry concerns itself with the importance of the dynamics of occupational group activities as these activities influence the attitudes and behavior of their members. As such it departs from more traditional emphases.

Sociological inquiries examining factors influencing the interaction between health professionals and lower-class or poor clients can be grouped into three traditional categories. The first includes studies explaining variations in orientations and behavior in terms of differences in the social class levels of those who provide services and those receiving the benefits of that service.[1] The second includes explanations of differences in orientations toward

Reprinted from the *Journal of Health and Social Behavior*, 9 (1968), pp. 16-28, by permission of the authors and the American Sociological Association.

The authors acknowledge assistance from General Support Grant FR 5451-04, National Institutes of Health and the University of Pittsburgh, Graduate School of Public Health, and GM 12367, The National Institute of General Medical Science.

1. See for example Robert Coles, "Psychiatrists and the Poor," *Atlantic*, 214 (July, 1964), 103-106; Lewis Coser, "The Sociology of Poverty," *Social Problems*, 13 (Fall, 1965), 140-148; Kingsley Davis, "Mental Hygiene and the Class Structure," *Psychiatry*, 1 (1938), 55-56; J.M. Ellis, "Socio-Economic Differentials in Mortality from Chronic Diseases," *Social Problems*, 5 (July, 1957), 30-37; August Hollingshead and Frederick Redlich, *Social Class and Mental Illness* (New York: John Wiley, 1958); Lorraine Klerman and P. H. and Camille Lambert, "Attitudes of Private Dentists Toward a Public Dental Care Program," *The Journal of the American Dental Association*, 68 (March, 1964), 416-423; Dwight Macdonald, "Physical and Mental Illness and the Medical Care of the Poor," in Robert E. Will and

clients in terms of bureaucratic organizational factors.[2] The third refers to efforts to outline various characteristics of members of the lower socioeconomic classes making it difficult to provide effective health care to them.[3]

Recently, however, several studies have concluded that the traditional concentration on social class differences and organizational impediments to the service worker-client relationship do not always explain the problems adequately. Authors of these studies have presented evidence that other factors significantly affect this relationship.[4] These "other factors," however, have not been as intensively examined as have the three traditional groupings of factors and influences.

This paper traces the implications of one of these other factors as revealed in a study of professional striving among occupational groups within the field of public health. It is the purpose of the paper to demonstrate empirically that members of groups actively engaged in efforts to improve their status are more negative in their orientations toward lower-class or

Harold G. Vatter, eds., *Poverty in Affluence* (New York: Harcourt, Brace and World, 1965), pp. 173-175; Charlotte Muller, "Income and the Receipt of Medical Care," *American Journal of Public Health*, 55 (April, 1965, 510-521; Leonard Schneiderman, "Social Class, Diagnosis and Treatment," *American Journal of Orthopsychiatry*, 35 (January, 1965), 99-105; Charles V. Willie, "The Social Class of Patients That Public Health Nurses Prefer to Serve," *American Journal of Public Health*, 50 (August, 1960), 1126-1136; Alfred Yankauer, Kenneth Gross, and Salvatore M. Romeo, "An Evaluation of Prenatal Care and Its Relationship to Social Class and Social Disorganization," *American Journal of Public Health*, 43 (August, 1953), 1001-1010; and Alonzo S. Yerby and William Agress, "Medical Care for the Indigent," *Public Health Reports*, 81 (January 1966), 7-11.

2. See for example Joseph Ben-David, "The Professional Role of the Physician in Bureaucratized Medicine," *Human Relations*, 11 (1958), 255-274; Peter M. Blau, "Orientations Toward Clients in a Public Welfare Agency," *Administrative Science Quarterly*, 5 (1960-1961), 341-361; Coser, *op. cit.*, p. 146; Morris Janowitz and William Delany, "The Bureaucrat and the Public," *Administrative Science Quarterly*, 2 (1957-58), 141-162; Merton Kahne, "Bureaucratic Structure and Impersonal Experience in Mental Hospitals," *Psychiatry*, 22 (November, 1959), 363-375; William Kornhauser, *Scientists In Industry* (Berkeley: University of California Press, 1962); Thomas J. Scheff, "The Societal Reaction to Deviance: Ascriptive Elements in the Psychiatric Screening of Mental Patients in a Midwestern State," *Social Problems*, 11 (Spring, 1964), 491-413; and Harold L. Wilensky, "The Professionalization of Everyone?", *American Journal of Sociology*, 70 (September, 1964), 137-158.

3. See for example Jerome Cohen, "Social Work and the Culture of Poverty," *Social Work*, 9 (January, 1964), 3-11; Jules V. Coleman, "Therapy of the 'Inaccessible' Mentally Ill Patient," (Paper presented at the International Congress of Psychotheraphy, London, August 24, 1964), p. 1; Michael Harrington, *The Other America* (New York: Macmillan, 1962); Elizabeth Herzog, "Some Assumptions About the Poor," *Social Service Review*, 37 (December, 1963), 389-402; Lee Rainwater, *And the Poor Get Children*, (Chicago: Quadrangle Books, 1960); Jona M. Rosenfeld, "Strangeness Between Helper and Client: A Possible Explanation for Non-Use of Available Professional Help." *Social Service Review*, 38 (March, 1964), 17-25; and Alonzo S. Yerby, "The Problems of Medical Care for Indigent Populations," *American Journal of Public Health*, 55 (August, 1965), 1212-1216.

4. Katherine Laughton, Carol W. Buck, and G. E. Hobbs, "Socioeconomic Status and Illness," *Milbank Memorial Fund Quarterly*, 36 (1958), 46-57: Charles Kadushin, "Social Class and the Experience of Ill Health," *Sociological Inquiry*, 34 (Winter, 1964), 67-80, Elaine Cumming, "Allocation of Care to the Mentally Ill,

impoverished clients than are members of similar groups less active in this quest. The inquiry was facilitated by a theoretical framework drawing out similarities in the form and consequences of occupational group striving and some social movements.

Professional Striving as a Social Movement

This theoretical approach has been employed to examine the orientations of three "professional" occupational groups. The theory is not limited to professional occupational groups, however. It has relevance to occupational groups at all levels. Rather than enter the frustrating argument over what makes an occupation a profession or one profession "more professional" than another, we shall follow Becker and suggest that the label "profession" is no more than an everyday usage lending prestige and general approbation to occupational groups which have more or less "arrived." If an occupational group succeeds in winning for itself the title "profession," then it is a profession.[5] All work groups, then, can be placed in a continuum in that all are professional to some degree.[6] While the groups studied in this research are "professions" in Becker's sense, investigations of other human service occupations could be conducted in a similar fashion and in this report, therefore, the terms occupational group and professional group are used interchangeably.

Considering professional occupational groups as social movements is not a unique notion, even though social movement theory and research traditionally have been confined to discussions of far-reaching efforts to outline the processes of tension, growth, and change in a disparate collection of professional groups. The works of Bucher and Strauss, Borman, Eaton, and Elling can be noted.[7]

American Style," (Working Paper #26, Center for Social Organizational Studies, Department of Sociology, University of Chicago); Saxon Graham, "Socio-economic Status, Illness, and the Use of Medical Services," in E. Gartley Jaco, ed., *Patients, Physicians, and Illness* (Glencoe, Ill.: The Free Press, 1958), pp. 129-134; Ray H. Elling, Ruth Whittemore, and Morris Greene, "Patients' Participation in a Pediatric Program," *Journal of Health and Human Behavior*, 1 (Fall, 1960), 183-191; Edward A. Suchman, "Social Factors in Medical Deprivation," *American Journal of Public Health*, 55 (November, 1965), 1725-1733; Peter Kong-Ming New, "Communication: Problems of Interaction Between Professionals and Clients," *Community Mental Health Journal*, (Fall, 1965), 251-255; Blau, *op. cit.*; and Ben-David, *op. cit.*

5. Howard S. Becker, "The Nature of a Profession," *Sixty-First Year-Book of the National Society for the Study of Education, Part II, Education for the Professions* (Chicago: University of Chicago Press, 1962), pp. 27-46.

6. Peter Kong-Ming New, "Is Professionalization Necessary?" (Paper presented at annual meetings of the Pennsylvania League for Nursing, York, Pa., April 6, 1964).

7. Joseph W. Eaton, *Stone Walls Not a Prison Make* (Springfield, Ill.: Charles C. Thomas, 1962); Rue Bucher, "Pathology: A Study of Social Movements Within a Profession," in this volume. Rue Bucher and Anselm Strauss, "Professions in Process" *American Journal of Sociology*, 46 (January, 1961), 325-334; Leonard D. Borman, "A Revitalization Movement in the Mental Health Professions," (Paper presented at the American Orthopsychiatric Association, New York, 1965); and Ray H. Elling, "Occupa-

This perspective enables one to argue that work groups, in a manner similar to social movements, seek to enhance their positions vis-á-vis other occupational groups. Some health professionals are involved in group efforts to achieve a higher or more secure rung on the social ladder for the professional group of which they are members.[8] Goode characterizes these efforts as a struggle in a zero-sum game—one in which there is only a limited supply of power and income available. Therefore, as one group rises another must decline.[9]

Borrowing an argument as old as Durkheim,[10] Goode points out that an industrializing society is a professionalizing society. The process does not occur automatically, however. Struggle is inevitable, for as one group reaches out for a higher place, members of other professions react so as to maintain the integrity and position of their group.[11] This conception of occupational group behavior seems quite compatible with that of social movement theory and research describing the efforts of many groups to advance their ideology or to withstand challenges from new quarters.[12]

Suggesting the utility of this framework, Oswald Hall points out, "Practitioners of a profession become self-conscious about their work, develop collective concerns about their destiny, and take collective steps to fit their work and themselves into the social order.[13]

Considering some potential costs of these collective steps, this paper hypothesizes that as professional groups strive for increased power and prestige, compromises result in the orientations and behavior of members of these service groupings toward indigent or lower-class clients. The compromises can be expected from members of professional groups which are most actively involved in movements to enhance professional standing.

These compromises spring from many sources, of course, but the factor of professional striving seems to be of the utmost importance in efforts to

---

tional Group Striving and Administration in Public Health," in Mary Arnold, Vaughn Blankenship, and John Hell, eds., *Public Health Administration* (New York: Atherton Press, 1967).

8. Bucher and Strauss, *op. cit.*

9. William J. Goode, "The Librarian: From Occupation to Profession? *Library Quarterly*, 31 (October, 1961), 306-320.

10. Emile Durkheim, *The Division of Labor in Society* (Glencoe, Ill.: The Free Press, 1962), pp. 267-270. .

11. William J. Goode, "Encroachment, Charlatanism, and the Emerging Profession: Psychology, Sociology, and Medicine," *American Sociological Review*, 25 (December, 1960), 902-914.

12. See, for example, Sheldon Messinger, "Organizational Transformation: A Case Study of a Declining Social Movement," *American Sociological Review*, 20 (February, 1955), 3-10; Joseph Gusfield, "Social Structure and Moral Reform: A Study of the Women's Christian Temperance Union," *American Journal of Sociology*, 61 (November, 1955), 221-232; and D. Sills, *The Volunteers*, (Glencoe, Ill.: The Free Press, 1957).

13. Oswald Hall, "The Place of the Professions in the Urban Community," in S. D. Clark, ed., *Urbanism and the Changing Canadian Society* (Toronto: University of Toronto Press, 1961), pp. 117-134.

understand them better. As Everett Hughes pointed out, one of the means of identifying "highly professional" occupational groups is by the clients they serve.[14] Ideologically a professional is to serve all who have need of his skills. But, in the competition for a larger share of the professional prestige pie, it may be that one way to advance is to seek to serve a "higher"-class clientele rather than to risk being identified as a servant of the poor or the lower class. As is the case in some social movements, it may be that some professionals internalize certain values of the striving professional group to which they belong and these values affect their orientations toward lower-class or poor clients.

Simmons has lent support to Hughes' observation. He argues that "protestant ethic" values of cleanliness, industry, thrift, deferment of gratification, individual responsibility and rationality are often applied by health professionals assuming that they are universally meaningful and valid.[15] Wyllie carries his argument further by pointing out that such values may be conducive to evaluative approaches to indigent and lower-class clients.[16]

Willie offers some empirical support to this argument. On the basis of his research, Willie concluded that although public health nurses accept patients without regard for their social class positions, they would still prefer to work with patients from the middle class.[17]

Becker, too, has argued along these lines. He pointed out that the typical process of professionalization includes shedding "dirty work" and attempting to devote one's time and energies to other "more professional" activities.[18] We suggest that certain human service workers equate "dirty work" with dealing with undesirable clients. Efforts to advance the prestige and status of the group may, therefore, lead members to view dealing with the lower class or the poor as an obstacle to the quest for higher professional status. Attitudinal and behavioral differences in dealing with these clients may result.[19]

Coser, in an article based on Simmel's insights,[20] argues that the poor are "...Men who have been so defined by society and have evoked particular reactions from it."[21] Hence, the poor have not always been with us. Instead, like Durkheim's criminals,[22] they emerged when society elected to

14. Everett Hughes, "Comment to Roach," *American Journal of Sociology*, 71 (July, 1965), 75-76.

15. Ozzie G. Simmons, "Implications of Social Class for Public Health," *Human Organization*, 16 (Fall, 1957), 7-10.

16. Irving Wyllie, *The Self-Made Man in America: The Myth of Rags to Riches* (New Brunswick: Rutgers University Press, 1954).

17. Willie, *op. cit.*

18. Howard S. Becker, "Some Problems of Professionalization," *Adult Education*, 6 (Winter, 1956), 101-105.

19. Cumming, *op. cit.*

20. Georg Simmel, "The Poor," *Social Problems*, 13 (Fall, 1965), 118-140.

21. Coser, *op. cit.*, p. 141.

22. Emile Durkheim, *The Rules of the Sociological Method* (New York: The Free Press, 1950), p. 35.

recognize poverty as a special status and assigned specific persons to that category.[23] The assignment of people to the category "poor" is forthcoming only at the price of a degradation or stigmatization of the person so assigned.[24]

Perhaps some sort of transference of this stigma is feared by the professionals working with the poor. If so, shedding dirty work may include attempts or desires to be identified as working with a higher-level clientele. Perhaps some public health professionals feel their prestige suffers from too much contact with lower-class patients.[25] The theoretical perspective of this study leads us to suggest that this is exactly the case in certain of the more highly striving work groups.

Methods

To test the hypothesis of this research, 207 public health professionals in the health departments of two large Eastern cities were asked to respond to a 54-item interview schedule. Usable responses were obtained from 198 professionals, including 110 nurses, 72 sanitarians, and 16 M.D.'s. In order to avoid the possibility that different kinds of job tasks may have produced different orientations toward clients, the respondents selected for this study were limited to those who performed similar jobs. The nurses were those who had regularly worked in clinics and carried out home visits in both lower- and middle-class areas. The sanitarians were those whose jobs had involved field contacts with a variety of clients in situations ranging from restaurant and food inspections in both "good" and "greasy spoon" establishments, to answering nuisance complaints and inspecting substandard housing. The physicians were drawn from health officers with administrative duties but who had had clinical experience.

Respondents were chosen on the basis of availability. No random sampling was attempted, but a follow-up investigation of the extent to which the respondents compared with nonrespondents on the basis of age, race, income, and length of employment indicated that the respondents were representative of similar professionals employed in the two health departments.[26] Further comparisons with data gathered in a nationwide study of the public health profession also indicated that the respondents to this study and

23. Coser, *op. cit.*

24. Simmel, *op. cit.*

25. Another problem here is the possibility that the connotation of "public" is often that of being on welfare or otherwise disinherited. Suggestions have come forth that the field change its name to "Community Health" or some other more inclusive term rather than risk having its role become that of caring for but one segment of the total population.

26. These data can be found in James Leo Walsh, "Professional Group Striving and the Orientations of Public Health Professionals Toward Lower-Class Clients," Unpublished Ph.D. dissertation, Department of Sociology, The University of Pittsburgh, 1966, pp. 150-168.

those of the nationwide sample were similar in social background characteristics.[27] Table 18.1, for example, indicates that the social class origins of the respondents to this study and those from similar professions in the nationwide study are not significantly different.

Table 18.1. Social class of respondents to this and nationwide study

Professional Group	Sample Source	I-II (high) N	I-II (high) %	III N	III %	IV-V (low) N	IV-V (low) %	total N	total %
			Social Class of Origin						
M.D.'s	National[a]	327	45	184	26	204	29	715	100
	This study	10	62	3	19	3	19	16	100
	$X^2=1.772$, 2 degrees of freedom, not significant								
Nurses	National	187	14	365	26	825	60	1377	100
	This study	18	17	35	33	53	50	106[b]	100
	$X^2=4.002$, 2 degrees of freedom, not significant								
Sanitarians	National	80	14	161	29	313	57	554	100
	This study	16	22	13	18	43	60	72	100
	$X^2=5.407$, 2 degrees of freedom, not significant								

[a] Made up of industrial physicians, clinical physicians in public health, preventive medicine specialists, and health officers. Minor proportions of the health officers and preventive medicine specialists (epidemiologists) are non-M.D.'s and this may account for the slightly lower social class origins of the nationwide sample.

[b] The social class origins of four of the nurses could not be calculated.

Following the collection of the data, social class, religion, age, and organizational differences between the two health departments—all variables that have been demonstrated to affect orientations toward clients—were controlled and specific attention was paid to determining the influence of professional group striving on the dependent variable—orientations toward lower-class or poor clients. This involved clearing several methodological hurdles.

The first of these was the task of clearly specifying the meaning of "professional striving." The work of Hodge, Siegel, Rossi, and others indicates that the relative prestige of a wide range of occupations has remained remarkably stable over the past 30 years.[28] How, then, can one speak of something called "professional striving"?

27. Ray H. Elling, William P. Shepard, and C. W. Dean, "Study of Public Health Careers," Graduate School of Public Health, The University of Pittsburgh, Pittsburgh, Pa. Method and some findings are presented in William P. Shepard, Ray H. Elling, and Walter F. Grimes, "Study of Public Health Careers: Some Characteristics of Industrial Physicians," *Journal of Occupational Medicine*, 8 (March, 1966), 108-119.

28. Robert W. Hodge, Paul M. Siegel, and Peter H. Rossi, "Occupational Prestige in the United States, 1925-63," *American Journal of Sociology*, 70 (November, 1964), 286-302.

This finding is of little relevance to the theory advanced in this report. To those who put forth real effort to find ways to provide themselves with more pay, power, better working conditions, and a more secure sense of professional status, this finding may be unknown or, if known, it apparently means little or enthusiasm would soon dampen. Whether the objective chances for climbing higher on the prestige ranking are favorable or unfavorable may be irrelevant to some public health workers. Or, if it is relevant, there is nothing in the NORC data to preclude the argument that perhaps several occupational groups are rising in status and that a profession has to exert real effort just to maintain the prestige it currently enjoys.

In this study the concern rested not with the "real" status an occupational group enjoyed nor with the chances it had to raise its stature. The consequences of the act of striving were of concern, not the chances for success.

To rank the three occupational groups along the professional striving dimension, a set of eleven questions was developed from which a professional striving score was ascertained.[29] This score indicated that the public health nurses, with a median striving score of 24.3, were most vigorous in their professional striving. Sanitarians followed with a median striving score of 20, and the professional striving of the public health physicians was lowest at 15.5. The nurses, therefore, became the high strivers in the test of the hypothesis that members of occupational groups energetically striving for professional status will be less favorably oriented toward lower-class or poor clients than will be members of low-striving work groups. The high- and low-striving segments of each occupational group were also ascertained and similar results were predicted when the high-striving segments were compared with the low-striving segments.

Seven items of the professional striving score were subjected to Guttman scale analysis. A coefficient of reproducibility of .83 resulted. This coefficient, while not reaching the .90 level set for Guttman scales nevertheless indicates the presence of a quasi-scale and that our measure of professional striving approaches unidimensionality. In addition, the presence of the quasi-scale enabled us to utilize several items to measure professional striving, not merely one.[30]

29. The score utilized in this research used items from the following sources: Elling, "Occupational Group Striving and Administration in Public Health," *loc. cit.*; Goode, "The Librarian: From Occupation to Profession?" *loc. cit.*; and Wilensky, *op. cit.*, p. 153.

30. The characteristics of occupational group striving stressed in this research included: (1) delegating—or shedding—menial or unpleasant tasks to less highly trained personnel; (2) attempting to assume more responsibilities on a higher level, such as seeking more voice in setting policy or undertaking new and novel activities; (3) seeking to become better known among professional colleagues in order to advance or gain professional respect; and (4) developing or expressing willingness to join a local-level professional organization with close ties to a national professional association, whose purpose is to advance the professional status of the group involved.

Another methodological procedure that merits discussion is the manner in which we went about defining the concept "lower-class" client. Several approaches to this problem were combined. First, we accepted the estimates of the respondents as being most meaningful. Whenever descriptions of clients utilized adjectives such as "lower-class," "lower-income," "poor people," or "slum people," we concluded that the respondent was referring to a lower-class or poor client. When respondents failed to characterize their clientele so graphically, their descriptions of clients were examined for indications that a checklist of attributes developed by Herzog might enable us to determine whether clients described by the respondents could be called poor or lower-class.[31] Finally, if neither of these criteria yielded results, we probed for occupational and educational descriptions of clients and employed the Hollingshead two-factor Index of Social Position.[32]

Testing the assertion that public health professionals belonging to high-striving professional groups would be more negative in orientations toward lower class clients necessitated the utilization of a method to differentiate structural from individual effects. Studies of group-level variables such as professional group striving based on the responses of individuals who are members of these groups face the problem of determining whether the results obtained are a function of the group, the individual, or both.[33] Blau; Davis, Spaeth, and Huson; and Tannenbaum and Bachman have discussed this problem at some length and have introduced the concepts "individual effect," "structural effect," and "compositional effect" into the sociological vocabulary.[34]

The specific techniques for the determination of individual and structural effects vary somewhat but Tannenbaum and Bachman suggest that partial correlation facilitates the computation in research such as that reported in this paper. In this case a structural effect is measured in terms of the correlation between group striving and orientations toward lower-class clients with individual striving partialed out. An individual effect is determined by the correlation between individual striving and orientation toward lower-class clients with group striving partialed out. Insofar as both individual and group striving scores were computed in this research, Tannenbaum and Bachman's technique was employed in this study.

31. Herzog, *op. cit.*
32. A. B. Hollingshead, "Two Factor Index of Social Position," (Yale University, mimeographed).
33. Peter M. Blau, "Formal Organization: Dimensions of Analysis," *American Journal of Sociology*, 63 (1957), 58-69.
34. Peter M. Blau, "Structural Effects," *American Sociological Review*, 25 (1960), 178-193; James A. Davis, Joe L. Spaeth, and Carolyn Huson, "A Technique for Analyzing the Effects of Group Composition," *American Sociological Review*, 26 (1961), 215-225; and Arnold S. Tannenbaum and Jerald G. Bachman, "Structural Versus Individual Effects," *American Journal of Sociology*, 69 (May, 1964), 585-595. For another contribution to this mode of analysis see Paul F. Lazarsfeld and Herbert Menzel, "On the Relation Between Individual and Collective Properties," in Amitai

These calculations were obtained by utilizing the non-parametric Kendall partial rank correlation coefficient which was most appropriate for use with our data.[35] The primary drawback of the implementation of the Kendall test is that no test of significance is available for use with it. Hence, in the presentation to follow, the argument will be limited to stating that one correlation is higher than another without implying a significant difference.

Findings

The first measure of the interplay between professional group striving and orientations toward lower-class clients was a question asking the respondents to describe their most unpleasant experience with a client.

Table 18.2 presents data demonstrating that the actively striving nurses were significantly more likely to describe experiences with lower-class clients as having been unpleasant than they were contacts with middle-class clients. The negative orientation measured by this item decreases as professional group striving decreases. The same relationship was noted within each professional group with the highest striving segments of the nursing and sanitarian occupational groups being significantly more negative in their orientations toward lower-class clients than were the low-striving segments of the two professions.

Table 18.2.   Social class of most unpleasant client

	Social Class of Client Described as Most Unpleasant					
	lower class		*middle class*		*total*	
Professional Group	N	%	N	%	N	%
Nurses	81	85	14	15	95	100
Sanitarians	36	72	14	28	50	100
M.D.'s	5	42	7	58	12	100
Total	122	78	35	22	157[a]	100

$X^2 = 13.066$, 2 degree of freedom, significant at .05

STRUCTURAL EFFECT = .241
INDIVIDUAL EFFECT = −.080

[a] Forty-one respondents were excluded from this analysis due to their giving insufficient information concerning clients from which social class could be ascertained. These included 15 nurses, 22 sanitarians, and 4 M.D.'s. Differential contact with clients was not a problem here.

The relationship between group-level factors and negative orientations noted in this table provides evidence to support the argument that group-

Etzioni, ed., *Complex Organizations* (New York: Holt, Rinehart and Winston, 1961), pp. 422-440.

35. Sidney Siegel, *Nonparametric Statistics* (New York: McGraw-Hill, 1956), pp. 223-229.

level striving is most influential in the formation of negative orientations toward indigent clients. The structural effect denoting the degree of correlation between group striving and this measure of negative orientation is .241. The individual effect is -.080, indicating that the group influence is both stronger and more directly related to this particular measure of orientations toward lower-class clients.

Another measure of orientations utilized in this study was a set of quesions designed to ascertain descriptions of a respondent's "most difficult" and 'ideal" clients. The rationale behind such a measure was that if social class characteristics make no difference, most respondents would describe their difficult clients in terms of types of illnesses or problem, not in social class terms. Or, if the descriptions were to include social class characteristics, there would be no appreciable differences in the number of lower-class and middle-class clients described as most pleasant or most difficult by members of the various occupational groups. This was not the case, however. The respondents to this study described their clients according to social class characteristics with little or no probing. Furthermore, their preferences for clients of one class or another related clearly to different levels of professional group striving.

The data reported in Table 18.3 again provide support for our argument that members of highly striving work groups are more negative in their orientations toward lower-class clients than are members of less actively striving groups. The data also provide evidence to support the argument that it is the impact of group factors that more effectively shape these negative orientations. The partial correlation coefficient denoting the structural effect on the orientations of the professionals included in Table 18.3 is .100. The individual effect is only .004.

Again when the data from this measure were examined for differences between the more actively striving segments within the nursing and sanitation groups, trends in the predicted direction could be detected. These trends, however, were not statistically significant.

Serendipity played a role in providing additional empirical support for the argument of this research. During the pre-test of the interview schedule several respondents stated that they were concerned with the large number of middle-class persons whom they felt had need of their services but would not request assistance. The respondents blamed too much contact with the lower class and the poor for this reticence and stated that the middle class persons needing their help identified them as being a facility solely for use by the poor and would not, therefore, consider them as being a source of assistance.

On the basis of these comments, it was decided to determine whether the more active professional strivers would differ from the less active strivers when asked about the kinds of persons having the most difficulty understanding what they do. Remaining within the theoretical outlines of the research, it was predicted that members of highly striving groups would be more like-

Table 18.3.   Social class of most difficult client

Professional Group[a]	Middle Class		Social Class Makes No Difference		Lower Class		Total	
	N	%	N	%	N	%	N	%
Nurses	13	12	17	16	75	72	104	100
Sanitarians	19	32	7	11	34	57	60	100
Total	32	19	24	15	109	66	165[b]	100

$X^2 = 9.134$, 2 degrees of freedom, significant at .05

STRUCTURAL EFFECT=.100
INDIVIDUAL EFFECT=.004

[a]The small number of physicians would necessitate violation of the restrictions of the chi-square test if they were included in this analysis.

[b]Seventeen responses were unclassifiable. These included 5 nurses and 12 sanitarians.

ly to state that the middle classes had the most difficulty than would mem bers of the low-striving groups.

At first glance, one would expect respondents to name uneducated ot lower-class clients as the group most likely to have difficulties understanding the services a profession has to offer. Our respondents—and the high-striving nurses in particular—interpreted this open-ended question differently. To the nurses the clients with the most difficulty understanding their services were those who identified the public health worker with the lower class or disinherited elements of the society.

As the data in Table 18.4 indicate, the sanitarians and the M.D.'s, the two low-striving groups, are the occupational groups most likely to indicate that social class either is unimportant in describing the kinds of people most likely to have difficulties understanding services or that lower-class clients have the most difficulty. In more than half of the cases, however, the high-striving nurses indicated that middle-class clients have the most difficulty understanding their services.

It could be argued that the nurses responded this way because they lacked contact with middle-class clients. Our data, however, indicate that this is not the case. The Index of Social Position scores computed on the basis of occupational and educational descriptions of clients indicate that our respondents dealt with both middle- and lower-class clients. Those who stated that the middle-class client is least understanding of their work, .for example, actually had more contact with middle-class clients in the weeks prior to our field work than did the respondents who stated that lower-class clients have the most difficulty understanding the services offered by public health nurses. Professional group striving, not lack of contact with the middle class, appears to be the major variable to consider in explaining this difference in orientation.

The data presented in Table 18.4 also provide another instance in which the structural effect—professional group striving—is more influential in the formation of these negative orientations than is the individual effect—individual striving. The partial correlation coefficient computed between degree of professional group striving and the dependent variable with individual striving partialed out is .170 whereas the individual level effect is .150.

Table 18.4.   Social class of clients most likely to have difficulties understanding the services a profession has to offer

Professional Group	Social Class of Least Understanding Clients							
	middle class		class no factor		lower class		total	
	N	%	N	%	N	%	N	%
Nurses	57	54	11	11	37	35	105	100
Sanitarians	14	24	10	17	34	59	58	100
M.D.'s	6	40	3	20	6	40	15	100
Total	77	43	24	14	77	43	178 [a]	100

$X^2 = 14.431$, 4 degrees of freedom, significant at .05
STRUCTURAL EFFECT=.170
INDIVIDUAL EFFECT=.150

[a] The responses of 20 interviewees were unclassifiable on this measure. These included 5 nurses, 14 sanitarians, and 1 M.D.

These findings can be explained in social movement terms. The theoretical perspective of this research leads to the suggestion that members of striving work groups come to perceive the poor in a manner analogous to the dynamics through which social movements specify an individual group, or social institution as the source of the problems the movement seeks to solve. The poor are perceived this way because they are seen as impediments to the quest for high status.

One of the respondents to this study, a member of a highly striving work group, expressed this cogently stating, "People with higher-class clientele tend to have higher prestige than those with a lower-class clientele." The poor shoulder the blame for frustrated status quests and the striving work group, much like the propagandists of a social movement, passes this attitude on to the members of the group.[36]

The final measure of orientations toward poor or lower-class clients utilized in this research was based on behavioral data or, more exactly, reports of behavior. We have data from which we estimated the social class of the clients with whom the respondents to this study had dealings in the weeks prior to our field work. We also asked the respondents to indicate which of their contacts with clients were pleasant and which were unpleasant. The differences between the striving nurses and low-striving sanitarians on

36. Neil J. Smelser, *Theory of Collective Behavior* (Glencoe, Ill.: The Free Press, 1963), p. 83.

Table 18.5. Number of unpleasant clients, by social class, with whom respondents worked in week prior to our interview

| Professional Group | Number of Unpleasant Clients By Social Class | | | | | |
| | lower class | | middle class | | total | |
	N	%	N	%	N	%
Nurses	59	87	9	13	68	100
Sanitarians	30	63	18	37	48	100
Total	89	77	27	23	116	100

$X^2=7.96$, 1 degree of freedom, significant at .05.

this measure are presented as the final evidence to support the hypothesis tested in this research. Comparisons of the high- and low-striving segments of the various professional groups examined yielded comparable results.

Table 18.5 presents data on the basis of which statistically significant differences can be noted between the different levels of professional striving. The table compares the high-striving nurses with the low-striving sanitarians. The M.D.'s, due to lack of consistent contact with patients because of administrative duties, were dropped from this analysis.

Table 18.6. Proportion of clients, by social class, listed as unpleasant by nurses and sanitarians

| | Professional Group | | | | | |
| | nurses high strivers | | sanitarians low strivers | | total | |
	N	%	N	%	N	%
Number of clients contacted in week prior to interview[a]	183	60	120	40	303	100
Number and percentage of middle-class clients	86	47	55	46	141	47
Number and percentage of lower-class clients	97	53	65	54	162	54
Number and percentage of middle-class clients called unpleasant	9	11	18	31	27	19
Number and percentage of lower-class clients called unpleasant	59	61	30	46	89	55

[a] This total does not include all of the contacts with clients made by the respondents in the weeks prior to our interviews. Most listed what they called a "good cross-section" of their client.

The high-striving nurses, as predicted, were most likely to report contacts with lower-class clients to have been unpleasant. These data again provide empirical verification for the argument that has been developed throughout this report concerning the relationship between professional group striving and orientations toward lower-class clients.

One final table follows in which the data indicate that the finding noted in Table 18.5 may indeed be utilized as evidence supporting our argument and is not merely the result of lack of contact with middle-class clients by the public health professionals interviewed. As the data in Table 18.6 demonstrate, a similar number of lower- and middle-class clients were contacted by the respondents in the week prior to the interview. But closer examination of that table indicates that whereas the total number of lower-class clients encountered by the high-striving nurses was 97—or 53 percent of the clients visited—a total of 61 percent of the clients called unpleasant came from the ranks of the lower class. And, while 86 of the nurses' patients were middle class—or 47 percent of the total number of clients—only 11 percent of these middle-class clients were considered by the nurses to have been unpleasant experiences.

A picture of quite another color can be seen in an examination of the percentages of unpleasant clients by social class of the less actively striving sanitarians. Among the sanitarians, 55 clients were middle class and of the 55 over 30 percent were said to have been unpleasant. Of the 65 lower-class clients listed by the sanitarians—54 percent of the total number of clients reported by them—only 46 percent were said to have been unpleasant experiences. Similar findings can be reported following comparisons of the high- and low-striving segments within each professional group.

Discussion

These data, then, support the argument of this research that members of highly striving human service groups are more negative in their orientations toward lower-class clients than are members of work groups less active in such striving. The data presented here compared separate occupational groups but mention was made of findings obtained when the high- and low-striving segments within each work group were similarly compared. For reasons of space this supplementary data has not been included in this article.[37]

The implications of these findings are several. In the first place, similar studies of other occupational groupings as varied as the clergy, social work, psychotherapy, education, the police, and law would greatly enhance our understanding of the complex factors shaping the attitudes and behaviors of persons working with clients of various social class levels.

These studies, coupled with the one reported here, would be of value in theoretical understandings of the processes of occupational growth and development. They would also have implications for the education and training of new service personnel, for in addition to making clear the personal and social benefits of becoming identified as "more professional," such studies could identify the dysfunctions of such a pursuit.

37. More detailed presentation of these data can be found in Walsh, *op. cit.*

The service worker assumes a set of blinders throughout the course of his training and the process of identifying himself with a particular professional or occupational ideology.[38] It would serve the professional well to be aware of the existence and extent of these blinders and the impact they can have on his dealings with clients of varying social class backgrounds. A comparison of human service personnel involved in professional striving activities conducive to the assumption of negative orientations toward their less appealing clients and the behavior of participants in some social movements whose goals include raising social prestige may not be too extreme. As Hughes observed, collective protest enables people to identify the source of their problems and in so doing provides the protestors with an alibi for the past plus an agenda for the future.[39] Veblen's trained incapacity may be at least partially due to internalizing the status-climbing ideology of one's occupational group.

This research leads us to speculate that the class structure maintains itself in significant part through the efforts of work groups as a whole to establish themselves. In this process, the differential distribution of rewards effected by the class structure operates not only through the money market and its salaries and incomes, but through orientations and behaviors of members of work groups which aid them in avoiding identification or involvement with detracting or devalued elements of society. The depth of this human tragedy is suggested by the fact that those most in need of service are least likely to receive it.[40]

On the other hand, it could be argued that the relationship between professional striving and negative orientations toward the poor set forth in this report neglects an alternative possibility. Perhaps the causal sequence works in the other direction and that professional striving does not produce negative orientations toward the poor at all but is instead the result of negative orientations which spawn the organized efforts of the occupational group to seek to rise above the poor. Interesting longitudinal research possibilities can be seen in such an argument; but the explanation presented in this paper seems adequate when the implications of the structural versus individual effect results are considered.

Approaching the data in this fashion facilitated more than differentiating levels of group and individual influences. It also provided at least a partial answer to the problem of causal direction. While credibility should certainly be given the argument that professional striving may result from negative orientations, the explanation set forth in this report provides an adequate theoretical explanation demonstrating the similarities between professional

38. C. Wright Mills, "The Professional Ideology of Social Pathologists," *The American Journal of Sociology*, 49 (September, 1943), 165-180.

39. Everett C. Hughes, "Social Change and Status Protest: An Essay On the Marginal Man," *Phylon* (First Quarter, 1949), 58-65.

40. Norman V. Lourie, "Impact of Social Change on the Tasks of the Mental Health Profession," *American Journal of Orthopsychiatry*, 35 (January, 1965), 43.

striving and social movements. Those who were members of highly striving work groups may indeed have had negative orientations toward the poor prior to the initiation of the organized striving; but the professional striving of the work group accomplished for them what social movements have accomplished for their members in other contexts by providing a "bogey man" or a readily visible group on whom blame for dissatisfaction and frustration could be placed.[41] This "bogey man" becomes the indigent patient.

When the structural effect of group striving is more closely linked to such negative orientations than is individual striving, and when persons with low levels of individual striving who are members of highly striving work groups regularly assume significantly more negative orientations toward the poor than do even the high individual strivers in low-striving groups, the validity of the analogy between professional group striving as a social movement conducive to negative orientations appears quite appropriate. The social movement characteristics of the striving group focus the attention of the professionals on the potential impact the poor may have on professional stature.

Those who administer and plan the allocation of human services—be they health or welfare—would do well to note that, as this research indicates, those who strive are sometimes victims as well as victors in the mechanics of the class structure. In this very striving to "professionalize" a human service occupational group, the members of that group may be led inadvertently to subvert one of the nobler aspects of their work group's ethic: service to all in need. Part and parcel with the effort to advance is the attempt on the part of the striving professional group to avoid too close contact or identification with the lower social class. Members of these occupational groups may be gearing their services to the needs of the more powerful and influential middle and upper classes rather than exerting real effort to fulfill the needs of the persons on the lower rungs of the social status ladder whose problems generally are greater both in number and severity.

It may be, therefore, that in order to induce the best human service for those most in need of it, occupational group associations and work organizations may have to build into the system a greater form of reward for serving the impoverished or the lower class. One solution may be to build in greater financial and professional recognition for those with the skill and the will necessary to deal extensively with the poor. Given the strength of the American class system there is no certainty in such a proposal; but it or some alternative solution is badly needed if the health needs of the indigent and the lower class are to be satisfied.

41. Richard Hofstadter has described this process in political social movements in his article, "The Paranoid Style in American Politics," *Harper's*, 229 (November, 1964), 77-86.

Defining and Diagnosing Illness

Central to medical work is the idea of illness. In whatever he does, the medical man participates in some fashion in a process of diagnosing and treating what is believed to be illness or impairment. The idea of illness is generic to medical work and distinguishes the rationale of work by those in medically related occupations from those in other occupations. Central as the idea is, however, its substance is by no means self-evident. Illness is often used to refer to some objective state of the human organism, independent of human knowledge. Obviously, physical states do exist independently of human knowledge and custom, but the way people behave toward those states, namely, by diagnosing illness or not and by treating or not, obviously is not independent of human knowledge and custom. Given the fact that much of what is called illness varies from one historical period to another, one culture to another, and even one segment of society to another, it seems useful to attempt to delineate the meaning of the word independently of the states to which it may be applied. If such could be done, it would be possible to specify the social consequences of the application of that meaning to any particular physical state; the physical or biological consequences can of course be analyzed separately in the light of contemporary medical knowledge. The first few papers in this section represent attempts to delineate the social meaning of the word "illness." In the course of doing so, they have occasion to discuss the implications of that meaning both for the way the medical man does his work, and for the way people called ill or sick are treated.

Several of the papers seek to clarify the broad dimensions of the problem by contrasting the idea of illness with the idea of crime, thereby continuing the comparison between medicine and law begun by Rueschemeyer earlier in this volume. The most sweeping comparison is made in the paper by Aubert and Messinger, where they discuss the analytical significance of issues like time and duration, isolation from "normal" society, and the imputation of responsibility to the individual for his manifestation of some undesirable state or behavior. By the nature of the case, they had to deal with the conceptions of both the man on the street and the professional.

Making the same comparison between law and medicine, Scheff extends it further by focusing on the characteristic stance which each profession takes toward its respective task. He notes that each uses a different "decision rule," medicine following the rule that it is better to wrongly diagnose illness and "miss" health than it is to wrongly diagnose health and "miss" illness, while law traditionally follows the opposite rule that it is better to wrongly "diagnose" innocence and overlook guilt than it is to wrongly "diagnose" guilt and overlook innocence. He points out the consequences for the patient when the rule to diagnose illness is invoked in medicine and suggests some of the qualifications one must keep in mind when attempting to isolate a typical "medical decision rule." Clifton Meador, whose paper directly follows Scheff's, suggests some of the medical sources of mistaken diagnoses of illness and, in a not entirely whimisical vein, delineates the social and medical status of "nondisease" for those whose diagnoses were discovered to be mistaken.

As Scheff pointed out in his paper, however, in some cases the subsequent status of the mistakenly diagnosed is not so easily converted to that of the specifically healthy person: in such cases, following the medical decision rule to diagnose illness in cases of doubt can lead to unfortunate social consequences. It is essentially an attempt to refine the various social meanings connected with the diagnosis of illness, and to connect with them the social consequences of assigning those meanings which the next paper addresses. Focusing on "impairments" or "disability" more than on acute illness, Freidson contrasts medicine with law, illness with crime, and attempts to suggest varied types of illness on a social rather than medical basis, dealing with the social characteristics attributed to them, the modes of managing them, and the consequences for the patient of the way the institutions of medical management are organized. Lay conceptions of illness, in interaction with the conceptions of the profession, lead to an individual's entrance into one of the "sick roles," but once in a treatment institution the professional conception dominates the subsequent "career" of the patient.

The remaining papers examine various problematic facets of the question of the diagnosis of illness. Szasz examines the concept of "malingering," which refers to instances when an individual's claim of illness is not accepted by diagnosticians and which, therefore, tends to lead to punishment or rejection. He points out how this denial of a claim of illness is commonly encouraged in particular kinds of practice settings, as in the military setting discussed by Daniels in an earlier paper in this volume. He also points out the curious procedure by which some diagnosticians come to consider the spurious claim to be ill as itself a special kind of illness!

And, consonant with his writings criticizing the nosology of psychiatry, he criticizes the logic upon which the use of the concept of illness in that context is based.

In the final paper Suchman analyzes the concept of "accident," which is sometimes considered a cause of illness or injury. He discusses the various meanings connected with it, the various approaches people have taken to the analysis of accidents, and the relationship of the concept to the idea of disease or illness. He suggests, in fact, as Scheff did in the case of mental illness, that the concept of accident is a residual category, and he indicates how one may approach it in such a way as to minimize the pertinence of the word to subsequent analysis.

In one way or another all the papers in this section point to the social values surrounding both the idea of illness and its diagnosis by layman and professional. The most elementary distinction is that of the deviant or devalued character of whatever is called illness, but, as we have seen, other meanings are also connected with the diagnosis. As the papers show, the social values connected with the concept of illness exist independently, and can be analyzed separately, from whatever physical reality may be referred to in any single time or place. And the diagnosis of illness has social consequences for the identity and life of the person which can be analyzed independently of physical or biological consequences. Confronted with the problem of studying medical work, the social scientist may therefore choose to analyze lay and professional diagnosis and its consequences on a purely social level, without great concern for the biophysical level which the physician deals with. Alternatively he may, like the socially oriented physician, choose to analyze the interaction between social life and the biophysical status of those authoritatively diagnosed by the members of the profession. The former approach is rather specific to sociology; the latter is in the tradition of social medicine, psychosomatic medicine, and social epidemiology.

BIBLIOGRAPHIC SUGGESTIONS

For a general discussion of conceptions of disease, see W. Riese, *The Conception of Disease: Its History, Its Versions and Its Nature* (New York: Philosophical Library, 1953). For a recent review of the problem in psychiatry, see Daniel Offer and Melvin Sabshin, *Normality, Theoretical and Clinical* (New York: Basic Books, 1966), and for a very broad and sophisticated discussion of the general problem see René Dubos, *Mirage of Health* (New York: Anchor Books, 1961). The many works of Thomas S. Szasz must also be examined, perhaps most usefully of all in the present context, Thomas S. Szasz, *Law, Liberty, and Psychiatry* (New York: Collier Books, 1963).

A number of sociological works must also be cited in this context. A now-classic discussion is that of Talcott Parsons, "Definitions of Health and Illness in the Light of American Values and Social Structure," in Talcott Parsons, *Social Structure and Personality* (New York: The Free Press, 1964), pp. 258-291.

A recent, extremely instructive review and discussion of the concept of deviance is that of David Matza, *Becoming Deviant* (Englewood Cliffs, N.J.: Prentice-Hall, 1969). A systematic discussion of the relation of the idea of deviance to that of illness, as well as an extensive discussion of sociological types of illness, is to be found in Eliot Freidson, *Profession of Medicine: A Study of the Sociology of Applied Knowledge* (New York: Dodd, Mead, 1970), pp. 205-243. A sociological theory of mental illness based on the idea of residual deviance is presented in Thomas J. Scheff, *Being Mentally Ill: A Sociological Theory* (Chicago: Aldine, 1966). A very stimulating analysis of the implications of one of the social meanings which get connected with that of illness is Erving Goffman, *Stigma: Notes on the Management of Spoiled Identity* (Englewood Cliffs, N.J.: Spectrum Books, 1963).

19

VILHELM AUBERT

SHELDON L. MESSINGER

The Criminal and the Sick

This paper deals with the everyday philosophies of ordinary men and women, as they are applied to certain recurrent situations, in this case, misfortunes. It does so from a sociological point of view, attempting to establish a few regularities, invariances, in social phenomena. We try to exploit the notion that just as philosophers are often trapped by their premises and their sense of logic, so are ordinary people caught when they construct models aiming at the understanding of other persons. If they say *a,* they often "have to" say *b,* or even *c,* on the basis of a sort of "everyday logic." Although this "logic" often is far from logical in any strict sense, we all have some familiarity with it. No attempt will be made to spell it out here in any detail. What we shall consider as being highly problematical is, rather, how people choose their basic premises when applying one or the other of a few ready-made models for the classification of other people.

It is our assumption that this choice is socially determined, in the sense that factors irrelevant to a scientific observer describing a person's actions play their part in the choice of everyday models for the perception of the same person. Furthermore, we propose that such a choice of model often implies a stand on traditional philosophical issues. We deal as sociologists with "man as a philospher," thereby adding to the number of models of man which already range from "Zoon politicon," "economic man," etc. to "man as a personality," "man as an actor," "Homo Ludens." "Man as a philosopher" is no entirely new subject matter to the social sciences. We can refer to the precedent set by the anthropologists who have cultivated the study of

Reprinted from *Inquiry,* 1, No. 3 (1958), pp. 137-160, by permission of the authors and publisher.

This paper developed while the authors were Fellows of the Center for Advanced Study in the Behavioral Sciences, Stanford, California. Sheldon Messinger's contribution is partly based on research carried out on the California prison system (The California Department of Corrections) with the aid of a Social Science Research Council predoctoral Fellowship.

primitive theories of disease and other explanations of misfortune for a long time. They treat primitive man as someone who, in the face of tragedy, disaster, and surprise, musters his intellectual resources and brings them to bear upon the situation in an attempt to re-establish order in the social universe, and to find grounds on which to act.[1] In a tentative and limited fashion we propose a similar sociological approach to modern man.

Crime and Illness

One of the simplest sociological statements that can be made about the control measures invoked to deal with crime and illness is that they involve the exclusion of some sick persons and some criminals from the performance of their everyday social roles. When exclusion takes place we may view the control processes as having been initiated, and we may talk about entrance into the roles of the sick person and the criminal, since recognizable changes in rights and duties take place.

We are interested in exploring how a person gets into one of these roles rather than the other, and in the implications of the process of role-entrance for leaving the role. Although at first glance the way one enters the sick and criminal roles may seem too obvious to bear discussion, the patent fact is that in an increasing number of instances in modern society there is dispute over whether "criminality" or "illness" has led to a particular behavior sequence. This suggests the utility of holding as problematical the identification of a given deviant behavior as "crime" or "illness," and inquiring into the conditions of entering one role or the other in modern society.

Entering the Sick and Criminal Roles

One manner of approaching the assumptions involved in identifying a performance as a crime is to examine the criminal law. From the sociological point of view, the criminal law is one among several regulators of values. The criminal law either orders priorities between values (ends) or between roads (means) to values. It gives the value of life to A priority over the value to B of getting rid of A, say by killing him. It gives the owner's road to his property priority over the thief's road to the same property. Although this is not unique to the criminal law, any criminal law must necessarily give priority-norms about strivings related to values.

This inevitable characteristic of the criminal law bestows a necessary attribute upon any criminal. A criminal is someone who strives, or has

1. A social-psychological account of related problems in modern society is given in Army Medical Research and Development Board, Office of the Surgeon General, Washington (Research Staff: Dembo, T., Ladien, G., Wright, B. A.) *Adjustment to Misfortune*, Final Report, April 1, 1948.

been striving, toward a value. Whatever theories we may entertain about what he actually achieves, a necessary condition for his being a criminal is that he, in some fashion, was out to obtain a value. There are a number of ways to formulate this: that he was engaged in goal-directed behavior, that he made choices or decisions, or simply that he acted. The change that takes place in a person's situation when he becomes a criminal is due to a motivated act—a choice.

Medical science defines illnesses. It is no necessary condition of a definition of disease that it should be concerned with the interpersonal regulation of values and the ordering of priorities. The only necessary assumption about values in medical literature is that illness is negatively valued. Illness is against the individual's own good, at least from one point of view. One becomes sick by undergoing a change for the worse. Further, the presumption is that one becomes sick *in spite of* strivings for a value—attempts to stay healthy.[2]

Thus, to summarize and repeat: to become a criminal it is necessary to have appeared to be striving for a value. This is not necessary in order to become ill. In order to become ill it is necessary to undergo an apparent change for the worse.

Leaving the Sick and Criminal Roles

We have held that the excluded criminal and the excluded sick are at a certain time in a fairly similar position, but that the necessary assumptions on which they enter their respective roles differ in at least one important respect: the entrance criteria are *explained* differently. Now we shall investigate some of the implications of these necessary, and necessarily different, explanations for the termination of exclusion.

One principle which will always in part determine exclusion of the criminal is the elementary protection of the values with which he was interfering. If he is excluded at all, some part of the exclusion will consist in separation from the values toward which he was striving. In other words, the defining characteristic of his crime is removed when the exclusion takes place. This separation of the individual from his defining situation does not, however, constitute recovery. Rather, there seems to be an inverse relationship between the distance from the defining value-striving and the possibility of recovery. The relationship between the assumptions on which a criminal enters his role and the nature of his exclusion is such that his criminality cannot be falsified while he is in exclusion. One might say that in order to show any precise symptoms of recovery he must have recovered already.

2. For more detailed statements on the sociological concept of illness, cf. Talcott Parsons, *The Social System* (Glencoe, Ill.: 1951); Aubrey Lewis, "Health as a Social Concept," *The British Journal of Sociology*, 4 (1953), 109-124; Lester S. King,

There is no reason inherent in the qualifying characteristic of the sick person which makes it impossible for him to stay in proximity to the negative values defining his illness during the period of exclusion. On the contrary, it is necessary to remain in proximity to some of the negative values—fever, pain, etc.—as long as the exclusion is legitimate. When all signs of malfunctioning disappear, the sick person has recovered, and the role ceases to apply. The basis for falsifying the claims that the role criteria apply, or do not apply, is present throughout the period of exclusion.

Now, what we have been saying is not that it is more likely that a sick person will recover than a criminal. No general statement to this or to the contrary effect can be made on the basis of the above analysis. What we have implied, however, is that if the sick person recovers, the reality basis for consensus about the recovery is defined in such a way that it is relatively easy to obtain consensus. That is, role-entrance, recovery, and role-leaving are closely linked in the case of the sick. If the criminal recovers, on the other hand, there is no well-defined reality basis on which consensus can build.[3] This may hamper "recovery" of the criminal, but it presumably may also speed up "recovery." The essential point is that whatever criteria of recovery are applied to the criminal, they have no necessary relationship to the criteria of entrance into the role. Thus, it is not clear when—or if—the criminal role can be left once entered.

Recovery and the Criminal Law

Still, it may asked, do not man-made laws furnish the predictability and consensus about the criminal that natural laws provide in the case of the sick? Is not the absence of accurate predictability of recovery on the basis of the nature of the crime simply an imperfection analogous to the lack of scientific knowledge within certain areas of medicine?

Our analysis presupposes that the difference is of a more fundamental nature. The crux of the matter seems to be that the function of man-made laws is, above all, even when they mete out punishments, to order value priorities. When predictability operates at all it seems to be of the following nature: if A violates rule R, his crime is defined as being of a degree of badness B, which implies a time of exclusion T. As we know, this scheme of predictability has a limited application. It is limited to crimes handled by the courts, where court practices do not fluctuate very much, and only with regard to publicly administered exclusion. But the main point is that under any conditions the prediction seems unrelated to the problem of recovery, in the sense of disappearance of criminality.

"What is Disease?" *Philosophy of Science*, 21: 3 (1954), 193-203.

3. The problem is related to Festinger's distinction between "physical reality" and "social reality." Leon Festinger et al., *Theory and Experiment in Social Communi-*

The most convincing argument for the irrelevance of recovery predictions in the criminal law is that the law so readily substitutes fines for imprisonment, and that some modern systems of criminal law authorize imprisonment for periods far in excess of the life expectancy of any human being. In fines there is obviously no implication about the predicted time of recovery. Further, the idea of punishing people in terms of time-serving is a relatively new one; most systems of criminal law have done without sanctions meted out in time periods.[4] The criminal law draws upon the future merely because under modern conditions time is one of the dimensions along which sanctions can be ordered. But no system of healing can work without time.

We shall claim that the relationship which the law establishes between a criminal act and a future time period is essentially of the same nature as the relationship established between a criminal act and a sum of money or a certain degree of physical pain, as in flogging. If this relationship is the same in all these cases, the criminal law cannot be concerned with predicting future events. We would hold, in fact, that the criminal law is basically not concerned with processes over time at all.

Crime, Illness, and the Situation of Performance

We should like to present briefly what we take to be certain research implications of the above analysis. First, it follows from what we have said that where the entrance criteria of the sick and criminal roles are difficult or impossible to perceive, a deviant performance will be rendered ambiguous along the dimension of crime-illness. In other words, the understanding of a given deviant performance as crime or illness is linked to the situation in which the performance takes place, including the social characteristics of the performers and observers. This can easily be illustrated, although details of the process obviously await empirical investigation.

For example, in the case of the sick, or those claiming the right to enter the sick role, our thesis suggests the following: any situation in which an individual stands to gain from withdrawal is such as to render suspect his claim to illness. Of course, this sort of proposition must be stated "other things being equal," and among those "other things" is prominently found the visibility of symptoms. However, within this proviso several situations can be immediately located, which suggest the truth of the hypothesis. The army stands as a situation, in general, in which the value of withdrawal, particularly for enlisted men, is so patent as to render claims to illness routinely suspect.[5] Absences from schools, factories, etc., in short, any

cation (Ann Arbor: 1950). Cf. also Leon Festinger, "A Theory of Social Comparison Processes," *Human Relations*, 7 (1954), 117-140.

4. Georg Rusche and Otto Kirchheimer, *Punishment and Social Structure* (New York: 1939).

5. Roger W. Little, "The 'Sick Soldier' and the Medical Ward Officer," *Human*

situation in which the observer ordinarily assumes that the person claiming illness may be motivated to withdraw, is such as to render claims to illness ambiguous. The reverse situation may be seen to obtain as well—that is, it is easier to be categorized as ill when the situation points to significant deprivation following validation of a claim to illness. For example, the child on his way to a party is not suspect.

Our thesis also suggests that any situation in which ends of doubtful value to the performer of a deviant performance are achieved is such as to render the criminal basis of the performance suspect. Petty theft by the wealthy is of this sort. Arson, except where insurance is involved, is another example of a situation in which the basis of "crime" seems as likely to be "illness" as "criminality." No doubt other instances could be cited. But what seems called for instead is the careful investigation of the nature of those situations in which involved persons have difficulty in deciding the nature of the deviant performance. One excellent source of information should be court records of cases in which a decision of "insanity" was reached (or was sought but not reached). Another source of information yet to be exploited should be legislative records of discussions leading to changes in the law providing that certain crimes, e.g. sex offenses, become an occasion for sending the performer to the mental hospital rather than to prison. On a still broader scale, we need insight into the social conditions which lead some people to regard prisons as properly mental hospitals.

All of these investigations will perforce deal with the typical actors and typical motives we use in structuring our everyday worlds. And such work has yet to begin in earnest.

The Everyday Models of Crime and Illness

From what has been said it would seem that the sick and the criminal are constructed as members of two rather different worlds, and do not only represent variants of a common category of roles.[6] The sick person is constructed as someone with characteristics along a dimension of time, while the criminal is constructed without any time perspective. The defining characteristics of the sick person are located in space, but the defining characteristics of the criminal, partly because of this discontinuity, have no location in space either. Is criminality, then, a mere chimera? No, but it is not a characteristic which is built upon the model of "physical reality," as are modern ideas of sickness. Physical reality is not, however, the only model according to which social objects can be constructed. They can also be constructed on the basis of our other basic source of experience, the "inner world."

Organization, 15:1 (1956), 22-24.

6. For a somewhat different approach to the dichotomy, cf. Antony G. N. Flew, "Crime or Disease," *The British Journal of Sociology*, 5 (1954), 49-62.

The characteristics of this inner world are somewhat elusive, but a few of them stand out rather clearly. In our inner world the possibility of choice usually seems to be present. The relevant argumentation before the inner audience is in terms of good and bad, and not in terms of cause and effect until the means are to be chosen. The inner world is characterized, furthermore, by discontinuity in terms of time. The difference between the past, the present, and the future is not a question of degree, but a difference with qualitative implications. About the present and the future it is possible to make choices. About the past, as past, it is impossible. In contrast to this, basic schemes for conceptualizing physical reality apply to past, present, and future. Our inner world gives the present, the now, a unique significance, since it is the meeting point of a process over which we have no power of choice and one over which we have power of choice.[7]

From this it follows that the criminal is one among a very large class of social objects. The sick, on the contrary, seem to represent a much smaller, but probably expanding, class of social objects.

It seems commonly accepted that it is the "moral" model which gives to human beings their character of being social objects, or even of "being human." Only organisms to which actions, motives, rights, and duties are attributed constitute parts of the social system. From this point of view the sick person is not initially a social object at all. We shall not put great emphasis upon what is the proper way to delimit the concept of "social objects." Whether the sick person is conceived as a nonsocial object (until he becomes a patient) or as a social object constructed in naturalistic terms does not greatly matter. We prefer the latter terminology.

The Victim of a Crime Compared to the Sick

A comparison of the victim of a crime and the sick, the victim of a disease, may add to the preceding analysis. There is in any society, it seems, a persistent need to "explain" misfortunes. Theories of sickness, both primitive and modern, belong in this category of explanations. For the reasons already given, it seems feasible in terms of our prevailing values to explain sickness in naturalistic terms, as a process which is just happening. We have also seen some reasons why the naturalistic model is inappropriate to the criminal and his behavior as a criminal. But how does the problem of explanation look from the point of view of his victim?

Since the crime, by definition, implies misfortune on the part of the victim, a change for the worse, there will be little spontaneous tendency to look for acts or choices made by the victim. Nevertheless, the criminal law, unlike modern medicine, does reckon with willful choices or provocations, on the part of the victims, as extenuating circumstances. One may put the difference

---

7. Cf. Alfred Schuetz, "On Multiple Realities," *Philosophy and Phenomenological Research*, 5 (1944-45), 533-576; Hubert Griggs Alexander, *Time as Dimension and History* (Albuquerque: The University of New Mexico Press, 1945).

between the sick and the victim this way: in medicine it makes no difference (at least until the advent of psychosomatic medicine) whether a disease is "deserved" or not. From the point of view of the criminal law, it does make a difference whether the victim "had it coming to him" or not. And the reason is that the criminal law deals with interaction situations and that values desired by both parties are relevant. Under such circumstances a symmetrical application of models is natural. If the criminal is viewed in normative terms, so is the victim. The victim must be innocent for the criminal to be guilty; or rather: the guilt of the victim reduces the guilt of the criminal. Comparisons of merit and guilt are relevant.

Granted that the normative (moral) model is applied to the victim, it fails to give "explanation" where the victim's innocence is clear. If he did not deserve his misfortune, why did it happen? Now the question "why" (but probably not its underlying psychological tension) changes meaning and becomes causal-genetic. The tendency will be to make the causal explanation very brief: I lost my money because a dishonest person wanted it and took it. Whereas the normative model "explained" by *comparing* guilts, this explanation *refers back* to a state of guilt in another person as a cause.[8] We know there are other, longer causal chains by which the question "why" can be tentatively answered: thefts occur because there are people who, by deep-rooted social and psychological factors, are led to steal. This type of explanation has many merits, but it does not specifically explain why *I* became a victim. Criminological theories are theories of criminals and not theories of victims.[9] It seems that about the only available explanation is that the criminal *chose* me as his victim. The explanation is certainly a shallow one, but it does carry the causal chain one step outside myself, which seems necessary if I do not want to accept blame for the misfortune.

There exists an additional "explanation," consisting in the assumption that the misfortune is due to *bad luck,* that it is an accident from the victim's point of view. And there are good reasons why this explanation would be more likely to prevail in the case of a victim than in the case of the sick. It has less to do with the positive merits of the "explanation" itself than with the alternative explanations which it pushes aside. For the victim to ascribe his misfortune to bad luck excludes the explanation that he deserved it. Furthermore, it excludes or modifies the explanation that the criminal chose *him* as a victim, which might also be disturbing. It seems that the sick person has less to gain by such an explanation and is so much the more open for the application of causal-genetic schemes, even though they may be very tenuous.

8. Our theories of victims are closely parallel to a major type of theories of disease in primitive societies. Cf. Henry E. Sigerist, *A History of Medicine. Vol. 1: Primitive and Archaic Medicine* (New York: Oxford University Press, 1951).

9. Cf. however Hans v. Hentig, *The Criminal and his Victim* (New Haven: Yale University Press, 1948).

Interaction and Exclusion in Relation
To the Criminal and the Sick

Known sickness seems virtually impossible without some exclusion. In almost all cases where a person is classified as sick, there will be certain relatively well-defined things he is not supposed to do or things he is permitted to abstain from. This is sufficient to justify the application of the role concept to his situation. With crime, the situation appears to be somewhat different. There are vast groups of crimes (or delinquencies) in both primitive and modern societies, for which the criminal law prescribes no exclusion and where no social ostracism may be present. In a large number of preliterate and archaic societies the major sanction against crimes is the payment of damages.[10] Although the nature of the pertinent actions makes it reasonable to classify them as crimes, they are not supposed to be followed by exclusion; but in the same societies some crimes lead to death, banishment, or excluding mutilation. In our own society some crimes lead only to exclusion, death, imprisonment, custody, etc. Others (the majority) lead to fines; and social ostracism is obliterated by the relative secrecy of both the offense and the penal sanction. In other words, criminality does not in itself automatically imply exclusion; this can also be expressed by saying that not all crimes are related to a criminal role.

Why is sickness universally related to exclusion, although in varying degrees, while crime may or may not lead to exclusion? We shall sketch one possible element (among several) in an explanation of this difference.

The sick person is unable to be healthy for the time being; however much he chooses to be well, he cannot. Failure to perform the roles he previously performed, or normally would have been able to perform, is not his responsibility. Viewed from any Alter's side, this means: if Alter does not exclude him to some extent in his interaction, by cutting down his expectations, the sick person will disappoint him. And the important point is that the normal everyday response to such disappointment is inappropriate because of the irresponsibility of the sick. A normative reaction to the disappointment has no balancing effect; it cannot correct the sick person's behavior; and, which is significant here, this failure has to be taken on as Alter's responsibility. He would thus easily get himself into guilt-provoking situations. In other words, protection of Alter's vital interaction interests demands that he cut down on his expectations in accordance with his understanding of the sickness. Such a reduction of expectations does, however, imply exclusion. By underexpecting, proper performance would be made socially difficult or impossible, irrespective of somatic ability. It is known that the proper balancing and timing of exclusion-levels is essential to the recovery process of the patient, showing that the implications of a naturalistic view

10. E. Adamson-Hoebel, *The Law of Primitive Man* (Cambridge: Harvard University Press, 1954).

of the sick and a normative view of him are mutually dependent.[11]

The criminal is not perceived in terms of inability. On the contrary, he is usually perceived as having been able to act differently had he chosen to do so. This makes it easier in one respect to interact with a criminal without getting into an anomic state for which Alter has to take responsibility. Let us assume that someone who has committed, or is convicted of, an offense, is met in interaction without exclusion. Expectations are not reduced relative to what they would have been had no criminality occurred. Alter may be disappointed; although this is not likely to happen in the same way as with sickness, where stable expectations built up during a long time by close relatives, friends, and associates may become unrealistic after the onset of sickness. A crime is a different kind of change, which need not affect the realism of long-standing, expectations on the parts of close Alters. Whether it does or does not depends more upon the nature of the expectations themselves. Let us, however, assume that the criminality in some sense renders normal expectations false, e.g. the expectations of law-abidingness and trust-worthiness in the handling of agreements and contracts. Disappointment will ensue. But it is quite proper to react normatively to this disappointment, because no assumption of causal inability applies to the criminal. This also means that ignorance of the criminality does not vitally affect the appro-priateness of response in the way ignorance of sickness may do. Whether the normative reaction to the criminal will correct his criminality is doubtful. But, unless causal-genetic considerations intrude, there will be no occasion for Alter to feel guilt about having misunderstood the situation or for hav-ing chosen an inappropriate mode of response. The everyday normative attitude does not seem to lead to anomie in these cases, as it would in re-lation to illness.

We can put it this way: to react properly to illness, one must either under-stand the sickness naturalistically or one must know normatively what the patient "can" and "cannot" do. To react properly to the criminal one does not have to know more than in any other interaction-situation. We may also say that Alter always has the burden of proof in interaction with a sick person. In interaction with the criminal, Alter has no such burden of proof. In the case of conflicting definitions of the situation the criminal has the obligation to prove that Alter acted on false assumptions. Alter is sup-posed to act as if he had no knowledge of criminality, if the crime has been dealt with by the proper authorities. The function of the lay (nonprofessional) environment is reversed when we go from sickness to crime. The environ-ment is supposed to understand the sickness but forget the crime.

From what has been said it follows that the requirements of interaction necessarily demand some exclusion in the case of the sick but not necessarily in the case of the criminal. This lies in the naturalistic constitution of the

11. Cf. Fred Davis, "Definitions of Time and Recovery in Paralytic Polio Con-valescence," *The American Journal of Sociology*, 61 (1956), 582-587.

sick and in the normative constitution of the criminal. Although the *necessary* characteristics of a criminal are compatible with no exclusion, many criminals have additional characteristics that for different reasons demand exclusion, and sometimes more vigorously than in the case of any sick person. For one thing protection of values may demand removal of the criminal from the opportunity to approach them.

The Repercussions upon Social Status of Illness and Crime

We have so far dealt with the excluded state of the sick and of the criminal as if they were of a similar kind. They are similar insofar as both the role of the patient and the role of the convict or inmate are incompatible with other role performances. They differ, however, not only in entrance and termination criteria, but also in the *kind* of incompatibility implied.

When the criminal is excluded, especially when he is imprisoned, the criminal quality will tend to spread to the whole person in spite of the courts' tendency to deal specifically with the criminal act.[12] Prisons, unlike fines, demand the exclusion of the total person, irrespective of the specificity or generality of the judgment authorizing the imprisonment. Since the criminal is held responsible for his act, he will also tend to be blamed for his total criminal status. In other words, he is perceived to have chosen a criminal role in society. And this general choice (which is an imputation, not necessarily a fact) is considered to be more or less incompatible with a number of legitimate roles which the criminal may previously have held; with being a "good family man," "a citizen," "a political leader," "holding a responsible job," "being in a respectable business," "being an honest worker." It may be assumed that the feeling of incompatibility will be the stronger, the more highly desirable incumbency of a previously held role is supposed to be. In other words, to be a criminal is considered least compatible with the high status and high power positions in society.[13] The perceived incompatibility, if sufficiently strong, may result in one or both of two consequences: a) the individual criminal loses his status because of his incumbency of a criminal role; and b) the criminal throws doubt upon the moral quality on the basis of which the position of his status peers is founded.

Both of these consequences, but especially the latter, may disturb the system of stratification in a society; and remedial institutions are likely to arise. A simple solution is for laws or customs explicitly to define crimes and

---

12. Cf. Vilhelm Aubert, "Legal Justice and Mental Health," *Psychiatry*, (May 2¹, 1958), 101-113.

13. This problem is dealt with more extensively in Edwin H. Sutherland, *White Collar Crime* (New York: 1949); Vilhelm Aubert, "White Collar Crime and Social Structure," *The American Journal of Sociology*, 58 (1952), 263-271.

sanctions differentially for offenders of high and low status. Primitive customary law sometimes implies that what is forbidden for ordinary people may be permissible for the chiefs. Or it may state that what is proper sanction for an upper-class offender, differs from the proper sanction against a lower-class offender. The criminal laws of Europe during the late medieval ages stipulated different sanctions for high- and low-status offenders. Many codifications made it possible for the offender to negotiate about payment of damages instead of being punished. Only the upper classes were able to pay such damages. The consequence was that there existed one criminal law for the rich, where the fine was the major sanction, and another criminal law for the poor based upon capital and corporal punishment.[14] Schwarzenberg's *Peinliche Halsgerichtsordnung* from the 16th century states that criminals who were *"ehrbar"* (honorable) were to be fined, while those who were not, should be sanctioned with corporal punishment. The distinction was, as practiced, in terms of social status. English criminal law from the 16th and 17th centuries stipulated more severe punishment for those who could not read than for those who could.[15] As late as in the 19th century German criminal law instituted a privileged kind of imprisonment, *"Festungshaft,"* for offenders belonging to the upper classes.

With the growth and spread of democratic, egalitarian ideologies and of achievement as the predominant basis for status, explicit discrimination in the criminal law became untenable. One of the achievements of the great criminal law reformers of the period of enlightenment, Beccaria, Feuerbach, and Bentham, was to give everybody an equal opportunity, in principle, to become a criminal. "The criminal" became an open role, depending upon negative achievement. They left it to the agents of enforcement to cope with the problem suggested above. The problem has in part been taken care of by the increasing use of fines, which are usually meted out secretly (without public trial) and which tend to be viewed in specific terms, related to the act more than to the person.

We shall advance the hypothesis that another way to cope with possible conflicts between criminality and status is to institute individualizing treatment of serious offenders, culminating in the idea that criminals are often sick people, and should be dealt with accordingly. The development of this idea has many roots; and our hypothesis claims no more than that the need to cope with incompatibilities between criminal roles and certain status considerations has been a supporting factor in this development.

The sick criminal is not considered responsible for his crime, and probably even less for having chosen to become "a criminal." Although it has become apparent that he is incapable now of performing other roles, es-

---

14. Rusche and Kirchheimer, *op. cit.*
15. Leon Radzinowicz, *A History of English Criminal Law and its Administration from 1750* (London:1948), p. 140.

pecially the high status roles, he is not morally blamed for the incompatibilities in his situation. And the idea that he was "exploiting" his high status when committing the crime, an idea which easily may reflect upon his status peers, is not likely to arise. The secrecy which follows when mental sickness is indicated, further tends to protect the criminal and his environment from observations that might lead to status-challenging moral judgments. The assumption about sickness, that it is temporary and provides for a recovery process, means that for the sick criminal there is a definitive way back to his lost status, although he may not be able to fulfill this expectation of recovery.

If the historical hypothesis outlined above is correct, we should assume that in current criminal trials there is a tendency to label upper-class defendants as sick more frequently than lower-class defendants. Such a discrimination would also follow from the assumption that criminals are out to obtain values. Since the high status offender is characterized by the higher general accessiblity of values to him, it seems less natural to perceive him as somebody striving for a value through a crime. In addition to this, he appears to have more to lose by being caught, which renders his action even more irrational in terms of striving toward values.

If we think in terms of empirical comparisons of upper-class and lower-class offenders, however, we must take note of a factor which contributes to a discrimination in the opposite direction. In most modern societies there exists a group of offenders who outwardly are less characterized by specific illegal acts than by a general sordid state of existence, the hard core of which are the alcoholic vagrants. In terms of the criminal law they strive toward values by illegal means and interfere with the values of others. But they do so in a blurred way. What is highly visible about them is that they are generally unsuccessful in obtaining the values desired by most people, a home, decent clothes, regular meals, a good income, etc. They give the impression of being down and out, often showing signs of somatic malfunctioning due to drink and an unhealthy way of life. Small wonder, then, that this has been one of the first groups of offenders—in Norwegian law—to be defined as sick. Closer analysis has shown, however, that the legal authorities have failed to take full cognizance of the everyday logic of the models they deal with.[16] Alcoholic vagrants have been defined as sick in the sense of being in need of extensive, long-term "treatment." Since this treatment is in their own interest, certain guarantees of due process have been waived and so are ordinary considerations of proportionality between offense and sanction. But the vagrants are not treated as sick in the sense that they may choose whether they want to be treated or not, nor in the sense that they are submitted to medical intervention with a clear-cut thera-

16. We build here upon unpublished work by the Norwegian sociologist Nils Christie.

peutic rationale. As a matter of fact, they are put away for long periods of time in old-fashioned penal institutions.

The Transformation of Inmates to Patients

Another hypothesis about the evolution of the conception that criminals may be sick should be mentioned here. But let us again give a reminder that we are only dealing with partial, or supportive, explanations. Above all, we do not want to disparage the notion that the development of medicine, psychiatry, and psychology in itself furnishes an important explanation of the idea that criminals may be sick. With this in mind, however, we shall exploit the notion that application of a time perspective to the criminal is a relatively recent development. It had its origin in conditions unrelated to the evaluation of crimes as such.[17] Once it becomes usual, however, to sentence criminals to serve time periods in prison, it also becomes "natural" to deal with criminality as if it were a state capable of manipulation or modification over time. The criminal can be reformed. To be sure, the idea of reform was in the beginning conceived of as a moral change, a conversion or a gradual moral enlightenment. Solitary confinement was introduced with the rationale that it would give the criminal a chance to repent and think over his sins and make new and better plans for his future life, or prepare for the hereafter. It was inevitable, however, with increasing secularization and rationality that the process of reform should be viewed as a question of improvement or recovery in more ethically neutral terms. The analogy with the sick was near at hand, and probably the only one available.

Our hypothesis is, then, that the mere fact of criminals being held in confinement for specified periods of time, within rational systems of thought almost inevitably implies—in terms of everyday logic—a question of the functioning of time in prison as a process of recovery. Once this step is taken, it is inevitable that attempts should be made to apply the role of the patient to the inmate. The obvious suffering of the convict and his helplessness when confined make this step seem "rational" and "natural." That there are formidable obstacles to this development, however, has already been argued above.

It is hard to see how a hypothesis like the one cited above could be tested directly. Indirect evidence is found in the fact that no one seems to have proposed to turn those offenders whose behavior is customarily sanctioned by fines into patients.

Underlying these various reasons for defining crimes as symptoms of disease, we may discern a general need for predictability.[18] The criminal

17. Rusche and Kirchheimer, *op. cit.*
18. This need for predictability in relation to mental illness has been discussed in Elaine and John Cumming, *Closed Ranks: an Experiment in Mental Health Educa-*

law tells us nothing about what we can reasonably expect of a criminal in the future, unless it stipulates a death penalty or long-term imprisonment. Such sanctions are becoming increasingly unpopular, leaving us with more uncertainty concerning the future behavior of those who have once been convicted of a crime. In this situation we find the development of a whole new science, criminology, which attempts to link the individual criminal act to processes that have a time dimension, and which furnish measurable stages allowing predictions to be made. In terms of scientific premises and procedure, criminology is puzzling; but the puzzle is diminished if one assumes a social need for predictability in cases where the group has felt threatened or bewildered by a visibly deviant act.

The simplest way to link an offense to a predictable process is to connect it with relatively stable, although not necessarily unchangeable traits in the offender. The development in these schemes of interpretation has been from inborn organic traits, Lombroso's deformed and born criminal, toward personality defects or defects in enduring social stimulations. Since these theories get their support from a social need, they have blindly assumed the dictate of everyday logic that like causes like. A negative consequence (the offense) must have a negative cause, a defect in the offender. In other words: the offender must be sick or he must be in a state much like a disease. Such a definition brings his disturbing display of deviance in touch with elaborate schemes of prediction based upon naturalistic models of persons. In principle, his behavior is predictable. To what extent this "predictability in principle" will be achieved in practice by successful treatment and other precautionary devices, remains to be seen.

Implications for Modes of Decision—Making

We have discussed some differences between two classes of social objects as they are perceived by others, and we have indicated some consequences of these for the interaction between the deviant and his social environment. The decision concerning the entrance, termination, and type of exclusion and treatment is, however, often made by professionals on behalf of society. The doctor and the lawyer, especially the judge, are the roles to which is delegated the authority to make these decisions. Decision-making within medicine and law show some striking differences, which are related to the differences between the models around which the deviant roles of the sick and of the criminal are constructed. We shall briefly sketch some of these differences between medical and legal decisions. Such a juxtapositioning may throw some light upon more general problems of decision-making and upon the sociological conditions for the application of science, since medical decisions are derived from scientific,

---

tion (Cambridge: Harvard University Press, 1957).

utilitarian thinking, while legal decisions are not.[19]

MEDICAL DECISIONS

Most decisions of the scientific-utilitarian type concern interference with nature, the relationship of man to his nonhuman habitat. Decisions of this kind have indirectly had the broadest possible consequences for interpersonal relationships and for the whole structure of society. But our concern is that area of science which only deals with nature in the sense that within it man and human interrelationships are understood to be part of nature.

The decision to be made by a doctor is, as a rule, how the patient is to be treated. In this decision we can distinguish three elements: the diagnosis, prognosis, and choice of therapy. Let us consider the decision-maker's relationships of responsibility, to whom and for what he is responsible.

The doctor is primarily responsible to the patient. The patient normally comes voluntarily to the doctor and asks him to make a decision which it is in his own, the patient's, interest to obtain. The doctor is also responsible in other directions for the way in which he makes decisions. He is responsible to the medical association, and may incur its disciplinary measures. He may also be made responsible to a court of law in the case of gross neglect of duty, and may be punished. But the latter responsibility is almost entirely derived from his responsibility to one particular patient or to a general group of potential patients.

For *what* the doctor is responsible is not so easy to define. If we take responsibility in its widest possible sense, so that it includes everything that influences the doctor's reputation, salary, career, prestige, etc., one must conclude that the doctor is primarily responsible for the future effects of his decision. A cure will be a central indication for both doctors and patients that the doctor satisfied the expectations one had of him, although it is not the only criterion. In spite of exceptions and modifications, the doctor's responsibility is to a great extent linked with the results, the effects of his decision. This is shown above all in the fact that the doctor is considered in duty bound to check the effects by following the process of cure, and also possible negative developments.

It is characteristic of medical decisions of some importance that only those with a certain professional training have the right to make them. The law of quackery forbids others to make such decisions, although it is not rigorously enforced when lay healers deal competently with minor ailments. As soon as more important decisions in serious cases are taken by people without medical training, however, a hue and cry is raised which shows clearly that central norms for methods of decision-making have been ignored.

19. For a more extensive treatment, see Aubert, "Legal Justice and Mental Health," *op. cit.*

Medical decisions are secret, and this is laid down by law in the rule concerning a doctor's pledge of secrecy. This applies to the publicizing of diagnosis and therapy in concrete cases, but it is also up to the doctor's judgment as to how much he will tell the patient about the basis for his decision.

Medical decisions are limited to problems of health. The doctor cannot include in the appraisal of his decisions any other effects they may have. Neither is he responsible for any effects beyond the state of the patient's health. This is clearly brought out in the doctor's duty to help enemy soldiers in the time of war. It also holds good in cases when it is necessary to give medical help to condemned criminals or dying persons who have little to look forward to. Nor can it be considered his right or duty in such cases to assess the patient's total sum of happiness. His decisions concern the patient's health; and it is the effect on his health for which the doctor is responsible. Problems may arise here if the doctor, in his capacity as medical officer of an industrial plant or any army camp comes up against conflicting pressure from considerations of health and of the organization's efficiency. There seems to be a strong tendency among doctors to insist on limiting their responsibility to matters strictly concerning health.

A doctor's decisions in a particular case of illness do not need to be similar to decisions taken in other cases. Each individual case must be judged according to its own peculiarities. A doctor may know that a number of cases presenting particular symptoms, stomach pains, constipation, etc. have been diagnosed as catarrh and been given treatment accordingly with unfavorable results; but this is no reason for not diagnosing cancer and treating it as such. Or to put it more precisely, other similar cases are only to be treated as material for experience, data for generalization, but they do not have the character of precedent. The doctor must do his best in each individual case for each individual patient without taking into account whether other patients, attending other doctors, or in other circumstances, are not being given similarly thorough diagnoses and equally good treatment. When the doctor is dealing with a patient, justice is not a particularly relevant consideration. Equality before medicine is not an ideal of the same kind as equality before the law. It is the duty of the health authorities, not of medical science nor of the doctor, to think of justice. From the point of view of the doctor every patient has, in principle, the right to unlimited good service, irrespective of whether other patients can obtain the same.

LEGAL DECISIONS

"Juridical man," man as the organs of the law regard the parties in a case, is not an organism which goes through processes of change over a period of time. His criminality is not something that can be established by investigating him at the moment of the decision. The criminal's qualification for being a criminal depends entirely on an historic fact, his guilt.

This brings us to the question of the responsibility of the legal decision-makers. Toward *whom* are they responsible and for *what?* The judge is not only responsible toward his immediate "clients." That is quite obvious. His responsibility toward them is almost entirely derived from other relationships of responsibility. He has no particular responsibility for their welfare if its furtherance does not coincide with the judge's duties toward other instances. The judge's relationships of responsibility are somewhat abstract, and are linked with the law more than with the persons who make laws.

There is naturally a connection between this relationship and the fact that people may become the objects of legal decisions without having asked for them, indeed, if necessary against the strongest opposition. This is the situation, with few exceptions, in criminal cases; and in civil disputes also it is fairly usual for one of the parties not to desire any legal decision. But in the latter case the situation is nevertheless such that at any rate one of the parties, the plaintiff, asks for a decision in the same manner as a sick person. This does not, however, create any particularistic responsibility for the judge. The plaintiff does not become the client of the judge in the same way as the sick person becomes the patient of the doctor. And while the doctor receives a fee from his patient, similar fees from the plaintiff are called bribes, and represent a punishable relationship.

For *what* is the judge responsible? What features of the decision influence the judge's legal and social status? The judge is responsible to a much lesser degree than in medical decisions for the decision's future consequences. The judge's responsibility is primarily retroactive, linked with factual conditions in the past. He has the responsibility of describing these in a true fashion; and he has the responsibility of forming a reasonable estimate of the degree of probability of the presence of guilt or of other legally relevant characteristics of past actions. If this probability is not sufficiently strong, he must avoid building on his interpretation of the facts, and decide the case instead on the basis of rules concerning the burden of proof, rules concerning which of the parties is to bear the risk if a fact remains insufficiently clarified.

Along with the responsibility for describing correctly certain facts which belong to the past, the judge is responsible for the correct choice of rules under which the facts are to be subsumed. There is here more certainty and less room for individual judgment than in the doctor's choice of medical text under which he can subsume a case. If the judge gives a correct description of certain facts in the past and applies the right rules to those facts, he is safeguarded quite independently of the factual consequences of his decision.

That the judge has little responsibility for the effects of a legal decision is based on the philosophic principles on which our legal thinking builds. While the action of the doctor is often assumed to create health and to be the cause of the patient's cure, it not usual to assume that the judge creates law, rights, and duties. The parties in a legal case have themselves already created their rights and duties by actions in the past. The judge only *establishes* the content of these rights and duties which are assumed to have existed before the judge was called upon. We might also say that responsibility for the real consequences of his decision, if it is formally correct and retro- actively plausible, is assumed to lie on the parties to the case. The judge merely establishes what they have done, and how this is judged by abstract rules of law. The real consequences are implicit, from the legal point of view, in the parties' own actions. We might perhaps say that medical ethics takes the responsibility for the future from the patient, the sick person, and places a considerable amount of it on the doctor. But legal ethics places the responsibility for the future on the law-breaker or on the litiga- ting parties, and exempts the judge from it to a very great degree.

Contrary to cases of medical decision, laymen play a fairly large part in legal decisions. There are even countries where permanent judges are ap- pointed by election, and these can be persons who do not have a legal training. To the same extent as quackery is condemned in medicine, so the institution of the lay judge is honored in the administration of justice. It doubtless has something to do with the element of force in law. In medi- cine "the people" sanction decisions directly, in that the patient agrees to be treated. Since this direct agreement is lacking in many legal situations, another, indirect, form of control by "the people" is necessary. Because the law is an aspect of the state, the judicial process has come to be in- fluenced by general political developments, where representation and democ- racy are ideologically basic demands.

The principle of the lay judge naturally has a number of consequences for legal decisions. As long as the lay judges are included the courts cannot draw much on specialized knowledge. This also means that legal thinking and terminology have to maintain the possibility of communication with laymen. It may also have the effect, which is its expressed purpose, of preventing judges' decisions from being too strongly influenced by the special attitudes and ways of thought which obtain among jurists. Tradi- tionally, jurists have been a somewhat unpopular professional group. The profession cannot under any circumstances measure up to "the men in white" who have been strongly romanticized.

The element of the layman in law is not only apparent in the institution of the lay judge. The professional judges are also more or less lay persons in a scientific or technical sense as regards most of the questions put before them. Few judges in Norway are specialized as to factual area of compe- tence. One and the same judge will usually function in cases which stem from a number of highly varied walks of life, and which are perhaps linked with several different sciences.[20]

The demand that the law shall be *one,* the same for all, becomes more dif-

20. When the Chief Justice of the Norwegian Supreme Court retired this spring, he mentioned the manifold of diverse cases, ranging over the total span of human existence, as one of the greatest attractions of the Bench.

ficult to meet, the more specialized the courts are. One could perhaps go a step further, beyond the administration of justice itself, and maintain that, because they are nonspecialized, the courts provide a point of contact for problems arising from areas of dissimilar specialists. In this way the lawyers become a link between the many professional "subcultures" which are to be found in a modern industrial society. The lawyers, and in the last resort the courts, help to prevent these special cultures from becoming too greatly isolated from each other, an eventuality which would cause the social structure to creak at the joints.

Oddly enough it is perhaps also true that professionals are not always most suited to making certain decisions even in their own field of specialization. Here we are thinking of those decisions in which there is a strong element of doubt, and legal decisions often belong to this category. This doubt would often make it impossible for a professional to reach a decision at all. His special insight and professional interest might make it psychologically exceedingly difficult to maintain that a particular decision, which in addition has to be reached quickly, is *the right one*. Lawyers are a professional group trained in making decisions, regardless of whether their scientific foundation is well worked out or whether they find themselves in an area where science is silent. Lawyers answer the need of society for a group of persons who can, and who are willing to, make—and justify—decisions in cases where the possibility of reaching a "scientifically correct" result is very small.

Medical decisions are on the whole secret, legal decisions are in principle public. This is to a great extent a consequence of the same considerations which support the institution of the lay judge. Since the individual can be forcibly exposed to legal decisions, there is little control in the fact that the accused himself knows the basis for the decision. Others must know it and make up their minds. In the same way as with the principle of the lay judge, the publicity surrounding legal cases also prevents too specialized and scientific a method of decision-making. There are three characteristics of scientific methods of approach which do not harmonize with complete publicity concerning decisions: the technical language of science, which is difficult to understand; its lack of engagement in important values at certain stages of the investigations, and finally its probabilistic character which openly warns against certainty and faith. As long as publicity is regarded as an important value in connection with legal decisions, it will be difficult for these decisions to take on these characteristics. And this means that it is difficult for them to take on a scientific character.

Legal decisions are not factually limited in the same way as medical decisions. But they too have a limitation, often a very narrow limitation. The judge can ignore everything which is "legally irrelevant." He does not have the duty of stressing all those factors which he believes to be important for the consequences of his decision, but only those which the law—legislation, custom, and precedent—have indicated as relevant. These factors may belong to the most varied professional areas, but, in that their limitation simplifies reality and makes it possible to act, they have something in common with an empirical theory.

In legal decisions precedent is of great importance, and comparisons are relevant to the highest degree. Equality before the law is a basic legal value in the sense that similar cases are to be treated similarly, even though several investigations have demonstrated the difficulties of realizing this ideal in legal practice. That the judicial system is built up as *one* pyramid, with *one* highest legislative instance and *one* supreme court, serves the purpose of guaranteeing a certain uniformity in legal practice. Nothing completely similar exists, and especially not in principle, with regard to medical or other scientific decisions. Scientific ethics rejects the idea of *one* supreme scientific authority. The centuries-long fight against the authority of Aristotle has created an exceedingly strong conviction on this point.

20

THOMAS J. SCHEFF

Decision Rules and Types of Error, and Their Consequences in Medical Diagnosis

Members of professions such as law and medicine frequently are confronted with uncertainty in the course of their routine duties. In these circumstances, informal norms have developed for handling uncertainty so that paralyzing hesitation is avoided. These norms are based upon assumptions that some types of error are more to be avoided than others; assumptions so basic that they are usually taken for granted, are seldom discussed, and are therefore slow to change.

The purpose of this paper is to describe one important norm for handling uncertainty in medical diagnosis, that judging a sick person well is more to be avoided than judging a well person sick, and to suggest some of the consequences of the application of this norm in medical practice. Apparently this norm, like many important cultural norms, "goes without saying" in the subculture of the medical profession; in form, however, it resembles any decision rule for guiding behavior under conditions of uncertainty. In the discussion that follows, decision rules in law, statistics, and medicine are compared, in order to indicate the types of error that are thought to be the more important to avoid and the assumptions underlying this preference. On the basis of recent findings of the widespread distribution of elements of disease and deviance in normal populations, the assumption of a uniform relationship between disease signs and impairment is criticized. Finally, it is suggested that to the extent that physicians are guided by this medical decision rule, they too often place patients in the "sick role" who could otherwise have continued in their normal pursuits.

Reprinted from *Behavioral Science*, 8 (1963), pp. 97-107, by permission of the author and publisher.

This paper was written with the financial support of the Graduate Research Committee of the University of Wisconsin. Colleagues too numerous to list here made useful suggestions. David Mechanic was particularly helpful. An earlier version was presented at the Conference on Mathematical Models in the Behavioral and Social Sciences, sponsored by the Western Management Science Institute, University of California

Decision Rules

To the extent that physicians and the public are biased toward treatment, the "creation" of illness, i.e., the production of unnecessary impairment, may go hand in hand with the prevention and treatment of disease in modern medicine. The magnitude of the bias toward treatment in any single case may be quite small, since there are probably other medical decision rules ("When in doubt, delay your decision") which counteract the rule discussed here. Even a small bias, however, if it is relatively constant throughout Western society, can have effects of large magnitude. Since this argument is based largely on fragmentary evidence, it is intended merely to stimulate further discussion and research, rather than to demonstrate the validity of a point of view. The discussion will begin with the consideration of a decision rule in law.

In criminal trials in England and the United States, there is an explicit rule for arriving at decisions in the face of uncertainty: "A man is innocent until proven guilty." The meaning of this rule is made clear by the English common-law definition of the phrase "proven guilty," which according to tradition is that the judge or jury must find the evidence of guilt compelling *beyond a reasonable doubt.* The basic legal rule for arriving at a decision in the face of uncertainty may be briefly stated: "When in doubt, acquit." That is, the jury or judge must not be equally wary of erroneously convicting or acquitting: the error that is most important to avoid is to erroneously convict. This concept is expressed in the maxim, "Better a thousand guilty men go free, than one innocent man be convicted."

The reasons underlying this rule seem clear. It is assumed that in most cases, a conviction will do irreversible harm to an individual by damaging his reputation in the eyes of his fellows. The individual is seen as weak and defenseless, relative to society, and therefore in no position to sustain the consequences of an erroneous decision. An erroneous acquittal, on the other hand, damages society. If an individual who has actually committed a crime is not punished, he may commit the crime again, or more important, the deterrent effect of punishment for the violation of this crime may be diminished for others. Although these are serious outcomes they are generally thought not to be as serious as the consequences of erroneous conviction for the innocent individual, since society is able to sustain an indefinite number of errors without serious consequences. For these and perhaps other reasons, the decision rule to assume innocence exerts a powerful influence on legal proceedings.

TYPE 1 AND TYPE 2 ERRORS

Deciding on guilt or innocence is a special case of a problem to which statisticians have given considerable attention, the testing of hypotheses.

at Los Angeles, Cambria, California, November 3-5, 1961

Since most scientific work is done with samples, statisticians have developed techniques to guard against results which are due to chance sampling fluctuations. The problem, however, is that one might reject a finding as due to sampling fluctuations which was actually correct. There are, therefore, two kinds of errors: rejecting a hypothesis which is true, and accepting one which is false. Usually the hypothesis is stated so that the former error (rejecting a hypothesis which is true) is the error that is thought to be the more important to avoid. This type of error is called an "error of the first kind," or a Type 1 error. The latter error (accepting a hypothesis which is false) is the less important error to avoid, and is called an "error of the second kind," or a Type 2 error.[1]

To guard against chance fluctuations in sampling, statisticians test the probability that findings could have arisen by chance. At some predetermined probability (called the alpha level), usually .05 or less, the possibility that the findings arose by chance is rejected. This level means that there are five chances in a hundred that one will reject a hypothesis which is true. Although these five chances indicate a real risk of error, it is not common to set the level much lower (say .001) because this raises the probability of making an error of the second kind.

A similar dilemma faces the judge or jury in deciding whether to convict or acquit in the face of uncertainty. Particularly in the adversary system of law, where professional attorneys seek to advance their arguments and refute those of their opponents, there is often considerable uncertainty even as to the facts of the case, let alone intangibles like intent. The maxim, "Better a thousand guilty men should go free, than one innocent man be convicted," would mean, if taken literally rather than as a rhetorical flourish, that the alpha level for legal decisions is set quite low.

Although the legal decision rule is not expressed in as precise a form as a statistical decision rule, it represents a very similar procedure for dealing with uncertainty. There is one respect, however, in which it is quite different. Statistical decision procedures are recognized by those who use them as mere conveniences, which can be varied according to the circumstances. The legal decision rule, in contrast, is an inflexible and binding moral rule, which carries with it the force of long sanction and tradition. The assumption of innocence is a part of the social institution of law in Western society; it is explicitly stated in legal codes, and is accepted as legitimate by jurists and usually by the general populace, with only occasional grumbling, e.g., a criminal is seen as "getting off" because of "legal technicalities."

DECISION RULES IN MEDICINE

Although the analogous rule for decisions in medicine is not as explicitly stated as the rule in law and probably is considerably less rigid,

1. J. Neyman, *First Course in Statistics and Probability* (New York: Holt, 1950), pp. 265-266.

it would seem that there is such a rule in medicine which is as imperative in its operation as its analogue in law. Do physicians and the general public consider that rejecting the hypothesis of illness when it is true, or accepting it when it is false, is the error that is most important to avoid? It seems fairly clear that the rule in medicine may be stated as: "When in doubt, continue to suspect illness." That is, for a physician to dismiss a patient when he is actually ill is a Type 1 error, and to retain a patient when he is not ill is a Type 2 error.

Most physicians learn early in their training that it is far more culpable to dismiss a sick patient than to retain a well one. This rule is so pervasive and fundamental that it goes unstated in textbooks on diagnosis. It is occasionally mentioned explicitly in other contexts, however. Neyman, for example, in his discussion of X-ray screening for tuberculosis, states:

"[If the patient is actually well, but the hypothesis that he is sick is accepted, a Type 2 error] then the patient will suffer some unjustified anxiety and, perhaps, will be put to some unnecessary expense until further studies of his health will establish that any alarm about the state of his chest is unfounded. Also, the unjustified precautions ordered by the clinic may somewhat affect its reputation. On the other hand, should the hypothesis [of sickness] be true and yet the accepted hypothesis be [that he is well, a Type 1 error], then the patient will be in danger of losing the precious opportunity of treating the incipient disease in its beginning stages when the cure is not so difficult. Furthermore, the oversight by the clinic's specialist of the dangerous condition would affect the clinic's reputation even more than the unnecessary alarm. From this point of view, it appears that the error of rejecting the hypothesis [of sickness] when it is true is *far more important* to avoid than the error of accepting the hypothesis [of illness] when it is false."[2]

Although this particular discussion pertains to tuberculosis, it is pertinent to many other diseases also. From casual conversations with physicians, the impression one gains is that this moral lesson is deeply ingrained in the physician's personal code.

It is not only physicians who feel this way, however. This rule is grounded both in legal proceedings and in popular sentiment. Although there is some sentiment against Type 2 errors (unnecessary surgery, for instance), it has nothing like the force and urgency of the sentiment against Type 1 errors. A physician who dismisses a patient who subsequently dies of a disease that should have been detected is not only subject to legal action for negligence and possible loss of license for incompetence, but also to moral condemnation from his colleagues and from his own conscience for his delinquency. Nothing remotely resembling this amount of moral and legal suasion is brought to bear for committing a Type 2 error. Indeed, this error is sometimes seen as sound clinical practice, indicating a healthily conservative approach to medicine.

2. *Ibid.*, p. 270. Italics added.

The discussion to this point suggests that physicians follow a decision rule which may be stated, "When in doubt, diagnose illness." If physicians are actually influenced by this rule, then studies of the validity of diagnosis should demonstrate the operation of the rule. That is, we should expect that objective studies of diagnostic errors should show that Type 1 and Type 2 errors do not occur with equal frequency, but in fact, that Type 2 errors far outnumber Type 1 errors. Unfortunately for our purposes, however, there are apparently only a few studies which provide the type of data which would adequately test the hypothesis. Although studies of the reliability of diagnosis abound,[3] showing that physicians disagree with each other in their diagnoses of the same patients, these studies do not report the validity of diagnosis, or the types of error which are made, with the following exceptions.

We can infer that Type 2 errors outnumber Type 1 errors from Bakwin's study of physicians' judgments regarding the advisability of tonsillectomy for 1,000 school children. "Of these, some 611 had had their tonsils removed. The remaining 389 were then examined by other physicians, and 174 were selected for tonsillectomy. This left 215 children whose tonsils were apparently normal. Another group of doctors was put to work examining these 215 children, and 99 of them were adjudged in need of tonsillectomy. Still another group of doctors was then employed to examine the remaining children, and nearly one-half were recommended for operation."[4] Almost half of each group of children were judged to be in need of the operation. Even assuming that a small proportion of children needing tonsillectomy were missed in each examination (Type 1 error), the number of Type 2 errors in this study far exceeded the number of Type 1 errors.

In the field of roentgenology, studies of diagnostic error are apparently more highly developed than in other areas of medicine. Garland, in his study, summarizes these findings, reporting that in a study of 14,867 films for tuberculosis signs, there were 1,216 positive readings which turned out to be clinically negative (Type 2 error) and only 24 negative readings which turned out to be clinically active (Type 1 error)! This ratio is apparently a fairly typical finding in roentgenographic studies. Since physicians are well aware of the provisional nature of radiological findings, this great discrepancy between the frequency of the types of error in film screening is not too alarming. On the other hand, it does provide objective evidence of the operation of the decision rule "Better safe than sorry."

BASIC ASSUMPTIONS

The logic of this decision rule rests on two assumptions:
1. Disease is usually a determinate, inevitably unfolding process, which,

3. L. H. Garland, "Studies of the Accuracy of Diagnostic Procedures," *American Journal of Roentgenology, Radium Therapy, Nuclear Medicine.* 82 (1959), 25-38.

4. H. Bakwin, "Pseudodoxia Pediatrica," *New England Journal of Medicine.* 232 (1945), 693.

if undetected and untreated, will grow to a point where it endangers the life or limb of the individual, and in the case of contagious diseases, the lives of others. This is not to say, of course, that physicians think of all diseases as determinate: witness the concept of the "benign" condition. The point here is that the imagery of disease which the physician uses in attempting to reach a decision, his working hypothesis, is *usually* based on the deterministic model of disease.

2. Medical diagnosis of illness, unlike legal judgment, is not an irreversible act which does untold damage to the status and reputation of the patient. A physician may search for illness for an indefinitely long time, causing inconvenience for the patient, perhaps, but in the typical case doing the patient no irradicable harm. Obviously, again, physicians do not *always* make this assumption. A physician who suspects epilepsy in a truck driver knows full well that his patient will probably never drive a truck again if the diagnosis is made, and the physician will go to great lengths to avoid a Type 2 error in this situation. Similarly, if a physician suspects that a particular patient has hypochondriacal trends, the physician will lean in the direction of a Type 1 error in a situation of uncertainty. These and other similar situations are exceptions, however. The physician's *usual* working assumption is that medical observation and diagnosis, in itself, is neutral and innocuous, relative to the dangers resulting from disease.[5]

In the light of these two assumptions, therefore, it is seen as far better for the physician to chance a Type 2 error than a Type 1 error. These two assumptions will be examined and criticized in the remainder of the paper. The assumption that Type 2 errors are relatively harmless will be considered first.

In recent discussions it is increasingly recognized that in one area of medicine, psychiatry, the assumption that medical diagnosis can cause no irreversible harm to the patient's status is dubious. Psychiatric treatment, in many segments of the population and for many occupations, raises a question about the person's social status. It could be argued that in making a medical diagnosis the psychiatrist comes very close to making a legal decision, with its ensuing consequences for the person's reputation. One might argue that the Type 2 error in psychiatry, of judging a well person sick, is at least as much to be avoided as the Type 1 error, of judging a sick person well. Yet the psychiatrist's moral orientation, since he is first and foremost a physician, is guided by the medical, rather than the legal, decision rule.[6] The psychiatrist continues to be more willing to err on the

5. Even though this assumption is widely held, it has been vigorously criticized within the medical profession. See, for example, W. Darley, "What Is the Next Step in Preventive Medicine?" *Association of Teachers of Preventive Medicine Newsletter* (1959), p. 6. For a witty criticism of both assumptions, see H.M. Ratner, *Interviews on the American Character* (Santa Barbara: Center for the Study of Democratic Institutions, 1962).

6. Many authorities believe that psychiatrists seldom turn away a patient without finding an illness. See, for example, the statement about large state mental hospitals

conservative side, to diagnose as ill when the person is healthy, even though it is no longer clear that this error is any more desirable than its opposite.[7]

There is a more fundamental question about this decision rule, however, which concerns both physical illness and mental disorder. This question primarily concerns the first assumption, that disease is a determinate process. It also implicates the second assumption, that medical treatment does not have irreversible effects.

In recent years physicians and social scientists have reported finding disease signs and deviant behavior prevalent in normal, noninstitutionalized populations. It has been shown, for instance, that deviant acts, some of a serious nature, are widely admitted by persons in random samples of normal populations.[8] There is some evidence which suggests that grossly deviant, "psychotic" behavior has at least temporarily existed in relatively large proportions of a normal population.[9] Finally, there is a growing body of evidence that many signs of physical disease are distributed quite widely in normal populations. A recent survey of simple high blood pressure indicated that the prevalence ranged from 11.4 to 37.2 percent in the various subgroups studied.[10]

It can be argued that physical defects and "psychiatric" deviancy exist in an uncrystallized form in large segments of the population. Lemert[11] calls this type of behavior, which is often transitory, *primary deviation.* Balint,[12] in his discussion of the doctor-patient relationship, speaks of similar behavior as the "unorganized phase of illness." Balint seems to

---

in Esther L. Brown, *Newer Dimensions of Patient Care* (New York: Russell Sage Foundation, 1961), n. p. 60, and D. Mechanic, "Some Factors in Identifying and Defining Mental Illness," *Mental Hygiene* 46 (1962), 66-74. For a study demonstrating the presumption of illness in psychiatric examinations, see T.J. Scheff, "The Societal Reaction to Deviance," *Social Problems* 11(1964), 401-413.

7. "The sociologist must point out that whenever a psychiatrist makes a clinical diagnosis of an existing need for treatment, society makes the social diagnosis of a changed status for one of its members." (K. T. Erickson, "Patient Role and Social Uncertainty—A Dilemma of the Mentally Ill," *Psychiatry* 20[1957], 263-274).

8. J. S. Wallerstein and C. J. Wyle, "Our Law-Abiding Law-Breakers," *Probation* 25 (1947), 107-112; A. L. Porterfield, *Youth in Trouble* (Fort Worth, Texas: Leo Potishman Foundation, 1946); A. C. Kinsey, W. B. Pomeroy, and C. E. Martin, *Sexual Behavior in the Human Male* (Philadelphia: W. B. Saunders, 1948).

9. A. J. Clausen and M. R. Yarrow, "Paths to the Mental Hospital," *Journal of Social Issues* 11 (1955), 25-32, and R. J. Plunkett and J. E. Gordon, *Epidemiology and Mental Illness* (New York: Basic Books, 1961).

10. P. M. Rautahargu, M. J. Karvonen, and A. Keys, "The Frequency of Arteriosclerotic and Hypertensive Heart Disease in Ostensibly Healthy Working Populations in Finland," *Journal of Chronic Diseases* 13 (1961), 426-439; J. Stokes and T. R. Dawber, "The 'Silent Coronary': The Frequency and Clinical Characteristics of Unrecognized Myocardial Infarction in the Framingham Study," *Annals of Internal Medicine*, 50 (1959), 1359-1369; and J. P. Dunn and L. E. Etter, "Inadequacy of the Medical History in the Diagnosis of Duodenal Ulcer," *New England Journal of Medicine*, 266 (1962), 68-72.

11. E. M. Lemart, *Social Pathology* (New York: McGraw-Hill, 1951), p. 75.

12. M. Balint, *The Doctor, His Patient, and the Illness* (New York: International Universities Press, 1957), p. 18.

take for granted, however, that patients will eventually "settle down" to an "organized" illness. Yet it is possible that other outcomes may occur. A person in this stage might change jobs or wives instead, or merely continue in the primary deviation stage indefinitely, without getting better or worse.

This discussion suggests that in order to know the probability that a person with a disease sign would become incapacitated because of the development of disease, investigations quite unlike existing studies would need to be conducted. These would be longitudinal studies of outcomes in persons having signs of disease in a random sample of a normal population, in which no attempt was made to arrest the disease. It is true that there are a number of longitudinal studies in which the effects of treatment are compared with the effects of nontreatment. These studies, however, have always been conducted with clinical groups, rather than with persons with disease signs who were located in field studies.[13] Even clinical trials appear to offer many difficulties, both from the ethical and scientific points of view.[14] These difficulties would be increased many times in controlled field trials, as would the problems which concern the amount of time and money necessary. Without such studies, nevertheless, the meaning of many common disease signs remains somewhat equivocal.

Given the relatively small amount of knowledge about the distributions and natural outcomes of many diseases, it is possible that our conceptions of the danger of disease are exaggerated. For example, until the late 1940's histoplasmosis was thought to be a rare tropical disease, with a uniform fatal outcome. Recently, however, it was discovered that it is widely prevalent, and with fatal outcome or impairment extremely rare.[15] It is conceivable that other diseases, such as some types of heart disease and mental disorder, may prove to be similar in character. Although no actuarial studies have been made which would yield the true probabilities of impairment, physicians usually set the Type 1 level quite high, because they believe that the probability of impairment from making a Type 2 error is quite low. Let us now examine that assumption.

THE "SICK ROLE"

If, as has been argued here, much illness goes unattended without serious consequences, the assumption that medical diagnosis has no irreversible effects on the patient seems questionable. "The patient's attitude to his illness

13. The Framingham study is an exception to this statement. Even in this study, however, experimental procedures (random assignment to treatment and nontreatment groups) were not used. (T. R. Dawber, F. E. Moore, and G. V. Mann, "Coronary Heart Disease in The Framingham Study," *American Journal of Public Health*, 47: 2 [1957], 4-24).

14. A.B. Hill, ed., *Controlled Clinical Trials* (Springfield, Ill.: Charles C. Thomas, 1960).

15. J. Schwartz and G. L. Baum, "The History of Histoplasmosis," *New England Journal of Medicine*, 256 (1957), 253-258.

is usually considerably changed during and by, the series of physical examinations. These changes, which may profoundly influence the course of a chronic illness, are not taken seriously by the medical profession and, though occasionally mentioned, they have never been the subject of a proper scientific investigation."[16]

There are grounds for believing that persons who avail themselves of professional services are under considerable strain and tension (if the problem could have been easily solved, they would probably have used more informal means of handling it). Social-psychological principles indicate that persons under strain are highly suggestible, particularly to suggestions from a prestigeful source, such as a physician.

It can be argued that the Type 2 error involves the danger of having a person enter the "sick role"[17] in circumstances where no serious result would ensue if the illness were unattended. Perhaps the combination of a physician determined to find disease *signs,* if they are to be found, and the suggestible patient, searching for subjective *symptoms* among the many amorphous and usually unattended bodily impulses, is often sufficient to unearth a disease which changes the patient's status from that of well to sick, and may also have effects on his familial and occupational status. (In Lemert's terms the illness would be *secondary deviation* after the person has entered the sick role.)

There is a considerable body of evidence in the medical literature concerning the process in which the physician unnecessarily causes the patient to enter the sick role. Thus, in a discussion of "iatrogenic" (physician-induced) heart disease, this point is made:

"The physician, by calling attention to a murmur or some cardiovascular abnormality, even though functionally insignificant, may precipitate [symptoms of heart disease]. The experience of the work classification units of cardiac-in-industry programs, where patients with cardiovascular disease are evaluated as to work capacity, gives impressive evidence regarding the high incidence of such functional manifestations in persons with the diagnosis of cardiac lesion."[18]

Although there is a tendency in medicine to dismiss this process as due to quirks of particular patients, e.g., as malingering, hypochrondriasis, or as "merely functional disease" (that is, functional for the patient), causation probably lies not in the patient, but in medical procedures. Most people, perhaps, if they actually have the disease signs and are told by an authority, the physician, that they are ill, will obligingly come up with appropriate symptoms. A case history will illustrate this process. Under the heading "It may be well to let sleeping dogs lie," a physician recounts the following case:

16. M. Balint, *op. cit.,* p. 43.

17. T. Parsons, "Illness and the Role of the Physician," *American Journal of Orthopsychiatry,* 21 (1950), 452-460.

18. J. V. Warren and Janet Wolter, "Symptoms and Diseases Induced by the Physician," *General Practitioner,* 9 (1954), 78.

"Here is a woman, aged 40 years, who is admitted with symptoms of congestive cardiac failure, valvular disease, mitral stenosis, and auricular fibrillation. She tells us that she did not know that there was anything wrong with her heart and that she had had no symptoms up to 5 years ago when her chest was x-rayed in the course of a mass radiography examination for tuberculosis. She was not suspected and this was only done in the course of routine at the factory. Her lungs were pronounced clear but she was told that she had an enlarged heart and was advised to go to a hospital for investigation and treatment. From that time she began to suffer from symptoms—breathlessness on exertion—and has been in the hospital 4 or 5 times since. Now she is here with congestive heart failure. She cannot understand why, from the time that her enlarged heart was discovered, she began to get symptoms."[19]

What makes this kind of "role taking" extremely important is that it can occur even when the diagnostic label is kept from the patient. By the way he is handled, the patient can usually infer the nature of the diagnosis, since in his uncertainty and anxiety he is extremely sensitive to subtleties in the physician's behavior. An interesting example of this process is found in reports on treatment of battle fatigue. Speaking of psychiatric patients in the Sicilian campaign during World War II, a psychiatrist notes:

"Although patients were received at this hospital within 24 to 48 hours after their breakdown, a disappointing number, approximately 15 percent, were salvaged for combat duty . . . any therapy, including usual interview methods that sought to uncover basic emotional conflicts or attempted to relate current behavior and symptoms with past personality patterns seemingly provided patients with logical reasons for their combat failure. The insights obtained by even such mild depth therapy readily convinced the patient and often his therapist that the limit of combat endurance had been reached as proved by vulnerable personality traits. Patients were obligingly cooperative in supplying details of their neurotic childhood, previous emotional difficulties, lack of aggressiveness and other dependency traits. . ."[20]

Glass goes on to say that removal of the soldier from his unit for treatment of any kind usually resulted in long-term neurosis. In contrast, if the soldier was given only superficial psychiatric attention and *kept with his unit,* chronic impairment was usually avoided. The implication is that removal from the military unit and psychiatric treatment symbolizes to the soldier, behaviorally rather than with verbal labels, the "fact" that he is a mental case.

The traditional way of interpreting these reactions of the soldiers, and

19. H. Gardiner-Hill, *Clinical Involvements* (London: Butterworth, 1958), p. 158.
20. A. J. Glass, "Psychotherapy in the Combat Zone," *Symposium on Stress* (Washington, D.C.: Army Medical Service Graduate School, 1953), p. 228. Cf. A. Kardiner and H. Spiegel, *War Stress and Neurotic Illness* (New York: Hoeber, 1947),

perhaps the civilian cases, is in terms of malingering or feigning illness. The process of taking roles, however, as it is conceived of here, is not completely or even largely voluntary.[21] Vaguely defined impulses become "real" to the participants when they are organized under any one of a number of more or less interchangeable social roles. It can be argued that when a person is in a confused and suggestible state, when he organizes his feelings and behavior by using the sick role, and when his choice of roles is validated by a physician and/or others, that he is "hooked" and will proceed on a career of chronic illness.[22]

Implications for Research

The hypothesis suggested by the preceding discussion is that physicians and the public typically overvalue medical treatment relative to nontreatment as a course of action in the face of uncertainty, and that this overvaluation results in the creation as well as the prevention of impairment. This hypothesis, since it is based on scattered observations, is put forward only to point out several areas where systematic research is needed.

From the point of view of assessing the effectiveness of medical practice, this hypothesis is probably too general to be used directly. Needed for such a task are hypotheses concerning the condition under which error is likely to occur, the type of error that is likely, and the consequences of each type of error. Significant dimensions of the amount and type of error and its consequences would appear to be characteristics of the disease, the physician, the patient, and the organizational setting in which diagnosis takes place. Thus for diseases such as pneumonia which produce almost certain impairment unless attended, and for which a quick and highly effective cure is available, the hypothesis is probably largely irrelevant. On the other hand, the hypothesis may be of considerable importance for diseases which have a less certain outcome, and for which existing treatments are protracted and of uncertain value. Mental disorders and some types of heart disease are cases in point.

The working philosophy of the physician is probably relevant to the predominant type of errors made. Physicians who generally favor active intervention probably make more Type 2 errors than other physicians who view their treatments only as assistance for natural bodily reactions to

chaps. 3 and 4.

21. For a sophisticated discussion of role-playing, see E. Goffman. *The Presentation of Self in Everyday Life* (Garden City, N.Y.: Doubleday Anchor, 1959), pp. 17-22.

22. Some of the findings of the Purdue Farm Cardiac Project support the position taken in this paper. It was found, for example, that "iatrogenics" took more health precautions than "hidden cardiacs," suggesting that entry into the sick role can cause more social incapacity than the actual disease does (R. L. Eichorn and R. M. Andersen, "Changes in Personal Adjustment to Perceived and Medically Established Heart Disease: A Panel Study," paper read at American Sociological Association Meeting, Washington, D.C., 1962, pp. 11-15).

disease. The physician's perception of the personality of the patient may also be relevant; Type 2 errors are less likely if the physician defines the patient as a "crock," a person overly sensitive to discomfort, rather than as a person who ignores or denies disease.

Finally, the organizational setting is relevant to the extent that it influences the relationship between the doctor and the patient. In some contexts, as in medical practice in organizations such as the military or industrial setting, the physician is not as likely to feel personal responsibility for the patient as he would in others, such as private practice. This may be due in part to the conditions of financial remuneration, and perhaps equally important, the sheer volume of patients dependent on the doctor's time. Cultural or class differences may also affect the amount of social distance between doctor and patient, and therefore the amount of responsibility which the doctor feels for the patient. Whatever the sources, the more the physician feels personally responsible for the patient, the more likely he is to make a Type 2 error.

To the extent that future research can indicate the conditions which influence the amount, type, and consequences of error, such research can make direct contributions to medical practice. Three types of research seem necessary. First, in order to establish the true risks of impairment associated with common disease signs, controlled field trials of treated and untreated outcomes in a normal population would be needed. Second, perhaps in conjunction with these field trials, experimental studies of the effect of suggestion of illness by physicians and others would be necessary to determine the risks of unnecessary entry into the sick role.

Finally, studies of a mathematical nature seem to be called for. Suppose that physicians were provided with the results of the studies suggested above. How could these findings be introduced into medical practice as a corrective to cultural and professional biases in decision-making procedures? One promising approach is the strategy of evaluating the relative utility of alternative courses of action, based upon decision theory or game theory.[23]

Ledley and Lusted[24] reviewed a number of mathematical techniques which might be applicable to medical decision-making, one of these techniques being the use of the "expected value" equation, which is derived from game theory. Although their discussion pertains to the relative value of two treatment procedures, it is also relevant, with only slight changes in wording, to determining the expected values of treatment relative to nontreatment. The expected values of two treatments, they say, may be calculated from a simple expression involving only two kinds of terms: the probability that the diagnosis is correct, and the absolute value of the treatment (at its sim-

---

23. For an introductory text, see H. Chernoff and L. E. Moses, *Elementary Decision Theory* (New York: John Wiley, 1959).
24. R. S. Ledley and L. B. Lusted, "Reasoning Foundations of Medical Diagnosis," *Science*, 130 (1959), 9-21.

plest, the absolute value is the rate of cure for persons known to have the disease).

The "expected value" of a treatment is:

$$E_t = p_s v_s{}^s + (1-p_s)v_h{}^s.$$

(The superscript refers to the way the patient is treated, the subscript refers to his actual condition. *s* signifies sick, *h*, healthy.) That is, the expected value of a treatment is the probability *p* that the patient has the disease, multiplied by the value of the treatment for patients who actually have the disease, plus the probability that the patient does not have the disease $(1 - p)$, multiplied by the value (or "cost") of the treatment for patients who do not have the disease.

Similarly, the expected value of nontreatment is:

$$E_n = p_s v_s{}^h + (1-p_s)v_h{}^h.$$

That is, the expected value of nontreatment is the probability that the patient has the disease multiplied by the value (or "cost") of treating a person as healthy who is actually sick, plus the probability that the patient does not have the disease, multiplied by the value of not treating a healthy person.

The best course of action is indicated by comparing the magnitude of E_t and E_n. If E_t is larger, treatment is indicated. If E_n is larger, nontreatment is indicated. Evaluating these equations involves estimating the probability of correct diagnosis and constructing a payoff matrix for the values of $v_s{}^s$ (proportion of patients who actually had the disease who were cured by the treatment), $v_h{}^s$ (cost of treating a healthy person as sick: inconvenience, working days lost, surgical risks, unneccessary entry into sick role), $v_s{}^h$ (cost of treating a sick person as well: a question involving the proportions of persons who spontaneously recover, and the seriousness of results when the disease goes unchecked), and finally, $v_h{}^h$ (the value of not treating a healthy person: medical expenses saved, working days, etc.).

To illustrate the use of the equation, Ledley and Lusted assign *arbitrary* absolute values in a case, because, as they say, "The decision of value problems frequently involves intangibles such as moral and ethical standards which must, in the last analysis, be left to the physician's judgment."[25] One might argue, however, that it is better to develop a technique for systematically determining the absolute values of treatment and nontreatment, crude though the technique might be, than to leave the problem to the perhaps refined, but nevertheless obscure, judgment processes of the physician. Particularly in a matter of comparing the value of treatment and nontreatment, the problem is to avoid biases in the physician's judgment due to the kind of moral orientation discussed above.

It is possible, moreover, that the difficulty met by Ledley and Lusted is not that the factors to be evaluated are "intangibles," but that they are ex-

25. *Ibid.*, p. 8.

pressed in seemingly incommensurate units. How does one weigh the risk of death against the monetary cost of treatment? How does one weigh the risk of physical or social disability against the risk of death? Although these are difficult questions to answer, the idea of leaving them to the physician's judgment is probably not conducive to an understanding of the problem.

Following the lead of the economists in their studies of utility, it may be feasible to reduce the various factors to be weighed to a common unit. How could the benefits, costs, and risks of alternative acts in medical practice be expressed in monetary units? One solution might be to use payment rates in disability and life insurance, which offer a comparative evaluation of the "cost" of death, and permanent and temporary disability of various degrees. Although this approach does not include everything which physicians weigh in reaching decisions (pain and suffering cannot be weighed in this framework), it does include many of the major factors. It therefore would provide the opportunity of constructing a fairly realistic payoff matrix of absolute values, which would then allow for the determination of the relative value of treatment and nontreatment using the expected value equation.[26]

Gathering data for the payoff matrix might make it possible to explore an otherwise almost inaccessible problem: the sometimes subtle conflicts of interest between the physician and the patient. Although it is fairly clear that medical intervention was unnecessary in particular cases, and that it was probably done for financial gain,[27] the evaluation of the influence of remuneration on diagnosis and treatment is probably in most cases a fairly intricate matter, requiring precise techniques of investigation. If the payoff were calculated in terms of values to the patient *and* values to the physician, such problems could be explored. Less tangible values such as convenience and work satisfactions could be introduced into the matrix. The following statements by psychiatrists were taken from Hollingshead and Redlich's study of social class and mental disorder:

"Seeing him every morning was a chore; I had to put him on my back and carry him for an hour." "He had to get attention in large doses, and this was hard to do." "The patient was not interesting or attractive; I had to repeat, repeat, repeat." "She was a poor unhappy, miserable woman—we were worlds apart."[28]

26. It is possible that more sophisticated techniques may be applicable to the problem of constructing medical payoff matrices (C. W. Churchman, R. L. Ackoff, and E. L. Arnoff, *Introduction to Operations Research* [New York: John Wiley, 1957], chaps. 6 and 11). The possibility of applying these techniques to the present problem was suggested to the author by James G. March.

27. R. E. Trussel, June Ehrlich and Mildred Morehead, *The Quantity, Quality and Costs of Medical and Hospital Care Secured by a Sample of Teamster Families in the New York Area* (New York: Columbia University School of Public Health and Administrative Medicine, 1962).

28. A. B. Hollingshead and F. C. Redlich, *Social Class and Mental Illness* (New York: John Wiley, 1958), p. 344.

This study strongly suggests that psychiatric diagnosis and treatment were influenced by the payoff for the psychiatrist as well as for the patient. In any type of medical decision, the use of the expected value equation might show the extent of the conflict of interest between physician and patient, and thereby shed light on the complex process of medical decision-making.

21

CLIFTON K. MEADOR

The Art and Science of Nondisease

For the physician accustomed to dealing only with pathologic entities, terms such as "nondisease entity" or "nondisease" are foreign and difficult to comprehend. This paper will present the background for the development of this new science, a classification of nondisease and finally the important therapeutic principles based on this concept.

Since disease is an abnormal state that lends itself to classification into syndromes and entities, one tends to think of health or nondisease as all encompassing and without specificity. This is not the case, since it is now clear that "nondisease" may be used in quite a specific manner; furthermore, it can be subdivided and classified into syndromes and entities. If a diseased person can be specifically sick, why is it not logical to suggest that a nondiseased one can be specifically healthy?

Patients are frequently seen on referral with a specific disease diagnosis, and yet investigation fails to substantiate the referral diagnosis; in fact it may not reveal any disease. What, then, does the patient have? He must have something. The argument will be presented that he or she has a particular nondisease. This is certainly more reasonable than the common error of continuing to label such patients with nonexistent diseases.

In a review of the charts of patients referred to the Endocrine Division with a variety of diagnoses it became apparent that a large number also had no disease. They were not *just* healthy; they had specific nondiseases. The most common such example was the typical patient referred with a diagnosis of Cushing's disease.

CASE 1. The patient was a slightly obese, middle-aged woman with facial rounding, ruddy complexion, and prominent hair on the upper lip. Cushing's disease was excluded by the appropriate laboratory tests, and in fact *no* disease

Reprinted from the *New England Journal of Medicine*, 277 (1965), pp. 92-95, by permission of the author and the publisher.

I am indebted to Drs. J. A. Pittman, Jr., J. L. Worrell and W. B. Frommeyer, Jr., and Miss Courtney King for their critical review of this manuscript.

was found. Why hesitate and say, "Cushing's disease, not found"? The patient had non-Cushing's disease—the first described entity of nondisease. Nugent et al.[1] recently recognized this entity in their report of 73 cases of "not Cushing's syndrome."

Fifteen patients with similar findings were seen by me in the past year; therefore, a syndrome must exist. It was not a *disease* so it must have represented a *nondisease*. One might argue that this is ridiculous; the patient happened to have a combination of findings that represented normal variations so that Cushing's disease was only suspected.[2] To the physician unfamiliar with nondisease that is true, but not so for the serious student of health and its classification. Thus, a nondisease exists when a specific entity is suspected but not found. Students of disease only might then argue that all normal persons are suspected of having Cushing's disease, so how could they all have non-Cushing's disease? It is true that they all have nondisease in a general sense but the not the entity non-Cushing's disease. ("Latent nondisease," although having some pertinence at this point, is more appropriately discussed below.)

For those untrained in nondisease additional case histories might illustrate these more basic concepts before the complexities of the subject are gone into.

CASE 2. A deeply pigmented 40-year-old man was found to have a blood pressure of 100/60 on a routine insurance examination. The patient was seen with a referral diagnosis of suspected Addison's disease. The history revealed that the grandfather was a Cherokee Indian, thus explaining the pigmentation. Adrenal-function studies were within normal limits, and no disease was found.

It should be obvious that the patient was healthy—even specifically healthy; he had "non-Addison's disease." This is now a well documented syndrome of nondisease manifested at times only by a lower limit of normal blood pressure. (Six similar patients have been seen in the past year.)

CASE 3. The 20-year-old daughter of Italian parents was referred for evaluation of "excessive facial hair," and a diagnosis of "suspected adrenal tumor, virilizing" was made. The history revealed normal menses. The mother and 2 sisters of the patient also had "excessive facial hair" but commented that it was considered a mark of womanhood. Laboratory studies ruled out an androgen excess.

The diagnosis was "nonadrenal tumor, virilizing."[3] (In the present state of ignorance nonadrenal tumor cannot be distinguished from non-Stein-Leventhal syndrome or noncongenital adrenal hyperplasia; perhaps it is best to consider all such cases as examples of the nonvirilizing syndrome.)

1. C. A. Nugent, H. R. Warner, J. T. Dunn, and F. H. Tyler, "Probability Theory in Diagnosis of Cushing's Syndrome," *Journal of Clinical Endocrinology,* 24 (1964), 621-627.

2. In the older terminology nondiseases were often lumped under such terms as "normal variations" or included in long lists called "differential diagnoses." The terminology of nondisease promotes concise language and avoids such confusing phrases.

3. Those oriented only in diseases classify this erroneously as idiopathic hirsutism.

Suffice it to say, then, that a nondisease may exist when a specific disease is suspected and when the suspected disease is not found. A corrollary to this rule is that for every disease there is probably a nondisease. There are no absolute requirements for nondisease since it may exist without a corresponding disease as discussed below. It should be noted at this point that the presence of a disease does not in itself exclude the coexistence of a nondisease. Thus, one may have non-Addison's disease and also have the entities of cholecystitis, pyelonephritis, and so forth. Also, just as one may find multiple diseases, one may see multiple nondiseases (as pointed out below).

The extensive experience gained in endocrine nondiseases suggested that a more comprehensive investigation into general medical nondiseases would be profitable. Even though the field was relatively untouched it became apparent quite early that subspecialization had already occurred in this young science. I readily found physicians with experience and training in such areas as noncardiology, nongastroenterology, and nonhematology; persons with exhaustive knowledge and firsthand experience were found in nonradiology and clinical nonpathology.

Rather than attempt to make any comprehensive and monotonous listing of nondiseases, it was decided to attempt a classification along more rational lines (one might facetiously say that this is a nonpathophysiologic classification). Nomenclature is in its earliest and most awkward form, and one must apologize for this. As the science of nondisease finds acceptance, mixed Latin and Greek roots are sure to supplant the present cumbersome English terms.

Table 21.1 lists the major classes of nondisease with illustrative examples. If examples of endocrine nondisease predominate, it is because I lack more extensive exposure to other nondiseases. It should be obvious that a referring physician need not be involved in the sequence of events leading to a diagnosis of nondisease. Every physician in his own right happens onto these with alarming frequency. All the examples of nondisease listed have been documented, most by other physicians—unfortunately, some personally.

Mimicking syndromes require a combination of findings (usually detected merely by inspection) that suggests a corresponding entity. Endocrine diseases readily lend themselves many times to diagnosis by inspection; therefore, endocrine nondiseases predominate in this syndrome. The entities listed (Table 21.1) are those most commonly seen. Rarer representatives of this syndrome observed were nonacromegaly, non-Turner's syndrome, and noncretinism. Non-Cushing's disease, non-Addison's disease, and the non-virilizing syndrome have already been discussed in detail.

Upper-lower-limit syndromes are perhaps the most common of all nondiseases. What physician has not treated in desperation "hypothyroidism" (serum protein-bound iodine of 4.1 microgm. per 100 ml.), only later to establish the correct diagnosis of nonhypothyroidism? Nonanemia (hemoglobin of 12.5 gm. per 100 ml.), nonpolycythemia vera (hematocrit of 50 percent), and nonhypertension (blood pressure of 150 systolic,

80 diastolic) are seen almost daily in busy clinics. Any medical or laboratory value subject to a lower and an upper limit of normal can lead one into this syndrome. Combinations within this syndrome are not rare; in fact nonhypotension ("low blood pressure" in the more precise vernacular of disease) and nonanemia occur together so frequently in neurotic females as to suggest a separate syndrome.

Table 21.1. Classification of nondisease

Syndrome	Clinical Examples	Clinical or Laboratory Manifestations
Mimicking drome	Non-Cushing's disease	Obesity; facial rounding; facial hair
	Non-Addison's disease	Pigmentation; "low blood pressure"
	Nonvirilizing syndrome	Facial hair (usually familial)
Upper-lower-limit syndrome	Nonanemia	Hemoglobin, 12.5 gm/100 ml.
	Nonpolycythemia vera	Hematocrit, 50 %
	Nonhypothyroidism	Protein-bound iodine, 4.1 microgm./100 ml.
	Nonhypercalcemia	Serum calcium, 10.6 mg./100 ml.
	Nonhypertension	Blood pressure, 150/80
Normal-variation syndrome	Nondwarfism	Short patient—short parents
	Nongigantism	Tall patient—tall parents
Laboratory error syndrome	Nonazotemia	Blood urea nitrogen, 50 mg./100 ml.
	Nonhyponatremia	Serum sodium, 110 milliequiv./liter
	Nonanemia	Hemoglobin, 4 gm./100 ml. (all in error)
Roentgenologic-overinterpretation syndrome	Suprarenal nonmass	Suprarenal "mass" on x-ray study; not found at surgery
	Colonic nonpolyps	"Filling defects" on air-contrast bariumenema study; not found at colectomy
	Duodenal nonulcer	"Crater" on gastrointestinal series; not confirmed at surgery
Congenitally-absent-organ syndrome	Nonfunctioning kidney	Nonfunction on pyelogram: kidney not found at surgery
	Nonfunctioning gallbladder	Nonfunction by cholecystogram: gallbladder not found at surgery
Overinterpretation-of-physical-findings syndrome	Nonaortic stenosis	Grade 1 basal systolic murmur
	Nonhepatomegaly	Low-lying liver
	Nonmitral insufficiency	Grade 1 apical systolic murmur
	Nonsigmoid carcinoma	Fecal mass in sigmoid colon

Normal-variation syndromes might be confused at times with the *mimicking syndrome* or the *upper-lower-limit syndrome*. They are distinct, however, in that laboratory values are not involved and combinations of findings are lacking. How else would one classify the child of short parents (nondwarfism) or the child of tall parents (nongigantism)?

Laboratory-error syndromes[4] are the delight of the alert nondisease clinician; one must add, however, only before therapy has been initiated. In this regard they are probably the most responsive to treatment of all entities —one merely has to repeat the test once or twice to see astounding results. For example, in what other nondisease or disease can one see a rise in the hemoglobin level from 6 to 14 gm. per 100 ml. in two hours with only 1 iron tablet?

The term "any-laboratory-test-available syndrome" is generally applicable. Documented cases of nondiseases run into the thousands. Combinations are frequent and bizarre. One rather curious syndrome recently seen was the coexistence of nonpolycythemia (hematocrit of 60 percent) and nonanemia (hemoglobin of 7 gm. per 100 ml.). The natural (or unnatural) course was fascinating and was manifested by a marked fall in hematocrit, a dramatic rise in hemoglobin to above-normal levels, and finally, a normal level for both. No entity known can present such a challenge to the physician.

In view of their marked tendency to occur at night paroxysmal nocturnal errors deserve mention as special variants. Entities in this class might then be preceded by "nocturnal," such as nocturnal nonanemia and nocturnal nonhyponatremia.

Roentgenologic-overinterpretation syndromes are difficult things indeed. Colonic nonpolyps and abdominal nonmasses, among others, have been encountered. Surgical exploration or even removal of an organ is often necessary to establish the true nature of the nondisease. These are not the delight of anyone and are therefore passed over briefly.

Congenitally-absent-organ syndromes, fortunately, are rare nondiseases. Nonfunctioning kidney and nonfunctioning-gallbladder syndromes, representatives of this group, have been documented. Surgical approach is always frustrating, particularly when directed at the allegedly paired functioning organ. It should be obvious that nondiseases in this group can be rapidly converted into diseases. (Many nondiseases are converted to diseases; this probably accounts for much of the ill-will directed at nondisease.) Iatrogenic diseases, or "diseases of medical progress,"[5] probably arise as

4. It has been suggested that the laboratory-error and roentgenologic overinterpretation syndromes be lumped into a mal-serendipity syndrome. Mal-serendipity is a subclass of serendipitomania (J. A. Pittman, Jr., personal communication), the common habit of ordering all the laboratory tests in hope of "falling onto" a disease. More often than not one "falls onto" a nondisease.

5. R. H. Moser, "Diseases of Medical Progress," *New England Journal of Medicine,* 255 (1955), 606-614.

often from treatment of nondiseases as from the treatment of diseases.

Overinterpretation-of-physical-findings syndromes are usually seen early in one's medical experience but tend to reappear later. Most of these entities are readily identified unless one becomes trapped into multiple nondiseases such as the *overinterpretation of physical signs*, leading to the *roentgenologic-overinterpretation syndrome* together with a touch of the *laboratory-error syndrome*—a nondisease often requiring fourteen days to run its diagnostic course. Common entities found in this group are nonmitral insufficiency, non-aortic stenosis, and nonhepatomegaly (often specifically designated).

Physicians, nurses, and patients contribute to the rising incidence of non-disease. Iatrogenic nonhyperthyroidism (elevated protein-bound iodine) is well known after a variety of iodinated contrast mediums. Nurses furnish an array of clinical material: nonfever, nonoliguria, nontachycardia, and even nonshock are examples for which the nondisease clinician must be on guard. Factitial nongastrointestinal bleeding, with tarry stools from iron salts, and factitial nonhyperthyroidism due to proprietary iodinated cough syrups are representative of the cunningness of the patient in this area.

The curious category of "pseudodisease" was not included in the present classification because of ignorance of this area. Pseudodisease at the present time appears to lie somewhere between disease and nondisease and often defies identification. Historically, medical science has witnessed the evolution of many pseudodiseases into nondiseases. Cascade stomachs, uterine suspensions of the "drooping womb" and nephropexies for the "sagging kidney" (now reviving itself) emphasize the enthusiasm that pseudodisease can enjoy and the grave error of not recognizing nondisease for what it is. One wonders how many such unrecognized nondiseases are still being treated as diseases today.

Latent nondisease was briefly mentioned earlier in relation to general non-disease. Latent nondisease lurks in every patient. It becomes overt as a specific entity usually in the hands of a physician, nurse, or technician, but occasionally through the lay press or "friends" of the patient. Latent non-disease is always desirable; manifest nondisease is usually due to error and is expensive, frustrating, and embarrassing to all concerned. Patients when told of their overt nondisease for some reasons tend to become hostile and difficult to manage. Nonanxiety becomes anxiety.

A short discussion of treatment and management is therefore necessary. (It might be better to say nontreatment to remain consistent.) As painful as it may be, the patient usually should be told of his nondisease, particularly if treatment for "the disease" has been instituted. Minor *laboratory-error syndromes* and so forth are so frequent that they can, of course, be overlooked. Treatment is always easy if the diagnosis is correct and nondisease clearly established. Stated simply, the treatment for nondisease is never the treatment indicated for the corresponding disease entity. In this statement lies the ultimate value of the science of nondisease.

22

ELIOT FREIDSON

Disability as Social Deviance

The institutions of the field known as rehabilitation may be said to carry on four activities. First, they specify what personal attributes shall be called handicaps. Second, they seek to identify who conforms to their specifications. Third, they attempt to gain access to those whom they call handicapped. And fourth, they try to get those to whom they gain access to change their behavior so as to conform more closely to what the institutions believe are their potentialities.

Logically, these four activities are sequential, each one being a necessary condition for what follows it. Furthermore, the universe embraced by these activities progressively diminishes: that is, in the first activity, a universe of people possessing a handicap is defined; in the second, since all of that logical universe cannot possibly be identified, those identified can only be a segment; the third activity involves a further diminution in the universe, for it is not likely that access can be gained to all those identified; similarly, "success" cannot be expected in the treatment of all cases, which further diminishes the absolute size of the sample of the universe originally defined. And finally, all four activities are predicated on a specific selective valuation of human attributes. They are guided by conceptions of what is proper and desirable behavior for the average person. They specifically single out some behaviors or attributes as undesirable, call them handicaps, and seek to rehabilitate them.

However, what is singled out as undesirable is often historically and culturally variable. While it is true that the loss of a limb is probably considered undesirable in every time and place, such is not the case for blindness, drug addiction, and many other traits we now believe to be unde-

Reprinted from M. B. Sussman, ed., *Sociology and Rehabilitation*, Washington: American Sociological Association, 1966, pp. 71-99, with permission of the author and publisher.

I am indebted to a number of people for their comments on an earlier version of this paper, but most particularly to Howard S. Becker, M. Elaine Cumming, and Stanton Wheeler for especially detailed criticism.

sirable. What is common to all acts of defining someone as handicapped and requiring rehabilitation, therefore, is not a set of physical attributes that always "are" handicaps, but rather *the act of definition itself*, which can be an imputation rather than a statement of fact. Since this is the case, it follows that the activities of rehabilitation institutions are determined at least as much by their conceptions (and the public's conceptions) of what a handicap is, as by the physical attributes they deal with. This is to say that social and cultural variables are in all cases at least as important as psychological and biological variables, and in some cases much more important.

What is a handicap in social terms? It is an imputation of difference from others; more particularly, imputation of an *undesirable* difference. By definition, then, a person said to be handicapped is so defined because he deviates from what he himself or others believe to be normal or appropriate. In this sense, the concept of *deviance* is central to rehabilitation activities.

As it happens, the past few decades of American sociology have seen an increasing tendency to find in the concept of deviance a focus for organizing thinking about one of the central questions of sociology—social control, or the source of order in human society. While there is more than one orientation toward the concept, in one form or another it has been appearing with increasing frequency in a number of seemingly disparate fields. In this paper, I shall bring together some of that material on deviance and try to show what kinds of questions it raises for sociological research in the field of rehabilitation. I shall attempt to do this by dealing with each of the four activities by which I have characterized the field of rehabilitation—the definition of the impaired as a special type of deviance, the determination and identification of the universe of deviance, the process of coming into contact with institutions devoted to the management of the deviant, and finally, most glancingly, the process by which it is sought to change the deviant. In each case, I shall try to show how social processes influence the outcome of the activity. Throughout I shall emphasize those features of social life that are external to the individual, that limit and channel his responses. I will not dwell on the more "psychological" elements of individual experience, largely because the external or structural approach, dreary and mechanical as it may seem, reflects a position that is less likely to be familiar to those in rehabilitation, and that has in fact been overneglected in research. It goes without saying that the orientation I shall stress by no means exhausts the variety that is contemporary sociology.

Definition of Deviance

What is meant by the term "deviance?" Or better, what is the most precise and pertinent way of defining the term? The most obvious definition is purely and simply statistical—any variation from an average. However, this is not a useful definition because it discriminates too little. Each one of us deviates from an average in many ways, but not all deviations have social consequences, and of those that do, some have more than others. This consideration leads us to a definition based on what is socially significant— "behavior which violates institutionalized expectations."[1] But this also is much too broad, for all of us in one way or another and at some time or another violate others' expectations of how we behave in our roles, and the casual interplay of everyday life with its subtle normative pressures is sufficient to bring us back into line without much self-consciousness.[2] Indeed, it is by such a constant interplay that we are learning what our roles and their limits are. While it is possible and perhaps logically necessary to define the general class in such terms, it seems most useful to discriminate between deviations that do not themselves constitute roles and those that do. The distinction that Lemert[3] makes between primary and secondary deviation is relevant here, for in the former case a man integrates his deviation into a "normal" role, while in the latter he has organized it into a deviant role. It is the latter I wish to focus on in this paper—conduct which violates sufficiently valued norms, that, if it is persistent, is assigned a special negatively deviant role, and "is generally thought to require the attention of social control agencies."[4] These are the forms of deviance that are often called "social problems," and that constitute the greatest challenge to rehabilitation agencies.

The concept of deviance has several implications worth pointing out here. First, it is a relative concept in that, from one culture and one historical period to another, what is singled out for attention and control varies considerably, as do the meaning assigned and the quality of control applied. Indeed, this is so even in our own present-day society, where the professional's conception of what needs his attention often varies from the layman's, and where one group's conception of the remarkable varies from another's. In this sense, deviance is socially defined and can vary independently of any physical or material circumstances. Insofar as it is secondary in Lemert's usage, what is important is its organization, not the attribute involved. It is an *imputed* condition, and the imputation may or may not rest on the physical reality. Not all handicapped people are called handicapped or act like handicapped people. Whatevever the reality may be, significance is established by the meaning *imputed* to it and

1. Albert K. Cohen, "The Study of Social Disorganization and Deviant Behavior," in R. K. Merton et al., eds., *Sociology Today* (New York: Basic Books, 1959), p. 462.

2. Cf. Talcott Parsons, *The Social System* (New York: The Free Press, 1951), p. 303.

3. Edwin M. Lemert, *Social Pathology* (New York: McGraw-Hill, 1951).

4. Kai T. Erikson, "Notes on the Sociology of Deviance," in H. S. Becker, ed., *The Other Side, Perspectives on Deviance* (New York: The Free Press, 1964), pp. 10-11.

5. In a personal communication, Stanton Wheeler points out that we actually know very little about the consequences of labeling, and should learn more.

the organization imposed on it, both of which can vary independently of it.

Second, insofar as the deviance constitutes a role, it implies a process of labeling and therefore the likely existence of a set of epithets connected with it. The process of labeling accompanies and may even produce[5] the assumption of a deviant role by providing the focus for stereotyping behavior.

Third, insofar as deviance is secondary, it is likely to be generally recognized as a "social problem," and thus, in complex societies such as ours, there will be connected with it a set of offices or organizations devoted to identifying and dealing with it—agents of social control. These organizations, however, are not always mere responses to general public recognition that some type of deviance exists and constitutes a problem. They come to have a life of their own and become active in labeling (or "discovering") deviance where none was recognized before and in persuading the public of its existence and importance.[6]

Types of Deviance

This paper is concerned with deviance sufficiently marked by society to be assigned a role to which a vocabulary of labels or epithets is attached, and with the control of which special organizations are "professionally" involved. But even stated so concretely, the concept is still insufficiently articulated in that there is no way of discriminating between the alcoholic and the criminal, the blind and the asthmatic. Since these are empirically quite different in many fateful ways, it would seem useful to be able to distinguish them as different types of deviance.

The most influential theoretical classification of deviance in modern sociology is that of Robert K. Merton,[7] elaborated by a number of writers[8] and woven by Talcott Parsons[9] into his own systematic theory.

Essentially, it is a classification of types of adjustment to situations in which there is some discrepancy between culturally emphasized goals and the means available to attain them: one may adopt, for example, a "rebellious" or a "ritualistic" stance. This type of classification, however, seems difficult to use for our present purposes. In Merton's case, it may classify variations in the way people perform everyday "normal" roles, and in Parsons', how people may be motivated to adopt deviant roles; but it does not seem able to deal with the structure of the deviant roles as such. For

6. Cf. Howard S. Becker, *Outsiders, Studies in the Sociology of Deviance* (New York: The Free Press, 1963), pp. 147-163.

7. Robert K. Merton, *Social Theory and Social Structure*, rev. ed. (New York: The Free Press, 1957), pp. 131-194.

8. These are summarized in Marshall B. Clinard, "The Theoretical Implications of Anomie and Deviant Behavior," in Marshall B. Clinard, ed., *Anomie and Deviant Behavior: A Discussion and Critique* (New York: The Free Press, 1964), pp. 1-56.

9. Parsons, *op. cit.*, pp. 249-325.

example, while it may be able to classify and explain variations in the way people perform such a deviant role as that of the blind, it cannot easily explain how the role itself comes to be. Furthermore, it seems hard pressed to explain in any but the most general terms how and why people end up in deviant roles even when, as in the case of the blind, they are not personally motivated to do so.

The problem seems to lie at too high a level of generality. More concrete distinctions are necessary here. I wish to suggest that a useful method of classifying deviant roles lies in the attributes imputed to them—in particular, the definition of the role with its implicit diagnosis, prognosis, and prescription for treatment, quite apart from the incumbent's motivation. By "diagnosis," I mean the cause imputed to the deviant behavior by others, and particularly its implication for the social identity of the person. Those conceptions of cause should not be considered necessarily true or objective, but rather conceptions of the nature of the deviance that contain within themselves directives for the way in which responses toward it will be organized. The actual conception of the cause of a particular form of deviance will in fact vary from time to time and place to place.

One critical dimension in imputing cause is that of personal responsibility, a dimension emphasized by Parsons' analysis of the sick role[10] and discussed in a broader framework by Aubert and Messinger.[11] It seems to be critical in that it bears closely on the moral identity of the person concerned and on the obligations others may feel toward him. It makes a great and real difference when the cause of deviant behavior is seen to lie in deliberate choice rather than in accident, inheritance, infection, or witchcraft. When the individual is believed to be responsible for his deviance, some form of punishment is likely to be involved in the way others respond to it. When he is believed not to be responsible, permissive treatment or instruction is used in his management. Thus, the dimension of imputed responsibility allows us to predict some of the elements of the way in which deviance will be managed or controlled by others.

To the dimension of responsibility, we may add the imputed prognosis—namely, whether the deviance is believed to be "curable" or "hopeless"; whether it need only be temporary with the proper management, or whether it cannot fail to be permanent. This dimension, too, bears on management or treatment. Since the management of all forms of deviance requires some form of segregation, the question becomes the quality of segregation. In "curable" cases, segregation is likely to be temporary and not far removed from community life. In "incurable" cases (such as being a newborn girl in ancient Sparta), it is likely to be permanent to the point of execution, or (as in the case of lepers in an earlier day) re-

10. *Ibid.*,p.440.
11. Vilhelm Aubert and Sheldon Messinger, "The Criminal and the Sick," in this volume.

moved to the point of banishment from the community.

These two criteria for classification are, as we shall see, oversimple, but they do throw into bold relief some of the differences to be found among the variety of all that is called deviance and suggest the relationship between qualities imputed to deviance and the form of management adopted for it. Table 22.1 is designed to throw them into bolder relief.

Table 22.1. Modes of managing deviance,
by imputation of responsibility and prognosis

Imputed Prognosis	Responsible	Not Responsible
Curable	Limited punishment	Treatment, education, or correction
Incurable	Execution; life imprisonment	Protective custody

One interesting difficulty with the table is the ambiguity of consequences in the case of "incurable" deviance, even when imputed responsibility varies. In some societies, negative sanctions as extreme as death are prescribed, not with a punitive intent, but rather to protect society at the expense of the individual or (as in the case of the aged in some Eskimo groups) to end a miserable and hopeless life. Incurability, whether or not responsibility is imputed, seems to pose severe problems to society. In our society, the "protective custody" of the severely mentally disabled in public institutions greatly resembles in some respects what is done to incorrigible criminals in maximum security prisons.[12] Even though we are less likely to hold the former than the latter responsible for their deviance, we can agree that the intent is in fact different and that "management" is also different in important ways.

The major deficiency of the table for our present purposes is its generality, for it may not be at all clear to the reader how present-day labels fit into it. This deficiency is a function of the peculiarly complex and confused world we live in, where there is organized dissensus. Let us take crime, for example, and, in order to simplify the case, adult rather than juvenile crime. We all know that there are a number of schools of thought about crime today. One, not so fashionable but nonetheless socially important, argues that a criminal act is one of personal choice and responsibility, and that punishment by loss of freedom is a price to be paid for such choice, to be calculated as a deterrent to future choices. Another school, the more "professional," argues that a criminal act does not occur as a rational and conscious choice, that personal responsibility is not to be clearly assigned, and that punishment as such is inappropriate: if the law requires imprisonment, prison should be an educational and treatment experience rather than merely punishment. And, of course, there

---

12. See Goffman's analysis of the "total institution": Erving Goffman, *Asylums* (Garden City, N.Y.: Anchor Books, 1961).

are yet other schools. Where, then, would you assign crime in our table?

Obviously, it depends on who is doing the assigning. The diagnosis of "responsibility" and the prognosis of cure are controversial in our society, which makes it difficult to assign particular types of deviance to any single cell of the table. Any concrete assignment is more likely to represent the view of one special segment of our society than a general consensus. Furthermore, it seems characteristic of our society (or at least of those who attempt to speak and assume responsibility for our society) both to press for diagnosing *all* forms of deviance as something for which the deviant should not be held entirely responsible, and to avoid the prognosis of "incurable." But this does not mean that most people are kind about motives and optimistic about outcomes. If we were to take the mythical man-in-the-street, we might guess that he would fill the cells with the following examples:

Table 22.2. *Types of deviance, by imputed responsibility and prognosis*

Imputed Prognosis	Responsible	Not Responsible
Curable	Juvenile shoplifting	Pneumonia
Incurable	Sex murder	Cancer

However, little more than casual inspection of the table and reflection on much of what may justifiably be called deviance leads to the conclusion that some important cases of deviance do not fit well into any of the four cells. First, a great many of the impairments dealt with by the field of rehabilitation are neither curable nor incurable, but something in between—"improvable," let us say. This fact represents not merely a matter of degree, which I am not attempting to discuss here, but a state quite distinct from the other two. Second, the simple moral dichotomy of responsibility does not allow for the halo of moral evaluation that in fact surrounds many types of deviance for which, theoretically, people are not held responsible, but which in some way damage their identities. Some diseases, such as syphilis, leprosy, and even tuberculosis, are surrounded with loathing even though they are all "merely" infections. And many forms of organic dysfunction or maldevelopment for which the sufferer is not held responsible occasion responses of fear or disgust—epilepsy, dwarfism, and disfigurement, for example. As Goffman has shown, these forms of deviance pose severe barriers to a normal social life because they serve as stigmata, isolating the individual and interrupting the flow of everyday interaction.

In order to take a number of forms of deviance into account, then, including those with which rehabilitation is concerned, I am suggesting the addition of stigma as a criterion, as well as the addition of the prognostic category of "improvable but incurable." We might thus revise our table, still using guesses about how the man-in-the-street would assign deviant behavior, and understanding that we ourselves and the professionals concerned with the management of deviance might fill the cells differently. Indeed, professionals are not supposed to impute stigma at all. In Table 22.3, two of the logically required cells of deviance for which responsibility is imputed but which are not stigmatized are left blank. This is so because deviance to which responsibility is imputed seems largely to be stigmatized by the man-in-the-street in our culture.

Table 22.3. *Types of deviance, by imputed responsibility, stigma, and prognosis*

Imputed Prognosis	Responsible		Not Responsible	
	no stigma	*stigma*	*no stigma*	*stigma*
Curable	Parking violation	Syphilis	Pneumonia	Leprosy
Improvable but Not Curable		Burglary	Hearing loss	Crippling
Incurable and Unimprovable		Sex murder	Cancer	Dwarfism

Sources of Deviance

The discussion thus far has attempted to indicate the character and range of the sociological concept of deviance, the as-yet-unresolved problems of classification it poses, and some elements of the concept that may be useful to hold in mind when considering the task of rehabilitation. Unsuccessful as these suggestions may prove to be, they would at least indicate the place of disability in the range of deviance and the special analytical problem disability poses to the sociologist.[13] That problem resides in the curious juxtaposition of stigma with the social legitimacy but incurability of disability.

In a now standard discussion, Talcott Parsons[14] treats sickness as a role by which a deviant at once finds legitmacy in his deviance and becomes subject to the control of others. By his definition, the sick role is one in which a deviant is not blamed for his deviance. But it is *conditionally* granted: one gains permissive (i.e., nonpunitive) treatment by others so long as he shows evidence of adopting the patient role and seeking the professional help that will allow him to return to normal. No one is allowed to use it as a permanent form of "retreatism." However, only in a very general way is this applicable to the analysis of the physical handicaps, particularly those that are stigmatized. It is true that the

13. For a more elaborate and abstract attempt, see Eliot Freidson, *Profession of Medicine* (New York: Dodd, Mead, 1970), pp. 244-277.
14. Parsons, *op. cit.*, pp. 297-321.

amputee, for example, may be treated permissively, in Parsons' terms, on the condition that he assume the role of the patient, allow himself to be fitted with prosthetic devices, and work at developing proficiency in their use, but when he has done that, he does not return to normal: upon working at ameliorating his impairment, he plays the role of the "good" amputee, but he still suffers acceptance by others that is conditional on not pressing them "past the point at which they can easily extend acceptance."[15] To put it crudely, he is pressed to be a "good Indian" rather than a bad, but good or bad, an Indian he remains, and, as everyone knows, the only really good Indian is a dead one. Thus, the concept of the sick role is severely limited in its capacity to facilitate analysis of stigmatized roles imputed with essentially incurable even though improvable deviance: it may deal with how improvement may take place, but not with the persistence of the role itself.

This limitation is reinforced by the concept's emphasis on "motivation," treating sickness as one of the number of alternatives open to an individual under pressure. Psychosomatic medicine notwithstanding, most illnesses, and certainly most impairments, are not motiviated: they are contingencies of inheritance, accidents of infection and trauma. In this sense, the individual is someone to whom something happens, who is then labeled by others and pressed to behave in a particular expected way quite independently of his own motives or desires. His motives may be involved in whether he rebels against the labeling, whether he falls into invalidism, or whether he becomes a showcase model of conformity to expectations, but the permanence and shape of the role he plays so badly or so well stand quite apart from his inclinations. Rather, the role may be constructed and maintained quite independently of him by the social responses of those surrounding him, responses that may be marked and organized by a process of labeling that places him willy-nilly into it. His motives may determine how he performs in that role, but not whether or not he is placed in that role. In this sense, the concept of deviance focuses as much attention on the lay and official "normals" who label deviance and carve out a role for it as it does on the individual deviant himself. And it precludes the easy assumption that the deviance is *necessarily* "caused" by the individual's characteristics rather than by the forces of society as such. Indeed, it points to a specifically and distinctly sociological mode of analysis that asks, first of all, about the mechanism by which deviant roles are defined and individual deviants identified.

The Identification of Deviance

In the discussion thus far, deviance has been treated as a social rather than necessarily behavioral or biological fact. This seems necessary in

---

15. Erving Goffman, *Stigma: Notes on the Management of Spoiled Identity* (Englewood Cliffs, N.J.: Spectrum Books, 1963), p. 120.

light of the fact that possession of a given trait does not always lead to assignment to a given deviant role. Indeed, socially structured biases seem to operate in the identification of deviants and their allocation into deviant roles. This may be understood when we recognize the implications of the fact that the true universe or rate of deviance, whether defined by behavioral or biological criteria, is difficult if not impossible to determine. In a practical sense, deviance consists in cases identified by agents or agencies concerned with controlling it—that is, the deviant is he who gets caught, whether he turns himself in or others do it for him, and the universe of deviance is that population of people delineated or defined by the agencies whose function it is to deal with those who get caught.[16] This seems true not only for "criminals," "perverts," or any other deviants who might be expected to hide themselves in order to avoid punishment, but also for the mentally ill, the blind, the deaf, or whatever. One does not play the role of the deviant until he has been so identified by others or by himself.

Formal control agents have become more and more important in making such identifications. In everyday life, precise delineations of classes of deviance are not made: vague and permissive stereotypes seem to be used, the tendency being in all areas, not merely mental illness,[17] to avoid segregating people into deviant roles in any but the most persistent and extreme cases. Control agencies in our society, however, have the business of defining deviance and must both solicit support for their activities and account for what support they have already gained: if only to account for themselves, they must calculate a general universe. They can, of course, as Mechanic feels has been the case for some medical investigation,[18] assume that what they see is in fact the total universe, but if they seek to maintain their level of support without implying that their method of control is ineffective, or if they seek to gain a higher level of support for their work, they are likely to consider the cases they see to be but a hint of the deplorable but as yet undiscovered state of things lying outside. If their orientation is punitive, they seek support to "root out" deviance lying outside their purview; if their orientation is therapeutic, they seek support to "reach out." In either case, they must define a universe outside of themselves.

In the course of defining and classifying the universe which they claim needs their services, all control agencies in effect become responsible for drawing clearer lines than in fact exist either in everyday life or in the processes by which people were originally led into their services, and agencies may come to define people as deviant who would not ordinarily have been so defined. Both professionalism and bureaucratization objectify

16. Cf. Becker, *Outsiders, op. cit.*, p. 10.
17. Elaine Cumming and John Cumming, *Closed Ranks* (Cambridge, Mass.: Harvard University Press, 1957).
18. David Mechanic, "Some Implications of Illness Behavior for Medical Sampling," in this volume.

deviance and reify diagnostic categories. In this sense, while such agencies may not actually *create* deviant roles, they do by the nature of their activities refine and clarify their boundaries and, by assuming responsibility for their control, add elements to the roles that may not have existed previously, and so encourage pulling new people into them.

These are general aspects of what Kitsuse and Cicourel called a "rate-producing process."[19] To this we may add some of the various circumstances responsible for producing different types of "representation" of the universe in the way by which control agencies "root out," "reach out," or "bring to book" their cases and establish the official rate of deviance.

Several circumstances seem especially important in determining how a rate is produced and what its bias will be. First, the degree to which a definition of deviance is so highly specialized that few people feel competent to assign it obviously limits the possibility of identifying cases. Second, the social distance of defining agents from the lay community obviously restricts access to cases to be identified. And the isolation of a defining agency from other agencies or agents also restricts access to possible cases to be identified.

Some agencies seem to find it difficult to make contact with the cases over which they presume jurisdiction. Agencies for the blind, for example, seem to be fairly isolated from others, and their definitions of blindness are comparatively technical, even if arbitrary. To "reach out" to all qualified cases, their discouragingly particularistic definitions must be disseminated to other agencies, running the gamut of independent and criticial valuation by such referring experts as school physicians, optometrists, and ophthalmologists. Given reluctance to impute stigma in both cases, a barrier composed of ignorance on the part of some potential referrers and of oversophistication and independence of judgment on the part of others is created by the very specialized character of the agency and discourages the ready transmission of cases. Therefore, the cases seen are markedly underrepresentative of the universe they presume by their definitions. Fewer people will be labled "appropriately" than in fact conform to the nominal definition of the deviance.[20] The cases that do come to their attention are likely to biased toward the most severe social and psychological handicaps, insofar as such can vary independently of visual acuity. In

19. John I. Kitsuse and Aaron V. Cicourel, "A Note on the Uses of Official Statistics," *Social Problems*, 11 (Fall, 1963), 131-139.

20. Howard S. Becker suggested in a personal communication that the very particularism of an agency can also lead to its gaining a virtual monopoly over dealings with people who fit its definition. An agency may develop the reputation of specializing in all people with a given impairment. People who have no particular difficulty with an impairment but who seek help for other types of difficulties at general, "normal" agencies may find themselves denied services and sent instead to the agency specially devoted to their impairment.

sum, the sampling bias is severe on both quantitative and qualitative grounds, making for disproportionately low rates.

In contrast to such specialized agencies are those that use definitions of deviance that are broad and vague enough to encourage an enormous variety of people to presume tentative identification and referral on the basis of an infinite variety of behavior presumed to be symptomatic. Many agencies devoted to mental illness fall there. Such key functionaries as teachers, social workers, and, to a considerably lesser but nonetheless important degree, policemen and physicians, have been encouraged to use the definition. And it is sufficiently nontechnical that virtually anyone so inclined can feel free to use it. It would follow that, stigma or not, agencies devoted to the control of those declared mentally ill are likely to obtain a fairer approximation of the universe of such cases outside. Indeed, "overrepresentation" can occur in the sense that many "mistaken" labelings are likely to be made, particularly among those segments of the population prone to use the label freely.[21] And insofar as the decision-logic of medical diagnosis described by Scheff [22] is involved in this rate-producing process, bias will be toward imputing pathology in cases of doubt just to make sure nothing is missed. This, too, produces "overrepresentation." More people will be labeled than conform to the definition, although in the case of mental illness, the shortage of facilities may mitigate the effect, as may reluctance to impute a stigmatized form of deviance.

Hopefully, these remarks have indicated the serious and interesting problem of analysis to be found in study of the process by which deviance comes to be known and rendered into statistical rates. However, so long as the agent or agency does not publicly label or segregate individuals, only a "rate-producing process" is involved, similar to that which occurs when a new census category is adopted. But if public labeling or visible segregation from which a labeling conclusion can be drawn occurs,[23] the process may be said to be deviance-producing in that, by labeling the individual, it may organize the responses of the community toward him as a stereotyped deviant. Whereas those around him might never have attained any consensus about his behavior before, each responding to him according to his individual relationship, public labeling establishes a common focus for uniform community responses that carve out a role for him. This lay process of retrospective selection of evidence confirming the label[24] is similar to the process in some official agencies of building up a case

21. "Overrepresentation" is likely to be greatest among groups prone to the use of the diagnosis. In this sense, the clinical insights of practicing psychiatry are "biased" toward middle-class values because of the practitioners see an overrepresentation of the literate and monied class in their "sample."

22. Thomas J. Scheff "Decision Rules, Types of Error, and Their Consequences in Medical Diagnosis" in this volume.

23. Cf. Becker, *Outsiders, op.cit.,* pp. 122 ff. for publicity.

24. Cf. John I. Kitsuse, "Societal Reaction to Deviant Behavior: Problems of Theory and Method," in Becker, *The Other Side, op. cit.,* pp. 87-102.

history or dossier observed by Goffman:[25] it is not a process by which evidence disconfirming the label is sought out and weighed against that confirming the label, but rather one by which the confirming evidence alone is recorded.

In the process of producing deviance, actual public degradation ceremonies are fairly rare, and in our society, as Garfinkel has noted,[26] are pretty much monopolized by law courts and their officers. However, insofar as "the public identity of an actor is transformed into something looked on as lower in the local scheme of social types," and insofar as that identity is "total," referring "to persons as 'motivational' types rather than as 'behavioral' types, not to what a person may be expected to have done or to do... but to what the group holds to be the ultimate 'grounds' or 'reasons' for his performance,"[27] some important elements of degradation ceremonies seem to be involved in fairly common instances of successful labeling, generally in those involving stigmatized roles, and more particularly in those bearing on what are seen as the essential human capacities of the individual—his sexuality, intelligence,[28] and self-control.

Producing Deviance by Management

Denunciation, and even organized publicity, are rare, however. The diffusion of a label usually occurs in more informal and indirect ways, generally without public announcement of the label so much as by the disposition of an individual in such a fashion that the public itself is led to apply a particular label. This may occur by requiring the acceptance of special treatment in a general community institution—the segregation into special classrooms of "exceptional" or handicapped children in public schools, for example.[29] Any special discriminatory device may come to imply an invidious label to the public and lead to consistent discrimination.

Another stimulus of labeling lies in the use of special segregated institutions in the community, which in themselves imply the structured seriousness of the problem as well as a label for it. Entering a mental hospital for treatment, and even seeing a psychiatrist rather than a physician,[30] seem to be critical events for changing public labels from, perhaps, "dif-

25. Goffman, *Asylums, op. cit., passim.*

26. Harold Garfinkel, "Conditions of Successful Degradation Ceremonies," *American Journal of Sociology*, 61 (March, 1956), 420-424.

27. *Ibid.,* p. 420.

28. Cf. Lewis Anthony Dexter, "On the Politics and Sociology of Stupidity in Our Society," in Becker, *The Other Side, op. cit.,* pp. 37-49.

29. For a study of the character of such decisions, see Aaron V. Cicourel and John I. Kitsuse, *The Educational Decision-Makers* (Indianapolis: Bobbs-Merrill, 1963).

30. See, for example, Derek L. Phillips, "Rejection, A Possible Consequence of Seeking Help for Mental Disorders." *American Sociological Review*, 28 (December, 1963), 963-972.

ficult" to "crazy." In more or less dramatic ways, the same seems to be the case for other special institutions, which may be why the more flexible treatment centers are likely to have changed their graphic nineteenth-century names to the bland, euphemistic, and, on occasion, utterly uninformative names of today. Name-changing, however, only temporarily confuses the labeling process: less attention seems to be paid by the public to the name of the institution than to the necessity for institutionalization. The latter fact, as well as the label involved, must be kept from the public so as to avoid reorganization of responses to the individual.

It should be clear that the management of deviance is quite capable of organizing deviant behavior in that labeling or implying a label for it stimulates the community to organize its response to the individual, to a degree segregating him by those special responses and encouraging him to behave the way the community has come to expect him to behave—to accept the role of the blind man, the village idiot, or the cripple. In this, the "treatment" process may be said to create organized or stereotypical behavior.

Such behavior is also created in quite a different way. It can be made "systematic," in Lemert's terms,[31] by bringing together a number of people who have all been labeled the same way, bum raps notwithstanding. Not merely prisons or mental hospitals, but also agencies for the physically handicapped have been observed to organize and stabilize deviant behavior into special roles, rather than eradicate it. In Erikson's words,

> Such institutions gather marginal people into segregated groups, give them the opportunity to teach one another the skills and attitudes of a deviant career, and often provoke them into employing those skills by reinforcing their sense of alienation from the rest of society.[32]

Paths Toward Deviant Roles

Thus far, we have dealt with some of the variables involved in the ways in which deviance is identified by agents of society, and in which the identification and disposition of individuals may lead to their assumption of deviant roles. Identification is not usually the first step in the path toward deviant roles, but was discussed first here because of its pertinence to our conception that such roles can be considered a creation of others independently of variations in the individual behavior involved. However, identification is often a rather late step, the extreme point at which, all other devices being exhausted, the individual is finally cast out symbolically and segregated into a special, non-normal role. Furthermore, it is not a step that is necessarily one in which the individual is a passive subject—

31. Edwin M. Lemert, *Social Pathology* (New York: McGraw-Hill, 1951), p. 44.
32. Erickson, *op. cit.*, p. 16.

he may cast himself out and segregate himself. And even when he is relatively passive, he is likely to undergo a series of changes in his conception of self, changes related to the way others interact with him. A whole sequence of events, even a career, may be seen to lead up to incumbency in a stable deviant role. Here the enormous variety of roles covered by the term "deviance" seems to be such that it is not possible to outline a single career with any adequacy.

One important variable in discriminating such careers, though, is the extent to which the deviant role is one that the individual wishes to avoid or not. In the case of at least some criminal or presumptively immoral acts, many of which are discussed by Becker,[33] the actors do not seem to devote themselves to avoiding the behavior or even its label so much as to avoiding the punishment that the official or unofficial world demands for the behavior. The career, by and large, is learning to enjoy the behavior, developing protective justifications for it, and creating ways of avoiding punishment. It is much the same for premarital heterosexual behavior and other "normal" forms of deviance as for smoking marijuana, practicing homosexuality, and other more or less exotic forms of deviance.

There is no general desire to be handicapped, however. This is a type of deviance people are inclined to avoid entirely—over which they feel no control, and therefore no responsibility, in the first place; from which they gain no pleasure; and which is stigmatized. There is no motivation to seek out the deviant role, except in unusual cases. In this type of deviance, then, the career may be said to consist in large part in an attempt to *avoid* the role (rather than play the role and seek to avoid punishment for it). But characteristically, the career consists in a progressive narrowing of alternatives until none but the deviant role remains. In the case of this career, upon the first perception of difficulty, the inclination is to explain it in very modest, everyday terms and to deal with it accordingly. Later, sometimes after a number of progressively less everyday attempts at solution, but sometimes, as Davis's findings exemplify,[34] quite shortly afterward, a serious, extreme explanation is contemplated. And even then, a considerable period of time may be necessary to accept others' definitions and initiate the process of organizing behavior to conform with or adjust to them.

One way of charting the potential course of such careers would seem to lie in constructing a kind of hierachy of the diagnoses that people try out, from the commonplace to the serious and truly deviant. In the particular case of children stricken with polio analyzed by Davis, the chronology might run from a cold or a sprain to polio infection from which recovery is expected, and finally to recovery or crippling paralysis of varied degrees.

33. Becker, *Outsiders, op. cit., passim.*

34. Fred Davis, *Passage Through Crisis, Polio Victims and Their Families* (Indianapolis: Bobbs-Merrill, 1963.)

It goes without saying, of course, that a cold may be the starting point for quite other final outcomes, but all the starting points in any one culture and all the outcomes are finite and have a patterned relationship. Insofar as diagnoses assume the form of labels or epithets, a vocabulary is involved: by the use of componential analysis, Charles Frake has shown us one way of tracing their patterning.[35]

Another way of organizing our view of the career leading up to deviance is to focus on the official or quasi-official agents and agencies with whom the prospective deviant comes into contact and through whom his status gets progressively focused, redefined, and then institutionally fixed. Often these agents and agencies are interconnected into a structure, joined together by an exchange of resources and clientele.[36] Because of the significance of the mechanism of the referral in directing subjects through this structure, I have elsewhere called that structure a referral system.[37] For our present purposes, we may ignore the lay participants in the referral process and observe that the structure of the career leading to deviance may be seen to be synonymous with that of the agents of social control he sees. And insofar as these agents are not merely passive recipients of those who fall into their hands, but define who those people are, what they should be, and what should be done to them, and are prone to have the power or influence to enforce those definitions, it is not impractically inaccurate to schematize the career of the deviant by reference to the agents he has run afoul of.

Such a career may be imagined as a progression through segments of a complicated maze, with many entrances and exits, and with a number of different labyrinths from which, once one enters, subsequent escape is improbable. At the branchings of the paths stand the agents of social control, who assume responsibility for holding or sending on the wayfarer. Critical to the career of the person traveling through this maze is the character of the agent he comes into contact with—his connection with other agents and his particular diagnostic and prognostic bias. Each agent having some discretionary power—to report or not, to put it in the books or not, to refer here or there—the sheer chance selection of agents can be of importance to the career. Some agencies, like the school, branch into a great variety of others, like the psychological clinic, the courts, and social agencies. Others, like that of the general medical practitioner, even when "fed" by a variety of sources including schools, courts, and social agencies, rarely reciprocate, instead referring cases to their own limited and parochial system.[38]

35. Charles O. Frake, "The Diagnosis of Disease Among the Subanun of Mindanao," *American Anthropologist*, 63 (February, 1961), 113-132.

36. Sol Levine and P. E. White, "Exchange as a Conceptual Framework for the Study of Interorganizational Relationships," *Administrative Science Quarterly*, 5 (March, 1961), 583-601.

37. Eliot Freidson, *Patients' Views of Medical Practice* (New York: Russell Sage Foundation, 1961).

38. Elaine Cumming, "Allocation of Care to the Mentally Ill, American Style," (unpublished manuscript).

Given the fact that every agent is not linked with every other but rather tends to operate within a subsystem consistent with his diagnostic and prognostic bias, contact with or choice of one may limit consequent moves accordingly. In areas of ambiguity, where a variety of agents may claim or be assigned jurisdiction, and where there are different, competing "schools," each with its own subsystem, a fateful element of the career is the particular agent and subsystem into which the individual may fall or be assigned or assign himself. In some instances, sheer accident may be involved—in the peculiar chaos of the American system of private and public agencies with competing resources and "philosophies," one may be led on a very long labyrinthine road merely by virtue of his first, accidental encounter with an agency representing one particular philosophy, with its own referral system and sense of certainty. In other instances, the selective bias of the agency itself may be involved in refusing or accepting a client—the notorious preference of most "treatment" agencies for clients who seem well-motivated, which is to say, relatively young and well-educated, with the demeanor of earnest cooperation and a functioning pocketbook,[39] or, to take a different context, the reluctance of police officers to book the white, middle-class boy of respectful and penitent demeanor.[40] What must be remembered here is that *while the same deviant act or attribute may be involved* in several cases —that is, the criminal offense, the personal problem, or an impairment—*the disposition or treatment of the individual can vary* solely because of the special preference (or biases) of the agency.

The most important point of the career of the prospective deviant lies in the events that establish his new role beyond any doubt—when he is trapped and cannot turn back. Prefatory to the point of no return, there seems sometimes to be one in which the possible course of the deviant's future is revealed to him, while he can still escape—for example, when the "snitch" is arrested by a private department-store officer, but nor formally charged with shoplifting and allowed to go free with a warning.[41] In many kinds of deviance, however, there is no such point of clear choice. Rather, one suddenly discovers that the cost of turning back is greater than that of continuing and that he is committed.[42] This may be a private experience, as when the addict first realizes he is addicted. Or it may be an official experience—when one is officially booked as a shoplifter, committed as legally in-

39. Richard A. Cloward and Irwin Epstein, "Private Social Welfare's Disengagement from the Poor: The Case of Family Adjustment Agencies," in Mayer M. Zald, ed., *Social Welfare Institutions* (New York: John Wiley, 1965), 623-644.

40. See, for example, the findings of Irving Piliavin and Scott Briar, "Police Encounters with Juveniles," *American Journal of Sociology,* 70 (September, 1964), 206-214.

41. Mary Owen Cameron, *The Booster and the Snitch, Department Store Shoplifting* (New York: The Free Press, 1964).

42. Howard S. Becker, "Notes on the Concept of Commitment," *American Journal of Sociology,* 66 (July, 1960), 32-40.

sane, or diagnosed irreversibly paralyzed. Here, deviance becomes indelibly fixed, and the individual's role is established in official records and, on occasion, in the public mind.

Up to the turning point, control agencies tend to be open diagnostic units—open in that they function to catch, attract, or receive prospective deviants, diagnostic in that they begin to discriminate among them, setting them on different management routes. Here is where the discrimination between the malingerer and the "really" sick occurs, where a troublesome child is set on the road to being delinquent, feeble-minded, emotionally disturbed, brain-damaged, or whatever. At such open diagnostic units, the clientele is heterogeneous and unorganized. At the turning point, however, the label is solidified and pressure is exerted on the incumbent to "accept" and "work with" a specific deviant role. Agencies at this point "work with" families, schools, and all significant community institutions in order to carve out a deviant role in the social space surrounding the individual. Subsequent to the turning point, the individual enters the jurisdiction of agencies that are prone to segregate him with his own kind, providing him with the social wherewithal to practice his deviance systematically.

The deviant career proper, being by definition a segregated one, is prone to be carried out in agencies segregated from the community at large—sheltered workshops, mental institutions, and the like. Insofar as the stigma attached to the role is strong, the segregation of the institutions may be sharp and extreme, physically as well as socially distinct from the everyday community. This is also true of the deviant's own organizations, some of which are, for this reason, secret and underground.

Throughout the careers of defining or diagnosing behavior and of passage through control agencies may be discerned a "moral career," a career in the course of which one's identity for others and one's image of self are deteriorating and being recast in another form. To deal with that element of the deviant's career requires concern with the complex process of social interaction in which people are not passive reflections of others so much as active manipulators of and negotiators with each other.

The Management of Stigma in Everyday Life

In studying the incumbent of a deviant role, particularly one that is stigmatized, it would seem useful to focus on his special problems of maintaining, if not normal, then at least smooth relations with "normals." In this sense, we focus not on the physically segregated deviant but on the deviant who is out in the world. The core of his problem has been justly stated by Goffman: "Those who have dealings with him fail to accord him the respect and regard which the uncontaminated aspects of his social identity have led them to anticipate extending and have led him to anticipate receiving.''[43] Assuming that his perceived deficiency is "incurable," even though it can be ameliorated or reduced in degree, and assuming that he does not or cannot withdraw into an entirely segregated world of his own kind, the essential problem of interaction is posed by occasions of "mixed contacts—the moments when stigmatized and normal are in the same 'social situation.'''[44] Thus, the problem is not essentially one of private or domestic relations, where over a period of time settled routines and relationships get established, even if on an "unrealistic" basis as far as the outside world goes,[45] but rather one of interaction on the streets, in the shops, and on the job, where he is likely to have to contend with people who are not accustomed to his impairments. These situations are strategic for us here, if only because of the goal of some forms of rehabilitation to equip the handicapped to operate in "normal" economic and social pursuits rather than remain in segregated and protected environments.

Insofar as a handicapped person can be taught to get around physically, the problem is teaching him to manage the social vicissitudes of doing so. The problem is to "pass" as a normal where he can, and where he cannot, to "cover." In the case of passing, Goffman brings together a variety of materials bearing on a wide range of stigmatized persons and, while he points out that some stigmata are on most occasions visible to others, he also points out that there are some normal occasions in which they may be overlooked entirely by others—such as when others meet a crippled person sitting behind a table, or a blind person seated in a poorly lit bar. It is thus possible for a person with very "obvious" deficiencies to mask them by selecting the situations and settings in which others see him, very often with the aid of confederates who are privy to his problem. In limiting much of his interaction with others to specially preselected situations, it may also be necessary to maintain a degree of distance from others, so as to avoid the obligation to divulge much information about himself or to meet frequently in unmanaged situations.

These devices connected with "passing" are in essence attempts to avoid playing the deviant role entirely. Where this is not possible, or where one chooses not to avoid the role, the deviant's relations with others will assume greater clarity and regularity if others cannot be caught napping, if they are made immediately and fully aware of his stigma so as to be able to adjust to it gracefully. Here, Goffman suggests, conventional forms of advertisement, like white canes, crutches, and the like, may be socially useful even when they are not physically necessary. Furthermore, interaction is made easier by "covering"—by attempting to turn attention away from the stigma in order to make it unobtrusive and so "to reduce ten-

43. Goffman, *Stigma, op. cit.*, pp. 8-9.
44. *Ibid.*, p. 12.
45. Cf. Davis, *op. cit.*

sion, that is, to make it easier for himself and the others to withdraw covert attention from the stigma, and to sustain spontaneous involvement in the official content of the interaction."[46] This includes the use of conventional aids for the disability (rather than exotic, attention-catching aids) and the development of social techniques that minimize the prominence of the impariment (such as the blind man turning toward the one he addressing).[47]

Questions for Rehabilitation Research

This paper has been devoted to reviewing and elaborating one distinctively sociological concept of deviance, hoping to convey both its special orientation and some of the ways its use can aid our understanding of both the institutions of rehabilitation and of the people with whom they attempt to deal. The discussion of the concept of deviance should clarify the profound sociological difference between the majority of the problems confronting rehabilitation and those confronting medical practice in general. The practicing physician usually deals with illness—a form of deviance for which the individual is not held responsible, which is not stigmatized, and which is often curable. Rehabilitation, however, seems to be involved with the consequences of illness or other misfortunes: while, by and large, the individual is not held responsible for his difficulties, they are nonetheless stigmatized and are considered essentially irremediable or incurable. What is at issue in rehabilitation is not that the blind should have functioning eyes, the amputee new living legs, but rather that the blind and crippled should be able to perform some "normal" tasks without "normal" equipment. The handicapped *remain* deviant, and the task of rehabilitation is to shape the form of their deviance, which is quite a different task than that of healing the sick or punishing or salvaging the delinquent.

This characteristic of rehabilitation poses moral problems that are even more severe and poignant than is the case with any other type of deviance control, for here, perhaps more than anywhere else, including the field of "mental hygiene," the idea of "adjustment" can be used in a mechanical and profoundly conservative way that rides roughshod over the unhappy individuals involved. Since Goffman describes the stereotyped adjustment of the "good deviant" eloquently, I can do no better than to quote him here:

> The nature of a "good adjustment" requires that the stigmatized individual cheerfully and unselfconsciously accept himself as essentially the same as normals, while at the same time he voluntarily withholds himself from those situa-

46. Goffman, *Stigma, op. cit.,* p. 102.
47. Cf. Fred Davis, "Deviance Disavowal: The Management of Strained Interaction by the Visibly Handicapped," in Becker, *The Other Side, op. cit.,* pp. 119-137.

tions in which normals find it difficult to give lip service to their similar acceptance of him...It means that the unfairness and pain of having to carry a stigma will never be presented to (normals); it means that normals will not have to admit to themselves how limited their tactfullness and tolerance is; and it means that normals will remain relatively uncontaminated by intimate contact with the stigmatized, relatively unthreatened in their identity beliefs...The stigmatized individual is asked to act so as to imply neither that his burden is heavy nor that bearing it has made him different from us; at the same time he must keep himself at that remove from us which ensures our painlessly being able to confirm his belief about him....A *phantom acceptance is thus allowed to provide the base for a phantom normalcy.*[48]

The danger is perpetuating the moral biases of such an expected adjustment, not deliberately, but unwittingly, by avoiding the examinations of those processes in our society that define deviance and what should be done about it. What kind of research will help us to avoid that danger?

1. The agency and the public. Throughout this discussion, the emphasis has been on how control agencies in general and rehabilitation agencies in particular can organize a deviant attribute into a deviant role by defining it as deviance where it was not so defined before and by organizing it in the course of identifying and managing it. These comments should not be misunderstood: treatment-oriented control agencies wish not to organize deviance into a role, but to eliminate it. Indeed, such agencies are inclined to adopt a "professional" approach to deviance that specifically denies attaching stigma and even the definition of deviance to them. Officially, even if not always in fact, stigma is an "unprofessional" assignment.

However, it seems that for the very reason that agencies do not concede stigma, they are too prone to ignore the fact that it does exist socially in the community, and so deny the consequences of their labeling for the individual's community life. Furthermore, agency personnel may see laymen's nonstigmatizing labels, e.g., "nerves" or "nervous" in the case of mental illness, "hard of hearing" in the case of technical deafness—as a form of denial of the seriousness of the problem. This may lead them deliberately to employ stigmatized labels as a form of public education. In either case, what happens to the individual as a result of agency policies occurs not through the knowing intent of the agency, but through the agency's preoccupation with its own "message" or "knowledge" to the exclusion of the significant social consequences of the public's views, no matter how enlightened or uninformed. By being labeled, the individual may be isolated from the lay community and given no other alternative than to fall into an organized deviant role. Thus, the critical problem of analysis might be called existential: what an impairment "really" is and what one's orientation to impairments *should* be (these being consciously

48. Goffman, *Stigma, op. cit.*, pp. 121-122.

formulated "professional" and agency positions) must be seen in the light of the real social consequences to the individual of the interaction between "ignorant" public definitions of impairment and agency policy. Obviously, we must know more about the components of such interaction.

2. The public. Surely we must learn more about the norms of the public, unprofessional as they may be. While Barker and his co-workers have brought together a great deal of material,[49] much remains to explore before we can feel truly well informed. There are significant differences in knowledge and attitude distributed differently through the population. It would seem well to explore public attitudes in detail, and above all comparatively across the various so-called disabilities, by means of carefully designed surveys. Which impairments are stigmatized most, which least, and by what segments of the population? How sharp are the boundaries between the normal and the handicapped? What are the ramifications of the stigma— in what cases does it play a role in casual encounters, in work relations, in social and sexual relations? What does the public think, if it thinks anything, about granting economic privileges to the handicapped? About excusing the handicapped from ordinary obligations? Recent national surveys of public attitudes toward mental illness can serve as precedent for both grossly descriptive studies providing us with detailed information we do not now have about the content of the various deviant roles involved, and for analytical studies that seek to explain that content.

3. The agency. There is probably greater awareness of the need for studying the lay public's contributions to the difficulties of rehabilitating the handicapped than there is for studying the contributions of the agencies which are prone to assume responsibility for them, which is one reason why I have emphasized the latter more than the former. It can hardly be denied that in our decentralized and mixed system, the conglomeration of competing agencies harbors many biases in orientation, many types of access to the population, and many types of special or vested interest.

Considering the agency's role in deviance leads to a number of research questions. What are the general biases in the system, and what are the special biases of those segments of the system addressed to specific disabilities? What is the "routine" or "normal" case of deviance they handle, and what is the consequence to treatment of developing the notion of a normal case and a routine way of treating it? Do policies of publicizing professional labels and definitions, leading people to be assigned them and creating special ways of managing them, actually encourage stigmatization by and segregation from the community at large, actually interfere with chances for success in everyday rather than institutional life?[50] What

49. Roger G. Barker et al., "Adjustment to Physical Handicap and Illness: A survey of the Social Psychology of Physique and Disability," *Social Science Research Council Bulletin*, 55 (Revised 1953). And see Beatrice A. Wright, *Physical Disability, A Psychological Approach* (New York: Harper & Row, 1960).

50. See the graphic discussion of stigmatization by the label "loco" and the con-

are the alternatives, if help is to be offered and people attracted? What is
the character of the process by which the agency comes to expand its definitions of those who need help to the point of defining new forms of deviance
and persuading the supporting public of their importance? What is the
process by which differential agency support is allocated by the community?
Are there elements in the setting in which rehabilitation agencies work, and
in the no-doubt-special-though-varied motives that lead people to support
and work in the rehabilitation movement, that in effect lead to systematic
irrationalities and failure being built into the system as a whole?

4. Another view. Finally, there is clearly need to explore the extent to
which the orientation used in this paper—one that sees the individual as a
pawn or victim of others' conceptions of him, and of the structure of agencies into which he happens to get pushed—is sufficiently true to be useful.
Clearly, reality is not wholly like that. Individuals do come to define
themselves in a particular way and to seek out the agencies at which they
present themselves. In this sense, the deviant population defined by agencies may not be that which the agency has picked out so much as that
which has picked itself out—"professional deviants," as it were, of special
characteristics.

This possibility implies that part of what goes on in the field of rehabilitation is a function, sometimes undesirable, of what goes on in the lay community, professional diagnoses merely giving validity to lay diagnoses.
Certainly control agencies depend to some extent on the cooperation of the
community, the police relying on individual confessions and on informers
from the underworld itself to gain material for processing, the psychiatrist
relying on individual self-definitions that motivate the seeking out of treatment. Not only, then, may individuals select themselves, but the lay
community also may select the problems that agencies work on by pressing
for something to be done. In both cases, the agency may be seen as a
relatively passive instrument of the lay world. This approach, too, is
oversimple, but if it, like the others, points to sharper questions to investigate, it can be more useful than determination to get "all the facts."
Here is the underlying point of this paper—that by taking a concept like
deviance and using it to ask questions about impairments and their social
organization, we can understand better which of the facts most requires
deliberate change to improve the tasks of rehabilitation.

trasting method of mobilizing community aid and support by nonprofessional practitioners in Lloyd H. Rogler and August B. Hollingshead, *Trapped: Families and
Schizophrenia* (New York: John Wiley, 1965).

23

THOMAS S. SZASZ

Malingering: "Diagnosis" or Social Condemnation?

According to Webster, malingering is the "feigning of illness or inability in order to avoid doing one's duty." It is consistent with this definition that in our actual daily life malingering is rarely an issue, except in the social framework of the military service. In civilian life, nowadays, the question of malingering is sometimes raised in cases involving litigations with insurance companies over alleged damages to the patient's health and in connection with criminal offenders who may plead "insanity." Accordingly, this (alleged) syndrome is discussed usually as a part of military psychiatry.[1] The concept of "malingering," however, has theoretical implications and significance which far transcend this framework.

Clarification of the problem of malingering is of interest for the following reasons: First, we touch here on a subject which has a clear and immediate relevance to the wide area of medicolegal matters. The relationship between psychiatry and law is currently a much-discussed subject. Analysis of our notions concerning "malingering" cannot fail to shed further light on this topic.

Second, inquiry into the nature and meaning of "malingering" makes it necessary to examine what we mean by the term "diagnosis." "Malingering" is often used as if it were a "diagnosis," much as in hysteria or schizophrenia. This is a grave error, and I shall try to show why and how malingering differs from our usual conception of a psychiatric diagnosis.

Finally, the problem of "malingering" provides an opening wedge into the large and currently also much-discussed problem of antisocial behavior.

Reprinted from *AMA Archives of Neurology and Psychiatry*, 76 (1956), pp. 432-443, by persmission of the author and publisher.

1. No attempt is made in this paper to present a review of the extensive psychiatric literature on the problem of "malingering." The reader's attention is called to K. R. Eissler, "Malingering," in *Psychoanalysis and Culture*, G. B. Wilbur and W. Muensterberger, eds. (New York: International Universities Press, 1951), pp. 218-253, which contains numerous references to the literature.

Indeed, no examination of "malingering" seems possible without touching on certain aspects of the sociopsychology of antisocial action ("psychopath," delinquency, criminality).

The purpose and method of this essay differ from those customarily encountered in studies of malingering. The latter usually take this label as a genuine diagnostic category and proceed to describe its (alleged) psychological characteristics. Instead of this approach, I propose to view "malingering" from a broader perspective. I shall question its meaning as "diagnosis," call attention to its legal and sociological implications, and, in general, try to examine and analyze the very concept of "malingering" from a point of view combining psychiatric, sociologic, and philosophic considerations.

Is Malingering a Diagnosis?

All psychiatric and psychoanalytic authors who use this term speak of "malingering" as if it were a diagnosis, on equal footing with concepts such as conversion hysteria, compulsion neurosis, or schizophrenia.[2] In my opinion, this is a logically unsupportable position, for it ignores (or denies) what is probably the most important element in the meaning of this word, namely, that it is applied to a bit of behavior which society, and presumably the psychiatrist himself, regards as morally despicable. In order to discuss the question, "Is malingering a diagnosis?" we cannot help also asking, "What is a diagnosis?" The posing and answering of these questions is by no means an exercise in pedantry. Diagnosis, Webster reminds us, is "the art or act of recognizing disease from its symptoms; also the decision reached." We might add that it has two important aims, one being to help the physician himself in selecting the proper treatment for the patient "afflicted" (so to speak, with the "diagnosis") and the second, to enable him to communicate with his fellow workers.

The communicative meaning of a diagnosis is, obviously, of great importance in connection with "malingering." Insofar as a diagnosis functions as a communication concept, it is clearly designed for the physician to communicate with his colleagues. We are familiar with the semantic and

2. It must be noted, in this connection, that the problem of what constitutes a "psychiatric diagnosis" is itself an exceedingly complicated matter, fraught with many difficulties from the point of view of scientific clarity and usefulness. For the sake of simplifying matters, in this essay we shall regard the conception of a "psychiatric diagnosis" as something definable and useful and shall focus on the sociopsychological meaning of this notion. It is important to remember throughout such a discussion that the overbearing motive behind this concept is a philosophical position (whether explicitly recognized or not) which insists on forcing social behavior into the framework of medicine and thus views some modes of action as "healthy" and others as "diseased." (T. S. Szasz, "Some Observations on the Relationship Between Psychiatry and the Law," *AMA Archives of Neurology and Psychiatry*, 75 [1956], 297.)

psychological complications which arise when diagnoses are communicated to patients, or their families, who do not "understand" them in the same way as they were intended.[3]

In military life, the implications of the communicative aspect or meaning of a diagnosis are far reaching. Any given diagnosis has, at the very least, the following three functions in this situation: 1. It represents the physician's (psychiatrist's) concept of what is "wrong" with the patient (e.g., fractured leg, acute appendicitis, schizophrenia). 2. It serves as a method of communication between him and other physicians. That is, each "diagnosis" calls for appropriate "treatment" (e.g., acute appendicitis is a command to the surgeon to operate, etc.). 3. It represents a method of communication between the physician (psychiatrist) and the military authorities who are the patient's superiors. Actually, similar considerations pertain also to civilian life, except that if the patient is an adult, the diagnosis is usually a private matter between him, his physician, and perhaps other physicians, and does not (or should not) involve the patient's social and professional organization.

For the present, we shall not be concerned with the first two meanings of a diagnosis (i.e., for the physician himself and as an intraprofessional concept) and shall concentrate on its third meaning (i.e., the patient's social or professional organization). If a diagnosis is going to be used in this way, it must fulfill, it seems to me, at least two important criteria. 1. The recipient of the message must receive from the "diagnosis" something closely approximating what was intended by the physician. 2. The diagnosis must carry a minimum of moral overtones; it must essentially be a clear description and explanation of behavior, not its praise or condemnation.[4] Now, as regards the first criterion, unambiguity of the communication, this is unsatisfactory, whether it is between psychiatrist and military authorities, or between psychiatrist and his civilian medical colleagues.[5] Since this is equally true, however, for all psychiatric diagnoses, it presents no distinct problem for any one syndrome. Clearly, it is the moral condemnation implicit in the term "malingering" that is of the greater relevance in this discussion. While this is obvious enough, it appears that its implications must be persistently overlooked or ignored, for otherwise this word would long ago have been dropped from the psychiatric "diagnostic" vocabulary (as have concepts like "demoniacal possession" or "falling sickness," which have now only historical significance).

A simple illustration will show that malingering cannot be rationally re-

3. G. Crile, Jr., "A Plea Against Blind Fear of Cancer," *Life*, 39 (October 31, 1955), 128.

4. K. M. Bowman and M. Rose, "A Criticism of Current Usage of the Term 'Sexual Psychopath,'" *American Journal of Psychiatry*, 109 (1952), 177.

5. K. Bowman and M. Rose, "Do Our Medical Colleges Know What to Expect from Psychotherapy?," *American Journal of Psychiatry*, 111 (1954), 401.

garded as a "diagnosis" in the military, or any other, setting. The categories of paranoid and catatonic schizophrenia are two good descriptive labels. Whether or not they are "correctly understood" by the nonmedical authorities, it is of no advantage or disadvantage for a person to be labeled with one of these diagnoses in preference to the other. Moreover, no moral connotations are attached to them (except that the patient may be "rewarded" for both by the payment of a disability compensation). In contrast to this, to the military authorities malingering means a bit of criminal behavior. This "diagnosis" is, in fact, nothing less than a covert command from the physician to the military judicial authorities to punish the patient.[6] The traditional "differential diagnosis" of malingering and hysteria is nonsense if it disregards this important fact. It seems to me that while the concepts of primary and secondary gain have much merit in this connection they retain a moralistic (and misleading) flavor, according to which primary gain is unconscious and beyond "willing," whereas secondary gain is conscious and therefore "willful." All facts considered, it appears necessary to conclude that malingering is so heavily impregnated with the moral condemnation of the behavior to which it is applied that its usefulness as a scientific, diagnostic term is completely vitiated.[7]

"Malingering" from the Viewpoint of Life as a Game

When a person calls another a "malinger," what does he tell us about himself? He tells us that the "malingerer" is, so to speak, "getting away with something." It is implicit in this judgment that the observer, as well those whom he is addressing, consider (even if not consciously) the duties which the malingerer is thought to shrink as oppressive, unpleasant, or dangerous, in brief, such that they, too, would like to free themselves from these duties. This social validation of the duty as something undesirable and oppressive, even though it may have many gratifying facets, too, is clearly illustrated by the example of compulsory military service. The slang term "goldbricking," which means malingering, would not be generally understood if it were not assumed that the *wish*

6. T. S. Szasz, "Psychiatric Expert Testimony: Its Covert Meaning and Social Function," *Psychiatry*, to be published.

7. We touch here on the nature and use of symbols. Langer's following comments explain further why "malingering" is such a "distracting" symbol. "Another recommendation for words is that they have no value except as symbols (or signs); in themselves they are completely trivial. This is a greater advantage than philosophers of language generally realize. A symbol which interests us *also* as an object is distracting. It does not convey its meaning without obstruction. For instance, if the word "plenty" were replaced by a succulent, ripe, real peach, few people could attend entirely to the mere concept of *quite enough* when confronted with such a symbol. The more barren and indifferent the symbol, the greater is its semantic power."

to not be in the service was not shared by everyone. It seems useful, therefore, to suspend our psychiatric tendency to view malingering in terms of "psychopathology" and psychical "mechanisms," and, instead, to look upon it from the viewpoint of life as a game. Malingering, then, is the same as *cheating*. The "game" in which the malingerer cheats (in this frame of reference) is, moreover, not a playful interlude in life, but is a segment of life itself. Its rules are defined by society—as laws, which are explicit, and as more subtle social conventions, which are usually implicit in the culture and are not formally stated. Certainly, the assertion that malingering in wartime is regarded as a form of "cheating" does not require documentation. Eissler has emphasized that "malingering nearly always shows us the individual in direct rebellion against society."[8] It must not be thought, however, that this constitutes a distinctive feature of "malingering," since we know that so-called criminal behavior, as well as illnesses of all types, may be so motivated, or, in any case, may be looked upon from this point of view. For example, not long ago all sorts of behavior now regarded as "psychiatric illness" was thought of as "malingering." Even today, those unsympathetic to the psychiatric mode of thought concerning human behavior tend to think (and speak) of deviant behavior as "malingering."

The point which I want to make is simply this: Insofar as we look upon life as a game—its rules consisting of modes of behavior prescribed by society—all behavior which violates the rules may be regarded as "malingering." Thus, the hysteric in Charcot's day was regarded as evading the "duties" of procreation and other adult female "responsibilities"— and was therefore thought of as a malingerer—a view by no means altogether obliterated by psychoanalytic discoveries. It is important to note that in this view the "rules of the game" are held inviolate and unchanging. Those who violate them incur the observer's moral opprobrium.[9] Freud's contribution, among others, was to focus attention on the "rules of the game" (civilization, the family situation, etc.) and thus to reveal the determinate and meaningful character of all modes of adaptation to these rules. He thus lifted "neurotic" behavior from the realm of morals into that of science. From the point of view of science, however, the social structure—whatever it might be—cannot be regarded either as fixed or as "good." From this line of thought, too, we arrive at the conclusion that "malingering" cannot be used in a scientific sense, since it embodies an unquestioning acceptance and approval on the part of the observer of the rules which are prevalent in society at any given time.

An example will perhaps clarify the foregoing assertion. During the

(S. K. Longer, *Philosophy in a New Key* [New York: Mentor Books, 1953], p. 61.
   8. Eissler, *op. cit.,* p. 218.
   9. K. A. Menninger, *Man Against Himself* (New York: Harcourt, Brace, 1938).

last war, approximately 10,000,000 Americans were drafted for service in the armed forces. The laws and regulations governing life in general, and acceptability in the military service in particular, were clearly set forth and were well known by the public. There were, among these regulations, certain standards regarding physical and "mental" health to which one had to measure up to be acceptable for service. The reasons for these standards of health had, on the whole, little or nothing to do with practical matters ("utility") and were governed, rather, by unconscious moral considerations. There is little in most military duties that requires a man to be any healthier than he would have to be to earn a living as a civilian. It is, rather, one of the social conventions of Western civilization that a man must be healthy before he can be conscripted for military service. There is a strong analogy here with the treatment accorded to "criminals" who are aged or ill; that is to say, they are treated more leniently than they would be if they were young and healthy. As I have suggested elsewhere,[10] the most probable explanation for this seems to lie in the assumption that assurance about the soldier's or individual's health serves to mitigate the guilt which society—and its representatives (judge, jury, draft board, etc.)—tends to feel when it damages (sentences) a criminal, or when it exposes a soldier to possible injury or death. Thus, matters of health constitute, in part, the rules of the game, which could be paraphrased as follows: "You must be healthy in order to be drafted and possibly be killed; if you are sick, you are excused from such onerous duties—indeed, you might even get financial compensation for your suffering." Considerations of the sociopsychology of so-called "service-incurred" disabilities would carry us too far afield. Suffice it to note, in this connection, that this entire problem, too, appears to me best understood when viewed as an attempt on the part of society to expiate its own feelings of guilt and responsibility in connection with the injured soldier's fate. It is not governed—and makes little sense when so viewed—by what "actually" happened to the alleged victim.

Let us return to the theme of the criteria of health as a part of the social rules governing military service.[11] This notion is of the greatest importance for our subject—malingering—chiefly for two reasons. First, it shows us that the rules themselves contain many proper, socially condoned "moves" (or ways of playing the game without cheating), which make it possible to evade an onerous duty. Second, it provides the essential clue for our understanding of the psychiatrist's role in this social structure.[12]

It is clear from the premise that one must be healthy in order to be ac-

---

10. Szasz, "Psychiatric Testimony," *op. cit.*, and "Some Observations," *op. cit.*

11. D. M. Schneider, "The Social Dynamics of Physical Disability in Army Basic Training," *Psychiatry*, 10 (1947), 323.

12. W. Caudill, "Applied Anthropology in Medicine," in *Anthropology Today: An Encyclopedic Inventory*, A. L. Kroeber, ed. (Chicago: University of Chicago Press, 1953), pp. 771-806.

ceptable for military service, that a premium is put upon illness for those who want to avoid such service. By being ill one can avoid being drafted and still play the game entirely according to the rules. Neglect of this facet of the problem, it seems to me, has led Eissler to pose the following problem:

> Reluctance to serve in the armed forces has been so general that the problem could be seen rather in the fact of millions not having malingered than in the few who did. Yet such an approach would lead us to overlook the specific combination of personality factors which make malingering possible.[13]

The fact is that millions upon millions were rejected because of physical or psychiatric "disability," and further millions avoided military duty by the appropriate selection of occupations. If "malingering" is a matter of motives, all these modes of behavior would qualify for this disparaging term. The traditional use of malingering, however, is more truly operational than are many concepts of motivational psychology. Accordingly, malingering is reserved for those modes of conduct which aim—and perhaps achieve—avoidance of an unpleasant duty by some mode of behavior *expressly disallowed by society*.[14] What are such modes of behavior in our present culture? The answer to this question brings us face to face with all of our philosophical preconceptions and prejudices about health and illness. Briefly, we can state that aches and pains not clearly attributable to somatic lesions are among the most disreputable "symptoms" which one can have today. This is particularly true in the military services. Accordingly, every soldier who complains of headache is suspected of "malingering" (in the sense of wanting to get out of an unpleasant situation). On the contrary, should such a headache lead to the diagnosis of brain tumor, he will be retired from the service and will receive financial compensation for it for the rest of his life.

It follows from the consideration that matters of health constitute in part the "rules of the game" of military service that the physician's role in this social structure is significantly different from his role in the private practice of medicine.[15] In the latter, his main concern is his patient, who—metaphorically speaking—hires the doctor to repair his damaged body. In the military situation, the physican is not "hired" by the patient at all. In the induction station, for example, his role is to determine who is ac-

---

13. Eissler, *op. cit.*, p. 218.

14. Thus "fraudulent enlistment" is not thought of as "malingering," since it constitutes a mode of escape from unpleasant duties (at the "home front"), which is expressly allowed by the morality of our society. (For further remarks concerning the difference between "malingering" and "fraudulent enlistment," see the last section of this article.)

15. T. Parsons, "Illness and the Role of the Physician: A Sociological Perspective," *American Journal of Orthopsychiatry,* 21 (1951), 452; and T. Parsons, "Social Structure and Dynamic Process: The Case of Modern Medical Practice," in *The Social System* (Glencoe, Ill.; The Free Press, 1951), pp. 428-479.

ceptable for service according to the criteria set forth. Similarly, in a military hospital or at the front lines, the physician is primarily an agent of the military service. Whatever his relationship to the body (or mind) of the soldier, he retains the important function of determining the patient's role vis-à-vis the military organization (e.g., evacuation from danger at the front, retention in or discharge from the service, etc.).

A confusion or clashing of the aforementioned two roles constitutes one of the most important sources of trouble in military medicine, and particularly in military psychiatry. Thus, civilian physicians drafted into the service have a tendency to identify with the patient in the latter's conflicts with the military authorities. They are then regarded as "poor officers." On the other hand, the career medical officer is expected to have his primary allegiance to the military organization. In all those situations, then, in which the needs of the individual and of the service cannot be harmonized, the physician is caught in a serious dilemma. This problem is, obviously, commonest in psychiatry, much less of a problem in surgery, and no problem at all in pediatrics. The pediatrician in military service never encounters a situation in which his patient's needs do not coincide with the needs of the service. The psychiatrist encounters many such cases. It is sheer hypocrisy to maintain that one can take an impartial position in the face of such conflicting needs and be able to do "justice" to both sets of obligations.[16]

In summary, then, from the point of view which we are now considering, it would seem that the physician's (and psychiatrist's) chief function is that of an umpire: He is an agent or representative of the social body (the game), and it is his duty to make sure that everyone plays the game according to the rules. Like the umpire in a tennis or football game, his duty is to watch,

---

16. An entirely similar clashing of roles occurs in present-day psychoanalytic training: The training analyst occupies the dual position of therapist vis-à-vis the institute or analytic society. Both roles clearly define his "responsibility." According to the former, it is to the candidate; according to the latter, it is to the professional group, of which the training analyst is a representative ("responsibility" is often further projected out into society, so that teachers generally feel that they are the representatives, or even the defenders, of the best interests of "society" in general, or of potential patients in particular, in the case of medicine and psychoanalysis). The conjoint form of the expressions "training-analyst" and "medical officer" is itself a statement of the double role described above. While all this is common knowledge, there remains a persistent belief in such situations of "double responsibility" that with sufficient skill and honesty it is possible to reconcile the two roles and to satisfy the needs of all the parties involved. I want merely to call attention to what appears to be a complex matter which requires careful attention and which does not permit of easy generalizations. It seems to me, further, that in psychoanalytic training, just as in military medicine, the training-analyst (physician) can function effectively only if there is no conflict between the needs of the candidate (soldier), on the one hand, and the needs (or what the analyst *thinks* are the needs) of the analytic community (military service), on the other hand. Should the needs of these two "systems" be, or appear to be, in conflict, the training-analyst's role readily becomes restructured, so that he becomes a "mediator" between two clashing systems with (apparently) mutually exclusive aspirations. In this role, his usefulness for either therapy or teaching is obviously vitiated.

apprehend, judge, and sentence those who "cheat" or otherwise violate the rules. It is clear, moreover, that he can do this job best by identifying psychologically both with those who set the rules and with the players. He must be "at one" with the rules—with the social structure, whatever it might be and however it might change—for what good would it do him, in the performance of his job, to question the rationality of the rules themselves? Such an attitude would obviously tend to interfere with his performance as "umpire." He must, however, also be identified with the players and must be familiar with the game as an active performer, or else he would be easily fooled by the "tricks of the game." Just as the umpire assumes that every player is out to win—by fair means or foul—so the military physician (insofar as he plays this particular role) assumes that everyone is ready to use illness for illegitimate purposes. If such assumptions were, indeed, not dominant features of competitive sports, why should there be umpires? Similarly, the universal premise in our culture that everyone is a potential malingerer accounts for the role of the physician as an expert arbiter who must decide whether a person is "ill" within or outside the rules which society sets for illness. Often enough physicians refuse to play this role and seek instead to alter the "rules of the game," that is, the standards by which society judges one mode of conduct as "illness," and therefore legitimate, and another as "criminality," and therefore reprehensible. We shall consider this phase of our subject in the following section.

"Malingering" from the Viewpoint of Psychopathology

Psychiatrists often are, or seem to be, committed to a point of view according to which they try to interpret all sorts of behavior in terms of "psychological illness" or "maladaptation," in brief, as psychopathology. This era was probably ushered in by Freud's study of Leonardo da Vinci[17] and led to numerous interesting psychoanalytic "pathographies" of famous people. Such studies contributed richly to our understanding of human behavior, including the psychology of artistic and scientific creativity.

It is one thing, however, to use a fruitful point of view, such as was opened up by psychoanalysis, as a frame of reference from which to examine all sorts of phenomena (such as art, religion, and education), and it is quite another to put forward the viewpoint itself as the *answer* to perplexing problems. Psychiatrists, particularly psychoanalysts, have at times done just this. Three areas of human living come to mind as illustrating this trend most clearly: criminality, the problem of malingering, and some aspects of political leadership. (These are, however, by no means the only ones.) It is common for psychiatrists to maintain that "crime" is an

17. S. Freud, *Leonardo da Vinci: A Study in Psychosexuality* (1910), authorized translation by A. A. Brill (New York: Random House, 1947).

"illness" and that the "criminal" is an "ill person." Balint, for example, stated clearly and simply, "Being a doctor, I propose to treat criminality as an illness." [18] This view not only is common today among psychiatrists, but is also considered to be "progressive," and especially meritorious on account of its alleged "humaneness."[19]

The problem of malingering is, in this respect, similar to that of criminality. Instead of asking exactly what is meant by this term—or instead of defining and scrutinizing the concept itself—psychiatrists have accepted "malingering" as an entity, much like pneumonia, and have proceeded to describe its characteristic "psychopathological" features. To proceed in this way amounts to a confusion of our mode of operation (i.e., our method of observation and communication) with which we approach a problem with the "explanation" of the problem itself. For a psychiatrist to maintain that he will approach the problem of crime as an illness is not very different than for a neurophysiologist to proclaim that he will approach the problem of neurosis in terms of cybernetics. Such statements are declarations of faith and explicit affirmations of one's mode of approach to a problem. If the method in question possesses much prestige, the very act of adherence to it may appear as a meritorious accomplishment. This is, however, sheer illusion. Thus, to maintain that criminality, malingering, or some aspects of political leadership are matters of "psychopathology" is to indulge ourselves in such an illusion. By so doing, we merely substitute the vague and all-inclusive notion of "mental illness" for all sorts of other problems.

Let us turn our attention now to a consideration of the specific pitfalls which entrap the psychiatrist who approaches malingering as if it were a "syndrome" which "exists in nature." What does he find? He finds that in which he is most interested.[20] Thus, Eissler, who has contributed much to our understanding of egopsychology and schizophrenia, arrives at a conception of "malingering" in line with these interests. His conclusion, at the end of his long and scholarly psychiatric essay on malingering, is as follows:

> It can be rightly claimed that malingering is always the sign of a disease often more severe than a neurotic disorder because it concerns an arrest of development at an early phase. Moreover, whereas in neurotic disorders the pathological process is limited and the functional capacity of the rest of the personality is at least potentially preserved, malingering is a symptom of a

18. M. Balint, "On Punishing Offenders," in *Psychoanalysis and Culture, op. cit.*, pp. 254-279.

19. Szasz, "Some Observations on the Relationship Between Psychiatry and Law," *op cit.*

20. "There is the problem of the psychology of the person who makes the diagnosis of malingering" (Eissler, *op. cit.*, p. 224). With these words Eissler cautioned against this danger, but did not pursue its implications. The fact that malingering as a psychiatric "syndrome" is undefined makes it particularly suitable for each psychi-

disorder which does not leave any single structure of the personally unaffected. It deserves special clinical interest because it is a disorder which is in between alloplastic and autoplastic disorders, and thus maintains an unique position in clinical classification. It is the result of a rigidity of the ego, of its loss of capacity to respond organically to stimuli. It is a disease which to diagnose requires particularly keen diagnostic acumen. The diagnosis should never be made but by the psychiatrist. It is a great mistake to make a patient suffering from the disease liable to prosecution, at least if he falls within the type of personality I have described here.[21]

Wertham's views[22] stand in interesting contrast to those of Eissler. He considers "malingering" in connection with criminality, specifically murder, a subject which is of special interest to him. Wertham's opinion is that some murderers are "sick," suffering from a syndrome which he carefully describes and calls the "catathymic crisis." Others, in contrast, commit murder and simply "malinger" insanity. He assumes without question that it is for the psychiatrist to make the distinction as to which murderer is "sick" and which is "not sick" and thus, in essence, to determine their subsequent fate. The following are excerpts from his writings relevant to our thesis:

> The topic of simulation, of the malingering or faking of mental disease, is unpopular in psychiatric circles. Not a single really good monograph exists on the subject. Beating the law through simulation of a mental disease is not merely a psychological phenomenon, it is also a social one. Crime does not pay, but criminals sometimes do.[23]. . .I have done research on the simulation of mental disease for a long time and found out a number of curious things. There is a strange, entirely unfounded, superstition even among psychiatrists that if a man simulates insanity there must be something mentally wrong with him in the first place. As if a sane man would not grasp at any straw if his life were endangered by the electric chair.[24]

In his book, "The Show of Violence,"[25] Wertham presents the story of several murders and murderers. Some murderers, as mentioned, he considers to have suffered from a "catathymic crisis," and are labeled "sick." Two of the men who committed murders, however, he states were "malingerers" (Martin Lavin and Forlino).

The case of Forlino is of particular interest in this connection. This man killed his 3-month-old nephew with a hunting knife. Prior to this, he had

atrist to find that sort of psychopathology characteristic of it in which he is most interested. This, I believe, accounts for the fact that the foremost men in our field have made quite diverse comments about this alleged syndrome; and each of these notions is reasonable and more or less valid for the material at hand.

21. *Ibid.*, pp. 252-253.

22. F. Wertham, *Dark Legend* (New York: Doubleday, 1949), and *The Show of Violence* (New York: Doubleday, 1949).

23. Wertham, *The Show of Violence*, p. 48.

24. *Ibid.*, p. 49.

25. *Ibid.*

been arrested for exhibitionism; he was also overtly homosexual. Still, Wertham writes:

> It was only too clear from his account that he had definitely and consciously been simulating a mental disease at the time he was in the psychiatric hospital. He had played crazy. But why? Long experience has convinced me that when criminals simulate insanity the charge against them is usually serious.[26] . . . However enthusiastic you may be about the use of psychiatry in jurisprudence, there should be little doubt that the Forlino case belongs to jurisprudence and not to psychiatry.[27] The whole story is an unending game of hide-and-seek between an individual and the authorities.[28] . . . Despite his glimmering of guilt feelings, Forlino is a personality of unheard-of moral callousness. No clinical psychiatry, no psychoanalysis, no biology can yet tell us the cause and cure for such a person. But the victims need protection.[29]

Quite aside from whether one agrees or not with Wertham's ideas about the "catathymic crisis," it seems clear that his conclusions concerning the Forlino case illustrate the personally arbitrary nature of what is considered to constitute a "mental disease." Forlino, who was arrested for exhibitionism, is "not sick." This implicit assertion of Wertham's and his plea that this case "belongs to jurisprudence" does not mean anything other than that he wishes the offender to be punished. Others, whom he does not consider to be "malingerers," should not be "punished," but should be "treated." However reasonable this may sound, it must be kept in mind that the psychiatrist, were he to function in this manner, would play two distinct and separate roles: first, the role of a scientist, an expert in the study of human behavior and, second, the role of an arbiter, a holder of social power, who decides which modes of behavior shall be punished and which rewarded.

The following excerpts are quoted to show further opinions about malingering. Here is what Glover says:

> In the majority of cases, particularly when a cluster of phobias is maintained, anxiety hysterics extract a considerable unconscious advantage from their symptoms. They usually dominate the household of which they are a member and can marshal their various phobias to meet every awkward emotional contingency. So marked is the factor of secondary gain that it has

---

26. *Ibid.,* p. 193.

27. Consider, in the way of contrast, the following statement by Max Radin (an eminent attorney and professor of law at the University of California): "The law, I have said, makes the humiliating discovery that it really has no subject matter of its own. Throughout the nineteenth century, men who busied themselves with the science of law, chiefly in Germany, thought they could isolate acts and facts which were characteristically legal. They called them 'juristic' acts or facts or else 'acts or facts in-the-law.' There really are no such things. Any act or fact can be juristic, no matter what it is, if it becomes necessary for some legal institution, a court or an administrative agency, to deal with it." (*The Law and You* [New York: Mentor Books, 1955], p. 78.)

28. Wertham, *Violence,* p. 208.

29. *Ibid.,* p. 210.

been regarded by some observers as an etiological factor. But this is to confuse hysteria with simulation and malingering. The continual exploitation of secondary gain is, however, a good diagnostic pointer.[30]

For Menninger some forms of "malingering," at least, constitute examples of "focal suicide." He wrote:

To the extent that a neurotic person consciously makes use of the secondary gains of his illness, he is of course a malingerer, and to just the extent that he is conscious of this does the neurotic patient deserve to share in the opprobrium that attaches to malingering.[31] . . . Malingering of the self-mutilative type may thus be described as a form of localized self-destruction which serves simultaneously as an externally directed aggression of deceit, robbery, and false appeal. The aggression is of such an inflammatory sort that it, in turn. obtains for the malingerer not only sympathy, attention, and monetary gain (at first), but, ultimately, exposure, reproach, and "punishment."[32]

Bleuler stated the opinion:

Those who simulate insanity with some cleverness are nearly all psychopaths and some are actually insane. Demonstration of simulation, therefore, does not at all prove that the patient is mentally sound and responsible for his actions.[33]

Henderson and Gillespie consider "simulation" in the differential diagnosis of "psychoneurotic reaction-types" and contrast it specifically with hysteria:

The dividing line between hysteria and simulation is often very difficult to draw. Simulation is the voluntary production of symptoms by an individual who has full knowledge of their voluntary origin. In hysteria there is no such knowledge, and the production of symptoms is the result of processes that are not fully conscious.[34]

Noyes's view of malingering[35] is the same as that of Henderson and Gillespie.

Reference to other authors shows still further divergences of opinion concerning the nature of "malingering."[36]

The foregoing quotations demonstrate the following two significant phenomena: 1. Psychiatrists regard "malingering" as a clearly identifiable

30. E. Glover, *Psycho-Analysis*, 2nd ed. (London: Staples Press, 1949), p. 157.

31. Menninger, *op. cit.*, p. 286.

32. *Ibid.*, pp. 295-296.

33. E. Bleuler, *A Textbook of Psychiatry*, trans. A. A. Brill (1924) (Macmillan, 944), p. 191.

34. D. Henderson and R. D. Gillespie, *A Textbook of Psychiatry*, 7th ed. (London: Oxford University Press, 1950), p. 196.

35. A. P. Noyes, *Modern Clinical Psychiatry*, 3rd ed. (Philadelphia: W. B. Saunders, 1948), p. 284.

36. W. R. D. Fairbairn, *Psychoanalytic Studies of the Personality*, with Preface by Ernest Jones (London: Tavistock, 1952); R. R. Grinker and J. P. Spiegel, *Men Under Stress* (Philadelphia: Blakiston, 1954); and J. H. Masserman, *The Practice of Dynamic Psychiatry* (Philadelphia: W. B. Saunders, 1955).

"clinical syndrome." 2. Many wholly dissimilar views—some diametrically opposed to others—are set forth as descriptions and psychiatric theories of "malingering." This state of affairs illustrates the epistemological confusion about the problem of "malingering," mentioned earlier. No amount of clinical psychiatric investigation alone will clarify this muddle.

It must not be thought, however, that the foregoing psychiatric opinions and descriptions are simply "wrong," for each contains valuable psychological observations. What is wrong with them is that they do not pertain to "malingering." Thus, to take the cases cited by Eissler—whose study is psychologically the most rewarding one—it is not clear why the two men whom he describes should be considered as having "malingered": The author himself describes one as a case of severe, near-psychotic personality disorder with long-standing symptoms, and the other as a case of manifest schizophrenic psychosis. If this is so, no additional "diagnostic" labels are required.

It is important to point out, in this connection, that many psychiatrists study "malingering" without their having made such a diagnosis themselves. (This is true, for example, for Eissler's case.) It follows, then, that someone other than the observer-author makes the diagnosis of malingering, with which the latter, in fact, might disagree, but which he accepts for purposes of classification. This is a wholly irrational procedure: It is as if a neurosurgeon were to publish a series of cases of "schizophrenia" (so diagnosed by others), all of whom proved to have suffered from various types of brain tumors.

Finally, there is a further consideration which shows us that the notion of "malingering" does not, and cannot, serve as a description either of a "psychopathological syndrome" or of a particular psychological mechanism. The foregoing assertion is made in view of the fact that in military life, for example, "malingering" is spoken of only in connection with a person's alleged intention to get out of the service (or combat, etc.). It seems to me that the reverse of this is equally as common, if not more. In other words, there are many persons who enlist in the armed forces in order to get away from painful situations in their civilian home life. Many falsify information about their age, past histories, symptoms, and the like, in order to meet the requirements for enlistment. This mode of behavior, interestingly enough, is never called "malingering." Sometimes it goes by the name of "fraudulent enlistment." Needless to say, persons who do this are never prosecuted. It is clear that this whole matter is colored by the fact that service in the armed forces is considered essentially "honorable," a "patriotic duty." Therefore, no matter how someone gets into a military organization, he and his behavior are regarded as "good." By the same token, any tendency in the reverse direction, that is, away from the military organization, is considered "bad," unless mitigated by one of the socially accepted "excuses." Similarly, the feigning of health by applicants for life insurance, or by victims of Nazi concentration camps, reflects first and foremost a social structure in which a powerful incentive is placed on health, not on disease.[37] It is true that such instances often go by the term "dissimulation," to indicate the similarity to "simulation." Yet here, too, further difficulties arise, since most psychiatrists would consider the dissimulation of symptoms by victims of Nazi concentration camps as eminently healthy. This was, after all, the only way to escape death. This is considered "healthy," however, only if the psychiatrist sides with the patient's value judgment. From the point of view of the Nazis, it would have had to be considered "malingering," since it violated the "rules of the game" which governed life and death in the concentration camps.[38] These considerations emphasize, once again, that the notion of "malingering" tells us more about the observer's agreement or disagreement with the value judgment of the social structure in which he and the patient live than it does about the latter's behavior.

Lastly, it should be noted that "malingering" is a term which has little or no meaning in the medical (psychiatric) situation limited to two people, physician and patient. In the private practice of psychiatry, the notion of "malingering" simply fails to arise. The "Ganser syndrome" and similar psychological observations pertain to the social structure of prisons. Here the psychiatrist functions in a multibody situation,[39] involving patient, guards, wardens, and other agents of society. Similarly, in matters pertaining to insurance, the social structure in which the psychiatrist operates comprises numerous persons, and often institutions, in addition to patient and doctor. Only in the light of such considerations can the meaning of "malingering" be approached in a rational, nonjudgmental, scientific manner.

Summary

Malingering is considered in every textbook of psychiatry, and in psychoanalytic writings, as if it were a scientific concept designating a distinct mode of behavior or a psychopathological syndrome. Observations in settings where the "diagnosis" of "malingering" is sometimes made, together with study and reflection on this subject, lead to the conclusion that the aforementioned conception of "malingering" is unsound from the points of view both of semantics and of psychiatric theory. The aim of this essay is to present an analysis of the concept of "malingering," not as an alleged syndrome but as a scientific abstraction.

The exposition of this theme is divided into three parts, based on three

37. S. Butler, *Erewhon (1872)* (Harmondsworth, England: Penguin, 1954).

38. E. A. Cohen, *Human Behavior in the Concentration Camp,* trans. M. H. Braaksma (London: Jonathan Cape, 1954).

39. J. Rickman, "Number and the Human Sciences," in *Psychoanalysis and Culture, op. cit.,* pp. 150-155.

more or less distinct frames of reference from which "malingering" may be viewed. We distinguish "malingering" as (1) a diagnosis; (2) a violation of a set of social rules, along the model of cheating in a game, and (3) a psychopathological syndrome characterized by special psychological features. An analysis of "malingering" in terms of each of these three points of view is presented. Particular attention is focused on an attempt to clarify, partly in terms of social structure, the various meanings of "diagnosis."

The principal conclusions of this study can be briefly summarized as follows: 1. Malingering is not a "diagnosis," in the usual sense of the word, and must be eliminated from psychiatric and medical writing as an item in the "differential diagnosis" of certain "diseases." 2. Malingering expresses the physician's moral condemnation of the patient in general, and of a specific pattern of behavior in particular. It thus tells us more about the observer (physician)—that is, his identification with the prevailing values of the social group in which he operates—than it does about the observed (patient). 3. No rational meaning can be given to "malingering" as an alleged psychopathological syndrome. It is suggested that "malingering" is best viewed in the frame of reference of the sociopsychology of games. Accordingly, this notion pertains to social situations in which the physician is a representative of some social body and plays a role analogous to that of an umpire in a competitive sport: It is his duty to make sure that no one cheats. The "malingerer" is one who cheats in a game which is a segment of "real" life.

24

EDWARD A. SUCHMAN

A Conceptual Analysis of
The Accident Phenomenon

Research begins with a description and, hopefully, a definition of the phenomenon to be studied. The term "accident" at present is not a scientific construct but rather a common-sense word generally used to describe some unforeseen or chance event that produces bodily injury or property damage. The major emphasis of most common-sense usage of the term "accident" seems to be upon the unexpectedness and undesirability of the phenomenon. An accident usually occurs swiftly with some sudden and unanticipated turn of events that takes the unfortunate and innocent victim by surprise. It is over quickly, and there is the general feeling that little can be done except to clean up the damage. And so, although accidents constitute one of the leading causes of death and disability, we find extremely little of the kind of research activity that characterizes modern medicine's attack upon such killers as heart disease and cancer, or such disablers as polio or cerebral palsy.

Much of this lack of research activity seems traceable to the current inadequacy of any systematic approach to the definition and conceptualization of the accident phenomenon. There is a need to examine accidental events in an attempt to remove them from the area of the unpredictable and uncontrollable. Our hope is that once accidents can be viewed as one aspect of human behavior, rather than the result of purely chance events, the full force of social and psychological theory and research might be brought to bear toward an increased understanding of them.

Problems of Definition

Research on accidents must begin with an attempt to define more clearly which events shall be called accidents. It is doubtful that any single defini-

Reprinted from Social Problems, No. 3 (1960-61), pp. 241-253, by permission of the author and The Society for the Study of Social Problems. Revision of a paper

tion will cover all types of events of interest to the student of accidents. Much will depend upon the objectives or special interests of the researcher. If we view an accident as the end product of a sequence of acts or events which result in some "unanticipated" consequence that is judged as "undesirable," we can immediately see that what is called unanticipated and undesirable may vary from individual to individual, from situation to situation, and even from culture to culture. These are subjective terms which are not easily amenable to rigorous definition.

Let us look briefly at some of the variations in meaning and emphasis which these terms can have. From the point of view of medicine and public health, accidents are listed among the various diseases as a cause of death. Certainly an accident is not a disease in the physiological sense, and it is not the accident but the "undesirable" injury that is the ultimate cause of death. In medicine and public health, therefore, the accent is upon the *consequences* of the event as determining whether or not that event will be called an accident. The same event, e.g., falling down stairs, will be called an accident if it results in an injury, but not called an accident if the individual picks himself up without any bodily injury. (But this event may still be labeled an accident if it subsequently produces some emotional disturbance such as a fear of heights.) Thus, from the medical point of view an accident may be viewed as a form of *injury-producing behavior*. The medical interest lies in preventing, lessening, or treating the injury (e.g., a good public health technique for preventing playground accidents might be to use sawdust under the swings—the child may still fall off, but there will be no accident as long as there is no injury). Accidents, therefore, from a medical point of view are of interest only as "causes" of injury or death. It is not the accident per se that is of interest, but like poor housing, or a polluted water supply, the accident is attacked because it produces an unhealthful condition.

Other points of view beside the medical are possible. For example, the field of law would probably be more interested in the antecedents than the consequences of the accident. Here the emphasis is upon the "unanticipated" variable in our definition of an accident. A legal analysis might attempt to determine to what extent an individual should be held responsible for the sequence of events leading to the accident. Homicide, for example, is an accident only if it is unpremeditated. Important distinctions are made between "acts of God" and "acts of man" in terms of liability. The focus of the undesirable consequences may also shift from individual injury to property damage. If our victim of the fall down the stairs escapes injury (and therefore a medical accident), he is still liable to a legal accident claim if in the course of his descent he damages the banister.

read at the Conference on Behavioral Approaches to Research on Childhood Accidents, October, 1960, for the Association for the Aid of Crippled Children.

A great deal of the present confusion in discussions about accidents stems from these quite legitimate differences in points of view. Our task will be to see to what extent we can separate the uses to which the term *accident* is put from its inherent distinguishing characteristics. How may we logically define the concept of accidents in such a way as to separate accident from nonaccident events, and then to develop a taxonomy of accidents which would permit us to classify the various forms of accidental events?

We begin with the two major attributes of accidents already noted in the common-sense definition of the term—unanticipated (i.e., chance) "causes" and undesirable (i.e., negative) "effects." These two factors do seem to constitute the major dimensions of most definitions of accidents. For example, Gordon and Aycock define accidents as "a chance event developing without foresight or expectation, and resulting in injury or loss."[1] (The *New International Dictionary* defines an accident as "1) an undesirable or unfortunate happening; casualty; mishap, 2) anything that happens unexpectedly, without design, or by chance."

We can, however, raise several challenging questions concerning these two characteristics. First, what do we mean by an unanticipated or chance event? The so-called "act of God," such as being hit by lightning or drowning in a flood, is generally considered as the most completely unavoidable and fortuitous event. At the other end of the scale would be an "act of man," where it is quite clear that the event was due to some man-made intervention. However, in a great many cases, this distinction between "acts of God" and "acts of man" becomes quite arbitrary. As science learns more about the "acts of God," they tend to become "acts of man." Furthermore, many behavioral (or man-made) events are even less predictable or controlled than natural phenomena (acts of God). It would seem to make much better sense from the point of view of definition to avoid this rather mystical distinction and instead to classify events according to their degree of predictability and control.

In a similar way, we can examine the dimension of "undesirable" effects and, once again, note the subjectivity of this appraisal. Physical injury in the medical sense can vary from minor cuts to crippling and to death. The assessment of the amount of property damage resulting from an accident may require the skills of a highly experienced insurance adjuster. Several research workers have questioned the validity of including the injury or damages altogether as an inherent part of the definition of accidents. "The resulting injury is a consequence of this unplanned event, and does not in itself constitute the accident—it follows afterward."[2]

If we relate these two dimensions of unpredictability and injury, we see

1. John E. Gordon and Lloyd W. Aycock, "Home Accidents as Community Health Problems," *American Journal of Medical Science* (March, 1949), 325-344.
2. A. G. Arbous, "Accident Statistics and the Concept of Accident Proneness, Part I: A Critical Evaluation," *Biometrics* (December, 1951).

that, to a large extent, these two variables are quite independent of each other. It is, for example, possible for an individual to fall down the stairs (the chance event) without hurting himself (the injury), just as it is possible for an injury to be the result of some "planned" event rather than a chance event. Although the presence of an injury or damage may be a necessary condition for a medical or legal interest in accidents, it does not appear to be an inherent part of the definition of the accident phenomenon.

The analysis above underscores some of the major problems involved in defining an accident. It seems apparent from the criticisms of much of the current data that we are dealing with a complex event for which we can only hope to develop a "range" definition rather than a "class" definition. We cannot define accidents as a simple, unitary concept: instead we must list a set of criteria for characterizing accidental events. In describing some event, the term "accident" is more likely to be used the more the event manifests the following three major characteristics:

(a) *Degree of expectedness*—the less the event could have been anticipated, the more likely it is to be labeled an accident.
(b) *Degree of avoidability*—the less the event could have been avoided, the more likely it is to be labeled an accident.
(c) *Degree of intention*—the less the event was the result of deliberate action, the more likely it is to be labeled an accident.

Thus, an accident may be defined as that class of event which involves a low level of expectedness, avoidability, and intention. This definition would therefore include as accidents not only those events that result in bodily injury (e.g., *medical* accidents) but also those unexpected, unavoidable, and unintentional acts such as losing things or forgetting appointments (e.g., behavioral accidents).

From this point of view, the definition of an event as an accident becomes a matter of setting up a cut-off point as to the degree of the unexpected, unavoidable, and the unintentional that is required before one is willing to accept an event as being an accident. It is obvious that this cut-off point will vary from group to group (e.g., a child's swallowing of poison is more likely to be accepted as an accident than would the same act by an adult) or from time to time (e.g., a person falling ill with malaria a hundred years ago may have been more readily viewed as the victim of an accident than would an individual today who deliberately enters a malarial mosquito-infested area without taking due precautions). Knowledge, in both cases, is assumed to reduce the unexpectedness and unavoidability and to make the subsequent negative consequences more the fault of the individual (i.e., intentional) than of the circumstances.

This definition of an accident clearly removes the presence or absence of an injury from the definition itself and makes it a consequence of the accident. Why the individual was injured becomes a separate question from why the accident occurred. Furthermore, there is nothing in our definition to limit accidental events to those with undesirable consequences. Whether the result of the unexpected, unavoidable, and unintentional act is an unhappy or a happy one remains independent of our definition. Our attempt here is to set up a class of events which can be studied quite independently of their consequences.

To our list of three defining characteristics, we may add certain corollaries which appear to be associated with the degree of expectedness, avoidability, and intention. To some extent these may be viewed as symptoms of accidents—the more they are present, the more likely is it that the event will be diagnosed as an "accident":

(a) *Degree of warning*—the less warning, the more likely the event is to be labeled an accident. (This characteristic is related to the degree of avoidability, since preventive behavior is more likely to occur if the individual is given enough time.)

(b) *Duration of occurrence*—the more quickly the event happens, the more likely it is to be labeled an accident. (An accident is usually over quickly, again reflecting a low degree of control.)

(c) *Degree of negligence*—the more recklessness or carelessness associated with the event, the less likely it is to be labeled an accident. (Negligence infers that the event was avoidable and therefore, "It was no accident.")

(d) *Degree of misjudgment*—the more mistakes in judgment associated with the event, the less likely it is to be labeled an accident. (Misjudgment implies a degree of predictability and, hence, the less likelihood of such an event being called an accident.)

In another sense these characteristics may be viewed as predicters or causes of accidents. We hypothesize that the more an event involves each of these characteristics, the more likely is it that the event will have the kind of consequence (i.e., injury or damage) which will lead one to label it an accident.

There is some degree of the unexpected and unavoidable in all events, and which of these events is called an accident depends upon the cutting-off point one wishes to use. For the researcher, this means that almost all events can be studied for their accidental qualities—and that all "accidents" must be studied in terms of their nonaccidental qualities. This approach opens up for analysis large areas of human activity which previously were not envisioned as being of interest to the accident researcher: losing articles, forgetting appointments, etc. Similarly it forces the accident researcher to challenge a great many of his current concerns (e.g., adult poisonings) in terms of their inherent accidental qualities.

To a large extent the labeling of an unexpected and unavoidable event as an accident is a matter of cultural definition, depending upon the value a society places upon the consequences of that event. Thus, in different societies and perhaps even among different groups in a single society, the same event may or may not be called an accident depending upon the society's judgment as to the degree of predictability, control, and damage involved. To the extent that the society views the event as unexpected or the damage as serious, it is likely to call the event an accident. Thus it also follows that knowledge of causation increases the predictability of an event and may serve to remove the event from the accident classification. (We have already noted the change in definition of an "act of God" to an "act of man" with an increase in knowledge of causation.) This has been illustrated repeatedly in medicine, where a disease may at first be viewed as an accident, but with increased understanding of the etiology of the disease and increased success at prevention, it is no longer viewed as an accident.

Thus the description of an event as an accident, we would maintain, is largely a matter of the degree of understanding of causal factors in the situation, the possibilities of control or prevention, and the seriousness of the damage involved. As our knowledge of causal factors increases, we are more likely to describe an event in terms of these causal factors and less likely to label it an "accident." The problem of defining an accident for research purposes becomes largely a matter of determining the "operational" indices for observing and measuring the amount of predictability, control, and damage associated with the event.

Problems of Operational Indices

By its very nature, an accident represents an ex post facto determination. It is only after the unanticipated event and an injury or damage have occurred that one in retrospect is able to call it an accident. Thus it is not until after the tire has blown and the car has swerved off the road into a tree and someone is hurt or the car damaged that we say that we have had an accident. If the driver manages to keep the car under control or no damage or injury results, no accident will be said to have occurred. It is only after the event that we proceed to reconstruct the degree of expectedness and avoidability associated with the accident. We now ask such questions as, "Could the blowout have been anticipated?" "Could the driver have controlled the car once the blowout happened?" "Would a seat belt have prevented injury to the driver?" "Should the road have had protective railings?" etc. All of these questions are aimed at determining the degree of control that might have been exerted over the car, the driver, or the road to have prevented the accident or averted the injury. To a large extent we identify accidents by the degree to which such control is present or absent.

An accident may be thought of as progressing through a series of stages. In describing the accident, we are likely to concentrate on the immediate events which produce the injury or damage. However, the accident began at some earlier stage, and just where to cut the developmental sequence is a problem of operational definition. We might divide the entire sequence into three broad segments. Working backwards from the accident, we have first the actual injury-producing event, preceded by the unsafe behavior in the face of some existing hazard or danger, in turn preceded by some predisposing characteristic of the individual involved in the accident. We shall discuss this type of sequence as an explanatory model in a later section of this paper.

Brody offers an interesting possibility of defining accidents not so much in terms of their outcome as in terms of certain "unsafe practices" which could lead to an accident ". . .the accident criterion is much weaker for analytic purposes than the criterion of unsafe practices or violations. By far the great majority of the latter never become accidents because other conditions necessary to precipitate an accident are not in play at the precise moment of time."[3] Thus, instead of describing accidents according to the type of resultant injury, we might concentrate upon the various forms of unsafe or accident-producing behavior. This approach would have the advantage of separating our dependent variable, the actual accident or injury, from the independent variable, the unsafe practice. Thus, we might talk about injury-producing behavior instead of accidents. This distinction could broaden research on accident prevention to include study of unsafe behavior which did *not* culminate in an accident or injury.

The determination of unsafe practices is largely a matter of subjective evaluation. We have to make judgments as to predictability and control, including an assessment of individual negligence or responsibility. It is doubtful that any set of objective operational criteria can be developed to separate accidental from nonaccidental events. From a research point of view, it appears much more promising to classify events according to the degrees of predictability and control and to speak about accident research as research aimed at determining those factors which increase or decrease the predictability or control of specific events. Research on traffic accidents would thus attempt to evolve a set of operational indices for such factors as reckless driving behavior, hazardous road conditions and dangerous car conditions according to which collisions, etc. (not "accidents") could be evaluated.

It has been claimed that accident research is difficult because accidents are rare and unanticipated events. What is really meant is that, out of the large number of unexpected and unavoidable events that involve any single individual, only one or two may result in an injury serious enough to require medical attention. It is our contention that any individual is constantly having accidents, and that we can learn a great deal about this phenomenon by studying all accidents rather than only those that result

3. Leon Brody, "Accidents and Attitudes," *Basic Aspects and Applications of the Psychology of Safety* (Center for Safety Education, New York University, 1959).

in a reportable injury. This point is especially relevant to accident prevention because we are interested in decreasing the lack of predictability and control in the situation quite apart from the element of injury.

It would be extremely interesting to compare accidents with other phenomena involving the unexpected and unavoidable, such as "accidents" in which one oversleeps or forgets an appointment or loses an object. In what respects can these forms of behavior be classed with accidents which produce bodily injury? Another important empirical question would involve the degree to which actual accidents are recruited from near-accidents. Are there other differences beside the injury between accidents and close calls?

From a research design point of view, it becomes important to reformulate our definitional characteristics in terms of predictive criteria (or else we run the danger of defining an accident in terms of its symptoms, leaving ourselves no way to then test the validity of these symptoms as predicters of accidents). Thus we would have to hypothesize that more unexpected, unavoidable, and unintentional acts will result in measurable consequences of an accident (i.e., injury or damage) than would expected, avoidable, and intentional acts. It becomes extremely important to study nonaccidental events for the presence or absence of these definitional characteristics or symptoms.

The following table indicates the various factors that need to be considered in research on accidents, using the above approach. This scheme anticipates our discussion in the next section on explanatory models, but we present it here, without detailed comment, because of its relevance to the problem of operational indices.

Table 24.1. *Major factors in the accident phenomenon*

Predisposing Characteristics	Situational Characteristics	Accident Conditions	Accident Effects
Susceptible host, hazardous environment, injury-producing agent	Risk-taking, appraisal of hazard, margin of error	Unexpected, unavoidable, unintentional	Injury, damage

According to this model, we may study injuries as the measurable indices of the accident but the "accident" itself is the unexpected, unavoidable, and unintentional act resulting from the interaction of host, agent, and environmental factors within situations which involve risk-taking and perception and judgment of danger.

Problems of Theoretical Models

As we noted above, an analysis of accident statistics indicates that most accidents do not seem to happen by chance. Certain individuals will consistently have more accidents than others; different situations will result in a higher or lower frequency of accidents; accidents are more likely to occur under certain conditions than others, etc. In other words, accidents do not occur at random.

Let us illustrate this highly significant point with a hypothetical example. Suppose we have a random population of men who cross a road regularly. If the men were all blindfolded, if the cars were all alike and driven automatically, and if the road were straight, we would expect that the distribution of men hit by automobiles might approximate a Poisson distribution. However, once the blindfold was removed and the men were asked to decide when, where, and how to cross the road, and once the cars were permitted to vary according to mechanical condition, and once the road conditions were not held constant, we would find that certain men, certain cars, and certain road conditions would *consistently* be more subject to accidents than others. In actuality, we do find that accident statistics present a picture of differential accident rates according to the three factors above. Thus we have an explanatory model which represents an interaction of individual susceptibility, agent potency, and environmental hazard. This model is only one of several that have been offered to account for the differential occurrence of accidents.

In this paper we wish to discuss two of the main approaches to the analysis of the accident sequence—one may be called the epidemiological or disease model and the other the behavioral or adjustive model. The first has its origins in medical and public health research, while the second stems from behavioral science research. The epidemiological model views accidents as a form of disease subject to the etiological factors of host, agent, and environment, while the behavioral model approaches accidents as a form of human behavior influenced by social and psychological factors. These two approaches are not incompatible, but differ in the relative emphasis they place upon the degree of human control.

THE EPIDEMIOLOGICAL MODEL

According to this approach, an accident may be compared to the occurrence of a disease. As a matter of fact, to a large extent, disease itself may be viewed as an accident, especially the acute communicable diseases. We may conceive of an environment in which is found a number of infectious agents and susceptible hosts. Which microbe will be inhaled by which individual is partly a matter of chance—or accident. Most illnesses are "unanticipated" events with "undesirable" consequences—the usual definition of an accident. A disease may strike the individual suddenly and without warning, and like an accident, the less we can attribute the disease to the individual's own negligence or misjudgment, the more likely are we to view the occurrence of this disease as an accident.

However, despite this similarity of characteristics, we do not approach diseases as if they were accidents. Medical research does not remain content with treating the consequences of the disease as it so often does the consequences of the accident, but instead it attempts to find out why this individual happened to catch this disease at this particular time. It assumes that despite universal risk, certain attributes will make some individuals more susceptible to catching the illness. and specific environmental conditions will promote both the potency of the infectious agent and the risk of exposure for the individual. Why should not the same approach toward understanding the etiology of a disease be applied to the study of accidents?

Certain other comparisons between accidents and disease are enlightening. A physician will usually treat a broken arm or a bruise without asking any questions about how the injury was incurred, while a sore throat or a fever may be the object of detailed questioning concerning antecedent events. This difference in approach probably reflects the greater readiness of the physician to accept accidents as "chance" events not subject to etiological inquiry.

Interesting comparisons between disease and accidents can be made in regard to prevention. A report of a few cases of polio will empty the beaches, but reports of many more deaths by automobile accidents on the roads to the beaches will have little effect. The mother who would not think of exposing her family to the risk of a polio "accident" does not apply the same logic to the risk of automobile accidents. Similarly, a great deal of effort and attention will be devoted to teach the child to brush his teeth or eat the right foods, but not to avoiding unnecessary risks in climbing, jumping, etc. One explanation for these differences may lie in the greater popular acceptance of accidents as inevitable and uncontrollable. Modern public health and preventive medicine have devoted much more attention to advocating polio inoculations than to promoting seat belts. Polio inoculation seems to be a proper matter for medical concern, while seat belts are considered more a question of consumer attitudes and behavior—a distinction which, incidentally, is undergoing rapid change in public health today.

This analogy of accidents to disease affords some interesting possibilities concerning the application of standard public health techniques for the prevention of disease to the prevention of accidents. To what extent can we apply such concepts as mass screening and early detection of "accident-liable" cases to accident prevention? Certainly industry has made successful use of such screening and detection programs to reduce dramatically industrial accidents. This seems to involve a question of social values. Society is not yet as willing to accept a screening program to limit who may drive an automobile as it is to accept a screening program for food handlers. When the public is willing to accept the same type of preventive program for accidents as it demands for the communicable diseases, we may expect to witness tremendous gains in removing accidents from its current position as one of the major causes of death and disability.

This public health point of view has recently led to the application of the epidemiological model for studying diseases to the analysis of accidents.[4] According to this model, we seek an explanation for the occurrence of accidents within those hosts, agent, and environmental factors associated with the differential rates of accidents. Although the agent factor is usually viewed as the more direct "clinical" cause of the accident, the emphasis is upon the interactions of all three factors in promoting the incidence of accidents.

By host factors are meant those factors present in the individual himself which makes him more or less susceptible to accidents. Thus we may analyze accident rates according to demographic group memberships (i.e., sex, age, race, socioeconomic status, etc.), personality characteristics (i.e., aggressiveness, sociability, nervousness, etc.), attitudes (i.e., risk-taking, attitudes toward law obedience, safety beliefs), physical status (i.e., health, body structure, reaction time, etc.) of those individuals who have or do not have accidents. These are the kind of factors which affect the individual's exposure to and his reactions within the accident situation.

Agent factors refer to the attributes of the object causing the accident or the injury. Thus we would list as possible agents of accidents—automobiles, airplanes, knives, poisons, water, fire, etc. These objects contain accident or injury potentialities and they may be analyzed in terms of the potency or the probability of their effectiveness. Thus, poisons may be rated according to lethalness, automobiles according to mechanical condition, speed of operation, etc., knives by sharpness, etc. These agents all constitute potential sources of injury to the host.

By environmental factors are meant the physical conditions surrounding the individual which constitute accident hazards themselves or which increase the susceptibility of the individual toward accidents or the potency of the agent for causing accidents. Thus, environmental hazards will include narrow roads, fire-trap tenement houses, unprotected roof ledges, unmarked poison bottles, etc. Environmental conditions increasing the susceptibility of the individual might include noise or other distraction factors, while agent potency might be affected by weather conditions, time of day, etc.

This model has proven to be quite successful in the study of causative factors in disease, especially where some specific agent or environmental factor could be identified and controlled as in the case of malaria, and it certainly should be applied to accident research. However, in the case of accidents, this is likely to prove to be more of a descriptive model than an explanatory one. It is probable that, in the case of accidents, these host, agent, and environment factors will prove to be only indirectly related to the actual causation of accidents, and the real need will be to study those

4. John E. Gordon, "Epidemiology of Accidents," *American Journal of Public Health*, 39 (April, 1949), 504-515, and Ross McFarland, "Epidemiologic Principles Applicable to the Study and Prevention of Child Accidents," *American Journal of Public Health* (October, 1955), 1302-1308.

forces underlying the observed differences in accidents according to these three factors in order to arrive at explanations of why the differences occur.

This has been found to be true in general of the use of this type of classificatory system for the understanding of human behavior. It is interesting to note the parallel development between this triumvirate of host, agent, and environment and the analysis scheme proposed by Lazarsfeld in his early work on tendencies, attributes, and influences. The host factors which reside in the individual may be compared to Lazarsfeld's tendencies within the individual, while the agent factors represent his *attributes* of the object, and the environmental factors his *influences* upon the individual. However, just as Lazarsfeld has found it desirable to drop this rather static descriptive scheme in favor of a more sophisticated "accounting" model approach to the explanation of social action, so is it likely that future epidemiological research will also move toward a more dynamic explanatory model for accident research.

Thus, while the epidemiological model serves a useful function as a simple descriptive scheme for classifying various factors associated with accidents, it is not too helpful for analyzing why accidents happen. Even on the descriptive level, this traditional classification of host, agent, and environment could be utilized with a great deal more sophistication than is currently found in the public health literature. For example, we could extend the host factors to include the personal relationships of the individual with his family and friends and his decision-making processes in risk-taking situations, the agent factors could be studied in more depth to include an analysis of the way in which the host controls the agent such as automobile driving or swimming habits, and the environmental factors might be expanded to include the cultural value system of the society concerning accidents and the social climate at the time of the accident. In addition, an attempt could be made to show the close interdependence of host, agent, and environmental factors upon each other. Agent factors are strongly affected by and dependent upon environmental and host factors. For example, the same drug may be both a killer and a saver of lives depending upon how it is administered or where it is kept. It is extremely difficult to separate the automobile from the driver or the driver from his interaction with other passengers in the car. Human engineering has shown that it is not so much man *versus* environment but man *in* environment which is important. Such increased sophistication would go a long way toward making current epidemiological research on accidents much more productive of knowledge concerning accident causation.

THE BEHAVIORAL MODEL

If we accept the basic premise that accidents represent one aspect of human behavior, we can then proceed to analyze the accident situation and the accident sequence in terms of related psychological and social factors.

We begin by assuming that the accident did not simply happen by chance, but that it developed through the same stages as any form of human behavior and was characterized by the same kind of social and psychological forces as determine other types of social action. Once viewed in this fashion, we may analyze the accident situation for the kinds of decision-making processes involved, the motivational forces, the cultural influences, the role of social interaction, etc. In other words, we can now approach accidents as behavior and apply the same explanatory models that the behavioral sciences have developed for understanding human behavior in general.

As an illustration of this approach to accidents, let us briefly note the analysis of suicide as a form of human behavior. A suicide for the purposes of this illustration may be viewed as a form of injury-producing behavior resulting in death. We tend to think of suicide as deliberate and of accidents as usually unintentional. However, we have already noted that accidents do not occur at random among different groups in the population. The "accident-prone" individual, it has also been hypothesized, may deliberately "cause" self-injury—in the same way that some individuals commit suicide. MacIver has postulated that accidents provide significant indices of dysfunctional aspects within the social order. This formulation reminds one of Durkheim's analysis of the relationship between anomie and suicide. The point we wish to make is that accidents may conceivably be subjected to the same type of sociological and psychological analysis as has been successfully applied to the phenomenon of suicide.

We have already discussed in some detail the behavioral approach to accident research in a previous report on childhood accidents.[5] In this report we have evaluated a number of different behavioral models for research on accidents. We do not feel that it is possible in the present state of knowledge to advocate any particular model as especially relevant for the study of accidental behavior. Certainly there is a need to examine learning models to understand why and how the individual does or does not learn from his previous experiences with accidents. This approach would be especially useful for understanding developmental factors in children as these affect the child's ability to handle sudden, unanticipated emergencies. As we have stated in the above report, "We can hypothesize that tfae child learns to avoid accidents on the basis of unfortunate personal exposure, I vicarious experiences, successful admonitions, and the learning of cognition, memory, productive thinking, and evaluation. We have very little ! knowledge about the mental or developmental factors that are involved in accidents—both in prevention and in behavior during accidents. Similarly, we know very little about personality development in relation to accidents, or about the role of parents' child-rearing attitudes and behavior."[6]

5. Edward A. Suchman, and Alfred L. Scherzer, *Current Research in Childhood m Accidents* (New York: Association for the Aid of Crippled Children, 1960).

6. *ibid., p.* 48.

We begin by assuming that the accident did not simply happen by chance, but that it developed through the same stages as any form of human behavior and was characterized by the same kind of social and psychological forces as determine other types of social action. Once viewed in this fashion, we may analyze the accident situation for the kinds of decision-making processes involved, the motivational forces, the cultural influences, the role of social interaction, etc. In other words, we can now approach accidents as behavior and apply the same explanatory models that the behavioral sciences have developed for understanding human behavior in general.

As an illustration of this approach to accidents, let us briefly note the analysis of suicide as a form of human behavior. A suicide for the purposes of this illustration may be viewed as a form of injury-producing behavior resulting in death. We tend to think of suicide as deliberate and of accidents as usually unintentional. However, we have already noted that accidents do not occur at random among different groups in the population. The "accident-prone" individual, it has also been hypothesized, may deliberately "cause" self-injury—in the same way that some individuals commit suicide. MacIver has postulated that accidents provide significant indices of dysfunctional aspects within the social order. This formulation reminds one of Durkheim's analysis of the relationship between anomie and suicide. The point we wish to make is that accidents may conceivably be subjected to the same type of sociological and psychological analysis as has been successfully applied to the phenomenon of suicide.

We have already discussed in some detail the behavioral approach to accident research in a previous report on childhood accidents.[5] In this report we have evaluated a number of different behavioral models for research on accidents. We do not feel that it is possible in the present state of knowledge to advocate any particular model as especially relevant for the study of accidental behavior. Certainly there is a need to examine learning models to understand why and how the individual does or does not learn from his previous experiences with accidents. This approach would be especially useful for understanding developmental factors in children as these affect the child's ability to handle sudden, unanticipated emergencies. As we have stated in the above report, "We can hypothesize that tfae child learns to avoid accidents on the basis of unfortunate personal exposure, I vicarious experiences, successful admonitions, and the learning of cognition, memory, productive thinking, and evaluation. We have very little ! knowledge about the mental or developmental factors that are involved in accidents—both in prevention and in behavior during accidents. Similarly, we know very little about personality development in relation to accidents, or about the role of parents' child-rearing attitudes and behavior."[6]

5. Edward A. Suchman, and Alfred L. Scherzer, *Current Research in Childhood m Accidents* (New York: Association for the Aid of Crippled Children, 1960).

6. *ibid., p.* 48.

traffic accident may be said to begin when a driver climbs into his car and drives off.''[12] While this analysis according to stages is more descriptive than it is explanatory, it does underline the need to view accidents as a gradually developing sequence rather than solely in terms of the immediate emergency situation.

There can be little doubt that the injury is only the end-point of a developing sequence of behavior surrounding the accidental event. From the behavioral point of view, the injury is actually of interest only as an indicator that an accident may have happened. The activity preceding the injury can be viewed as a segment of behavior and studied in much the same way as any segment of behavior. To be sure the focus will be upon those factors which determine the exposure of the individual to a hazardous situation and his reactions within the situation. This model would concentrate upon the determination of factors which make for unexpected, unavoidable, and unintentional acts involving situations with a potentiality of injury or damage.

Probably the most ambitious model for the analysis of accidents as part of a series of events has been developed in relation to research on automobile accidents. A number of projects are under way at Harvard and Cornell which involve the use of interdisciplinary teams of physicians, lawyers, engineers, and behavioral scientists who proceed to the scene of a traffic accident as soon as possible in an attempt to make an on-the-spot evaluation. Some efforts have also been made to simulate the accident sequence under experimental conditions. This type of systems analysis attempts to coordinate all three factors of host, agent, and environment into a single human-vehicle-environment system, including a series of controls affecting the driver, vehicle, and environment simultaneously. It is too early to evaluate the results of this approach, but this kind of systems model is a far cry from the simple classification of host, agent, and environmental factors associated with traditional epidemiological research on accidents.

CONCLUSION

It is to be expected that the kind of conceptual approach taken to the accident phenomenon will have a profound effect upon the type of research design used and the kind of data collected. Assuming that accidents are not simply chance events, but are differentially distributed according to some such classification scheme as host, agent, and environment, we may proceed to ask a great many significant research questions concerning the explanatory factors underlying these observed differences.

Our conceptual analysis of the accident phenomenon has led us to the conclusion that accidents are subject to the same form of causal analysis

12. Thomas Fanser, "The Dynamics of the Traffic Accident," *The Traffic Review* (September, 1959), 24-25.

as would be used to explain any nonaccidental event. For research purposes, we might define accidents as that type of event which consists of injury-producing behavior within situations characterized by a low level of expectedness, avoidability, and intent. We might then proceed to ask the research question, "How do host-agent-environment factors affect the degree of predictability, degree of control, and degree of injury of an event?"

According to this approach, we view accidents as social events—and as such, subject to the general model for studying social action or human behavior. This model permits us to study accidents using the same techniques and methods that have been developed for the study of other forms of human behavior or social action. We believe that this approach to accidents as events falling at one end of a continuum of unpredictable and uncontrollable behavior permits us to analyze these events in terms of current social theories of human behavior.

Producing Medical Knowledge

The papers in the preceding section dealt mostly with the broad social meanings and values underlying the definition and diagnosis of illness. Some of these meanings and values are shared by layman and medical man, but some are not. Where definitions of illness are not shared, the professional can impose his on the layman only in a situation where he is in complete authority. The converse situation, where the layman's values supersede the professional's, would make professional consultation unnecessary. The most common situation is somewhere in between—when interaction takes place between what the layman thinks is best for him and what the professional regards as important. In such situations, lay knowledge about illness is often influenced by interaction with professionals. However, in many important ways, professional knowledge is also influenced by interaction with laymen. The papers in this section show that lay perspectives have a strong influence on medical knowledge.

The working knowledge of the practicing physician comes not so much from medical textbooks as from his clinical experience with the patients he sees in medical school, in consulting rooms, and in hospitals. He is trained to believe his eyes, ears, and fingers in ferreting out the signs and symptoms of disease. His knowledge, therefore, is shaped by what kinds of patients he sees and how they present their symptoms to him. Should he want to do systematic medical research (which, along with clinical experience, forms much of the content of textbooks), he often uses patients in treatment for his study. The patients from which his sample is chosen, however, are not necessarily representative of the total population suffering from the disorder being investigated. Patients' perceptions of illness determine if, when, and how they present themselves to professionals for care. Not all who have symptoms come for treatment. Some ignore their symptoms, some define them as other than treatable illness, and some choose to treat themselves. Those "officially" diagnosed by a physician as

385

being ill with a specific disorder at any one time, therefore, are not congruent with all those having the signs and symptoms of the disorder.

What distinguishes patients from nonpatients is the choice of the former to seek professional help. Nonpatients are a more conglomerate group. They include those free of signs and symptoms of the disorder under study, those who have the same signs and symptoms but have not come for treatment, and, in the case of incurable disorders, those who have already been treated. Whether or not someone with pain or discomfort becomes a patient depends on the homely diagnoses and referrals of relatives and friends, previous experiences, cultural customs, financial competence, access to treatment facilities, norms of utilization of professional help, fear, shame, and so on. The push and pull of these social forces may direct the person with "something wrong" away from treatment as well as into treatment with one or another kind of professional. It is important to chart the devious paths into, away from, and out of treatment in order to determine the differences among patients and between patients and nonpatients. Those differences are often more important than biological similarities. Any physician in practice who sees mostly patients of one age, sex, class, or ethnic group will have a narrow view of illness highly influenced by the social characteristics of his patient population. His clinical experience is limited. In research too, any study of the epidemiology of a disorder based solely on patient populations is inherently biased by the social forces that have transformed nonpatients into patients. To say of a certain disorder that it is more prevalent in certain age groups, in one sex, or in a particular class or ethnic group is frequently saying that a person of such an age, sex, social class, or ethnic group is more likely to become a patient, not necessarily to have symptoms and signs of that disorder.

The first three papers in this section address themselves to the question of obvious and hidden variations in patient and nonpatient populations. Although only Zola discusses the implications of his findings for systematic research, the findings of the other two papers point in the same direction.

Zola's study of new outpatients of a clinic discovered that Italian and Irish patients reported and reacted to symptoms of the same disease in markedly dissimilar ways. The Italian patients, he found, dramatized and generalized their symptoms, while the Irish patients downplayed and delimited theirs. The perceptions of illness were so distinctly different as to lead Zola to try to trace their source in the different cultural values of these two ethnic groups. In his discussion of the implications of cultural interpretations of symptoms, Zola speculates that "illness, defined as the presence of clinically serious symptoms, is the statistical *norm*." That is, like other forms of deviance, physical pathology probably exists at fairly constant levels in all populations, but only some of this free-floating "dis-ease" is perceived as worth attending to, and even less is considered worth bringing to the attention of a professional healer. Zola's conclusion is that if illness is a learned experience shaped by cultural definitions, then variations in epidemiology of certain illnesses for certain populations are probably not the result of differences in physical condition, but in ways of attending to endemic symptoms.

In the next paper, Lorber argues that becoming a patient is not only the result of cultural influences, but can also be a calculated choice. She points out that an individual can deliberately present himself as ill in order to gain some advantage, such as to collect compensation for illness or injury, or to be excused from onerous duties. If illness will produce secondary gain, it will be more likely to bring people into treatment, since it is professional consultation which validates the sick role. Conversely, the desire to continue with normal everyday life could lead an individual to conceal the presence of symptoms that might be construed as illness. Hiding illness would occur most often in shameful and stigmatizing disorders, or those resulting from illegal activities, and people with these disorders would be underrepresented in the patient population. Again, the effect on medical knowledge is bias: from the point of view of the professional, diseases that bring secondary gain will seem more prevalent than ordinary undesirable illnesses, while diseases the layman wants to keep hidden will seem less prevalent.

The solution to the dilemma of inherent biases in patient populations would seem to be to use nonpatient populations as subjects of study. Mercer's paper shows that nonpatient populations, too, can have a built-in bias that is easily overlooked. Nonpatient populations include those who have been in treatment, but who have stopped being patients for one reason or another. The various reasons for leaving treatment stem from the same sort of social forces that get people into treatment—the advice of relatives and friends, financial ability to continue treatment, competition from other activities, cultural customs, norms of proper treatment for the age, sex, social class, and ethnic group of the patient, and lay definitions of "cure." Mercer's study describes the social class differences in the continuance of institutionalization for mentally retarded children. She found that high-status parents are likely to accept the diagnosis of their child as severely mentally retarded, to feel little can be done to change the condition, to rule out normal adult roles, and to continue "patienthood." Lower-status parents do not share the professional definition of the need for treatment of the mentally retarded. In addition, their expectations for education and career tend to be more minimal than those of high-status parents, so they feel the retarded child will fit in at home. They are more likely to take their child out of the institution, making him a nonpatient. One result of such social class bias in the institutionalization of mentally retarded children is that the "normal" lower-class population contains a higher proportion of people at the low end of the I.Q. curve than a "normal" middle-

or upper-class population. Any comparative studies of social class and mental retardation done on noninstitutionalized populations would thus have a built-in bias.

The last two papers in this section are specifically concerned with the question of bias in medical research. Mechanic's paper is on the biasing effect of the use of patient populations as subjects. He questioned previous research linking stress with certain disorders when his own research found that the inclination to use medical facilities, in part culturally determined, was an important factor in becoming a patient when stress was held constant. Since the research on stress and disease did not hold such social factors constant, he feels their validity is questionable. Mechanic's conclusion, similar to Zola's, is that "appearance in medical statistics may be a result as much of patterns of illness behavior and situational events as of the symptoms experienced." His recommendation is that subjects be drawn from general, or nontreated, populations in order to determine the true prevalence of pathology.

Phillips' paper is concerned with the effect of social biases of general populations on such "true prevalence" studies. Given the social nature of research conducted by human researchers on human subjects, Phillips asks whether respondents do not inevitably try to present themselves in the best possible light. He suggests that the contaminatory effect of giving socially desirable responses is particularly common in studies of mental illness, a shameful and stigmatizing disorder. If only those symptoms which are not considered undesirable will be admitted to, it is necessary to know what different respondents consider undesirable in order to assess the validity of their responses. It may be, Phillips says, that some ethnic groups seem to have more mental illness because they are not ashamed to admit to more symptoms. As in the other papers, the implication is that what is taken for objective differences in the prevalence of pathology for different groups is more likely a reflection of subjective differences in what the people of these groups think about this pathology.

The goal of every researcher is to know what is "out there." Cautioned not to trust what passes through his own hands as a sole source of knowledge the medical researcher is now warned that statistically impeccable information cannot be obtained in the field either, and he may despair of ever separating biological grain from social chaff. Perhaps the answer is that there is no such thing as "pure" medical knowledge, but that like all other knowledge, medical knowledge is a social product, created by researchers and their subjects, by practitioners and their clients. In producing medical knowledge, neither practitioners nor researchers may rule out social influences but must instead attend much more closely to the inextricable relationship between the physical and the social.

BIBLIOGRAPHIC SUGGESTIONS

There are many journal articles discussing social class and ethnic differences in reactions to signs and symptoms of illness. Stanislav V. Kasl and Sidney Cobb, "Health Behavior, Illness Behavior, and Sick Role Behavior," *Archives of Environmental Health*, 12 (February and April, 1966), 246-266 and 531-541, provides an extensive bibliography in this area. David Mechanic, to whom we are in debt for his emphasis on the phrase "illness behavior," discusses many of the problems referred to above in *Medical Sociology, A Selective View* (New York: The Free Press, 1968). Earl L. Koos, *The Health of Regionville* (New York: Columbia University Press, 1954), is a standard reference for different perceptions of illness by social class. Charles Kadushin, *Why People Go to Psychiatrists* (New York: Atherton Press, 1968), discusses the social aspects of entering treatment for a stigmatizing illness. For an interesting account of the subjective meanings of suicide, see Jack D. Douglas, *The Social Meaning of Suicide* (Princeton, N.J.: Princeton University Press, 1967). A more generalized discussion of the question of the implications of lay definitions of illness can be found in Eliot Freidson, *Profession of Medicine* (New York: Dodd, Mead, 1970), pp.278-301.

Many references to subjective reactions to pain as a symptom of illness exist in the medical literature. Henry K. Beecher, *Measurement of Subjective Responses* (New York: Oxford University Press, 1959), is an excellent source of these references, as well as a good introduction to the whole subject. There are fewer treatments of the social and cultural patterns of reactions to pain. Mark Zborowski, *People in Pain* (San Francisco: Jossey-Bass, 1969), is a book-length extension of his widely cited article "Cultural Components in Response to Pain," *Journal of Social Issues*, 8 (1952), 16-30. A review article containing a good bibliography is B. Berthold Wolff and Sarah Langley, "Cultural Factors and the Response to Pain: A Review," *American Anthropologist*, 70 (June, 1968), 494-501.

Two classic studies of the epidemiology of mental illness represent two major ways of doing field research in this area. The older work, August B. Hollingshead and Fredrick C. Redlich, *Social Class and Mental Illness* (New York: John Wiley, 1958), is a study of patients in treatment and provides an excellent description of differences in paths to treatment and the kinds of care given mental patients of different social classes. Leo Srole et al., *Mental Health in the Metropolis: The Midtown Manhattan Study,* vol. I (New York; McGraw-Hill, 1962), is the first volume of the report of a huge research project using the technique of interviewing nonpatients in an attempt to discover the true prevalence of mental illness. This volume is concerned with age, sex, and social class and the prevalence of symptoms of mental illness. A provocative book on researcher-produced results in experimental psychology in the laboratory is Neil Friedman, *The Social Nature of Psychological Research* (New York: Basic Books, 1967).

The question of the social nature of medical knowledge fits into the much larger area of the sociology of knowledge. An excellent introduction to this important area of study is Peter L. Berger and Thomas Luckmann, *The Social Construction of Reality* (Garden City, N.Y.: Doubleday, 1966).

25

IRVING KENNETH ZOLA

Culture and Symptoms — An Analysis of Patients' Presenting Complaints

The Conception of Disease

In most epidemiological studies, the definition of disease is taken for granted. Yet today's chronic disorders do not lend themselves to such easy conceptualization and measurement as did the contagious disorders of yesteryear. That we have long assumed that what constitutes disease *is* a settled matter is due to the tremendous medical and surgical advances of the past half-century. After the current battles against cancer, heart disease, cystic fibrosis and the like have been won, Utopia, a world without disease, would seem right around the next corner. Yet after each battle a new enemy seems to emerge. So often has this been the pattern, that some have wondered whether life without disease is attainable.[1]

Usually the issue of life without disease has been dismissed as a philosophical problem—a dismissal made considerably easier by our general assumptions about the statistical distribution of disorder. For though there is a grudging recognition that each of us must go sometime, illness is generally assumed to be a relatively infrequent, unusual, or abnormal phenomenon. Moreover, the general kinds of statistics used to describe illness support such an assumption. Specifically diagnosed conditions, days out of work, and doctor visits do occur for each of us relatively

Reprinted from the *American Sociological Review*, 31 (1966), pp. 615-630, by permission of the author and the American Sociological Association.

The data collection for this study was supported by the Departments of Psychiatry and Medicine of the Massachusetts General Hospital. The final writing and analysis was supported by the National Institute of General Medical Sciences Grant No. 11367. For their many substantive and editorial criticisms the author wishes to thank Margot Adams-Webber, Dr. Bernard Bergen, Anne Goldberg, Marlene Hindley, Dr. Philip E. Slater, and Dr. Mark Spivak. The greatest debt, however, is owed to Dr. John D. Stoeckle and Leonora K. Zola, who, together, read and criticized more drafts of this paper than the author cares to remember.

1. René Dubos, *Mirage of Health* (Garden City, N.Y.: Anchor, 1961). On more philosophical grounds, William A. White, in *The Meaning of Disease* (Baltimore: William and Wilkins, 1926), arrives at a similar conclusion.

infrequently. Though such statistics represent only treated illness, we rarely question whether such data give a true picture. Implicit is the further notion that people who do not consult doctors and other medical agencies (and thus do not appear in the "illness" statistics) may be regarded as healthy.

Yet studies have increasingly appeared which note the large number of disorders escaping detection. Whether based on physicians' estimates[2] or on the recall of lay populations,[3] the porportion of untreated disorders amounts to two-thirds or three-fourths of all existing conditions.[4] The most reliable data, however, come from periodic health examinations and community "health" surveys.[5] At least two such studies have noted that as much as 90 percent of their apparently healthy sample had some physical aberration or clinical disorder.[6] Moreover, neither the type of disorder, nor the seriousness by objective medical standards, differentiated those who felt sick

2. R.J.F.H. Pinsett, *Morbidity Statistics from General Practice,* Studies of Medical Populations, No. 14 (London: H.M.S.O., 1962); P. Stocks, *Sickness in the Population of England and Wales, 1944-1947,* Studies of Medical Populations, No. 2 (London: H.M.S.O., 1944); John Horder and Elizabeth Horder, "Illness in General Practice," *Practitioner,* 173 (August, 1954), 177-185.

3. Charles R. Hoffer and Edgar A. Schuler, "Measurement of Health Needs and Health Care," *American Sociological Review,* 13 (December, 1948), 719-724; Political and Economic Planning, *Family Needs and the Social Services* (London: George Allen and Unwin, 1961); Leonard S. Rosenfeld, Jacob Katz, and Avedis Donabedian, *Medical Care Needs and Services in the Boston Metropolitan Area* (Boston: Medical Care Evaluation Studies, Health, Hospitals, and Medical Care Division, United Community Services of Metropolitan Boston, 1957).

4. That these high figures of disorder include a great many minor problems is largely irrelevant. The latter are nevertheless disorders, clinical entities, and may even be the precursors of more medically serious difficulties.

5. See for example, Commission on Chronic Illness, *Chronic Illness in a Large City* (Cambridge: Harvard University Press, 1957); Kendall A. Elsom, Stanley Schor, Thomas W. Clark, Katherine O. Elsom, and John P. Hubbard, "Periodic Health Examination—Nature and Distribution of Newly Discovered Disease in Executives," *Journal of the American Medical Association,* 172 (January, 1960), 55-61; John W. Runyan, Jr., "Periodic Health Maintenance Examination—I. Business Executives, *New York State Journal of Medicine,* 59 (March, 1959), 770-774; Robert E. Sandroni, "Periodic Health Maintenance Examination—III. Industrial Employees," *New York State Journal of Medicine,* 59 (March, 1959), 778-781; C. J. Tupper and M. B. Becket, "Faculty Health Appraisal, University of Michigan," *Industrial Medicine and Surgery,* 27 (July, 1958), 328-332; Leo Wade, John Thorpe, Thomas Elias, and George Bock, "Are Periodic Health Examinations Worth-while?" *Annals of Internal Medicine,* 56 (January, 1962), 81-93. For questionnaire studies, see Paul B. Cornerly and Stanley K. Bigman, *Cultural Considerations in Changing Health Attitudes* (Department of Preventive Medicine and Public Health, College of Medicine, Howard University, Washington, D.C., 1961); and for more general summaries, J. Wister Meigs, "Occupational Medicine," *New England Journal of Medicine,* 264 (April, 1961), 861-867; George S. Siegel, *Periodic Health Examinations—Abstracts from the Literature,* Public Health Service Publication No. 1010 (Washington, D.C.: U.S. Government Printing Office, 1963).

6. See Innes H. Pearse and Lucy H. Crocker, *The Peckham Experiment* (London: George Allen and Unwin, 1949); *Biologists in Search of Material,* Interim Reports of the Pioneer Health Center, Peckham (London: Faber and Faber, 1938); Joseph E. Schenthal, "Multiphasic Screening of The Well Patient," *Journal of the American Medical Association,* 172 (January, 1960), 51-64.

from those who did not. In one of the above studies, even of those who felt sick, only 40 percent were under medical care.[7] It seems that the more intensive the investigation, the higher the prevalence of clinically serious but previously undiagnosed and untreated disorders.

Such data as these give an unexpected statistical picture of illness. Instead of it being a relatively infrequent or abnormal phenomenon, the empirical reality may be that illness, defined as the presence of clinically serious symptoms, is the statistical *norm*.[8] What is particularly striking about this line of reasoning is that the statistical notions underlying many "social" pathologies are similarly being questioned. A number of social scientists have noted that the basic acts or deviations, such as law-breaking, addictive behaviors, sexual "perversions" or mental illness, occur so frequently in the population[9] that were one to tabulate all the deviations that people possess or engage in, virtually no one could escape the label of "deviant."

Why are so relatively few potential "deviants" labeled such or, more accurately, why do so few come to the attention of official agencies? Perhaps the focus on how or why a particular deviation arose in the first place might be misplaced; an equally important issue for research might be the individual and societal reaction to the deviation once it occurs.[10] Might it be the differential response to deviation rather than the prevalence of the

7. Pearse and Crocker, *op. cit.*

8. Consider the following computation of Hinkle et al. They noted that the average lower-middle-class male between the ages of 20 and 45 experiences over a 20-year period approximately one life-endangering illness, 20 disabling illnesses, 200 nondisabling illnesses, and 1,000 symptomatic episodes. These total 1,221 episodes over 7,305 days or one new episode every six days. And this figure takes no account of the duration of a particular condition, nor does it consider any disorder of which the respondent may be unaware. In short, even among a supposedly "healthy" population scarcely a day goes by wherein they would not be able to report a symptomatic experience. Lawrence E. Hinkle, Jr., Ruth Redmont, Norman Plummer, and Harold G. Wolff, "An Examination of the Relation between Symptoms, Disability, and Serious Illness in Two Homogeneous Groups of Men and Women," *American Journal of Public Health,* 50 (September, 1960), 1327-1336.

9. See Fred J. Murphy, Mary M. Shirley, and Helen L. Witmer, "The Incidence of Hidden Delinquency," *American Journal of Orthopsychiatry,* 16 (October, 1946), 686-696; Austin L. Porterfield, *Youth in Trouble* (Fort Worth: Leo Potishman Foundation, 1949); James F. Short and F. Ivan Nye, "Extent of Unrecorded Delinquency," *Journal of Criminal Law, Criminology, and Police Science,* 49 (December, 1958), 296-302; James S. Wallerstein and Clement J. Wyle, "Our Law-abiding Lawbreakers," *Probation,* 25 (April, 1947), 107-112; Alfred C. Kinsey, Wardell B. Pomeroy, and Clyde C. Martin, *Sexual Behavior in the Human Male* (Philadelphia: W. B. Saunders, 1953); Stanton Wheeler, "Sex Offenses: A Sociological Critique," *Law and Contemporary Problems,* 25 (Spring, 1960), 258-278; Leo Srole, Thomas S. Langner, Stanley T. Michael, Marvin K. Opler, and Thomas A. C. Rennie, *Mental Health in the Metropolis* (New York: McGraw-Hill, 1962); Dorothea C. Leighton, John S. Harding, David B. Macklin, Allister M. MacMillan, and Alexander H. Leighton, *The Character of Danger,* (New York: Basic Books, 1963).

10. As seen in the work of Howard S. Becker, *Outsiders* (Glencoe, Iil.: The Free Press, 1963); Kai T. Erikson, "Notes on the Sociology of Deviance," *Social Problems,* 9 (Spring, 1962), 307-314; Erving Goffman, *Stigma—Notes on the Management of Spoiled Identity* (Englewood Cliffs, N.J.: Prentice-Hall, 1963); Wendell John-

deviation which accounts for many reported group and subgroup differences? A similar set of questions can be asked in regard to physical illness. Given that the prevalence of clinical abnormalities is so high and the rate of acknowledgment so low, how representative are "the treated" of all those with a particular condition? Given further that what *is* treated seems unrelated to what would usually be thought the objective situation, i.e., seriousness, disability, and subjective discomfort, is it possible that some selective process is operating in what gets counted or tabulated as illness?

The Interplay of Culture and "Symptoms"

Holding in abeyance the idea that many epidemiological differences may in fact be due to as yet undiscovered etiological forces, we may speculate on how such differences come to exist, or how a selective process of attention may operate. Upon surveying many cross-cultural comparisons of morbidity, we concluded that there are at least two ways in which signs ordinarily defined as indicating problems in one population may be ignored in others.[11] The first is related to the actual prevalence of the sign, and the second to its congruence with dominant or major value-orientations.

In the first instance, when the aberration is fairly widespread, this, in itself, might constitute a reason for its not being considered "symptomatic" or unusual. Among many Mexican-Americans in the Southwestern United States, diarrhea, sweating and coughing are everyday experiences,[12] while among certain groups of Greeks trachoma is almost universal.[13] Even within our own society, Koos has noted that, although lower back pain is a quite common condition among lower-class women, it is not considered symptomatic of any disease or disorder but part of their expected everyday existence.[4] For the population where the particular condition is ubi-

son, *Stuttering* (Minneapolis: University of Minnesota Press, 1961); John I. Kitsuse, "Societal Reaction to Deviant Behavior: Problems of Theory and Method," in Howard S. Becker, ed., *The Other Side* (Glencoe, Ill.: The Free Press, 1964) pp. 87-102; Edwin M. Lemert, *Social Pathology* (New York: McGraw-Hill, 1951); Thomas J. Scheff, "The Societal Reaction to Deviance: Ascriptive Elements in the Psychiatric Screening of Mental Patients in a Midwestern State," *Social Problems,* 11 Spring, 1964), 401-413.

11. Here we are dealing solely with factors influencing the perception of certain conditions as symptoms. A host of other factors influence a second stage in this process, i.e., once perceived as a symptom, what, if anything, is done. See, for example, Edward S. Suchman, "Stages of Illness and Medical Care," *Journal of Health and Human Behavior,* 6 (Fall, 1965), 114-128. Such mechanisms, by determining whether or not certain conditions are treated, would also affect their over- or underrepresentation in medical statistics.

12. Margaret Clark, *Health in the Mexican-American Culture* (Berkeley: University of California Press, 1958).

13. Richard H. Blum, *The Management of the Doctor-Patient Relationship* (New York: McGraw-Hill, 1960), p. 11.

14. Earl L. Koos, *The Health of Regionville* (New York: Columbia University Press, 1954).

quitous, the condition is perceived as the normal state![5] This does not mean that it is considered "good" (although instances have been noted where not having the endemic condition was considered abnormal)[16] but rather that it is natural and inevitable and thus to be ignored as being of no consequence. Because the "symptom" or condition is omnipresent (it always was and always will be) there simply exists for such populations or cultures no frame of reference according to which it could be considered a deviation.[17]

In the second process, it is the "fit" of certain signs with a society's major values which accounts for the degree of attention they receive. For example, in some nonliterate societies there is anxiety-free acceptance of and willingness to describe hallucinatory experiences. Wallace noted that in such societies the fact of hallucination *per se* is seldom disturbing; its content is the focus of interest. In Western society, however, with its emphasis on rationality and control, the very admission of hallucinations is commonly taken to be a grave sign and, in some literature, regarded as the essential feature of psychosis.[18] In such instances it is not the sign itself or its frequency which is significant but the social context within which it occurs and within which it is perceived and understood. Even more explicit workings of this process can be seen in the interplay of "symptoms" and social roles. Tiredness, for example, is a physical sign which is not only ubiquitous but a correlate of a vast number of disorders. Yet among a group of the author's students who kept a calendar noting all bodily states and conditions, tiredness, though often recorded, was rarely cited as a cause for concern. Attending school and being among peers who stressed the importance of hard work and achievement, almost as an end in itself, tiredness, rather than being an indication of something being wrong was instead positive proof that they were doing right. If they were tired, it must be because they had been working hard. In such a setting tiredness

---

15. Erwin W. Ackerknecht, "The Role of Medical History in Medical Education," *Bulletin of History of Medicine*, 21 (March-April, 1947), 135-145; Allan B. Raper, "The Incidence of Peptic Ulceration in Some African Tribal Groups," *Transactions of the Royal Society of Tropical Medicine and Hygiene*, 152 (November, 1958), 535-546.

16. For example, Ackerknecht, *op. cit.*, noted that pinto (dichromic spirochetosis), a skin disease, was so common among some South American tribes that the few single men who were not suffering from it were regarded as pathological to the degree of being excluded from marriage.

17. It is no doubt partly for this reason that many public health programs flounder when transported *in toto* to a foreign culture. In such a situation, when an outside authority comes in and labels a particularly highly prevalent condition a disease, and, as such, both abnormal and preventable, he is postulating an external standard of evaluation which, for the most part, is incomprehensible to the receiving culture. To them it simply has no cognitive reality.

18. Anthony F. C. Wallace, "Cultural Determinants of Response to Hallucinatory Experience," *Archives of General Psychiatry*, (July, 1959), 58-69. With the increased use of LSD, psychodelics, and so forth, within our own culture such a statement might have to be qualified.

would rarely, in itself, be either a cause for concern, a symptom, or a reason for action or seeking medical aid.[19] On the other hand, where arduous work is not gratifying in and of itself, tiredness would more likely be a matter for concern and perhaps medical attention.[20]

Also illustrative of this process are the divergent perceptions of those bodily complaints often referred to as "female troubles."[21] Nausea is a common and treatable concomitant of pregnancy, yet Margaret Mead records no morning sickness among the Arapesh; her data suggest that this may be related to the almost complete denial that a child exists, until shortly before birth.[22] In a Christian setting, where the existence of life is dated from conception, nausea becomes the external sign, hope, and proof that one is pregnant. Thus in the United States, this symptom is not only quite widespread but is also an expected and almost welcome part of pregnancy. A quite similar phenomenon is the recognition of dysmenorrhea. While Arapesh women reported no pain during menstruation, quite the contrary is reported in the United States.[23] Interestingly enough, the only consistent factor related to its manifestation among American women was a learning one—those that manifested it reported having observed it in other women during their childhood.[24]

19. For the specific delineation of this process, I am grateful to Barbara L. Carter, "Non-Physiological Dimensions of Health and Illness" unpublished manuscript.

20. Dr. John D. Stoeckle, in a personal communication, has noted that such a problem is often the presenting complaint of the "trapped housewife" syndrome. For detail on the latter see Betty Friedan, *The Feminine Mystique* (New York: Dell, 1963); and Richard E. Gordon, Katherine K. Gordon, and Max Gunther, *The Split-Level Trap* (New York: Dell, 1962). We realize, of course, that tiredness here might be more related to depression than any degree of physical exertion. But this does not alter how it is perceived and reacted to once it occurs.

21. This section on "female troubles" was suggested by the following readings: Simone de Beauvoir, *The Second Sex* (New York: Knopf, 1957); Helene Deutsch, *The Psychology of Women* (New York: Grune & Stratton, 1944), and Margaret Mead, *Male and Female* (New York: Morrow, 1949).

22. Margaret Mead, *Sex and Temperament in Three Primitive Societies* (New York: Mentor, 1950).

23. Mead, *op. cit.*, 1949. As far as the Arapesh are concerned, Mead does note that this lack of perception may be related to the considerable self-induced discomfort prescribed for women during menstruation.

24. Reported in Mead, *ibid.* The fact that one has to learn that something is painful or unpleasant has been noted elsewhere. Mead reports that in causalgia a given individual suffers and reports pain because she is *aware* of uterine contractions and not because of the occurrence of these contractions. Becker, *op. cit.*, 1963, and others studying addictive behaviors have noted not only that an individual has to learn that the experience is pleasurable but also that a key factor in becoming addicted is the recognition of the association of withdrawal symptoms with the lack of drugs. Among medical patients who had been heavily dosed and then withdrawn, even though they experience symptoms as a result of withdrawal, they may attribute them to their general convalescent aches and pains. Stanley Schacter and Jerome Singer, "Cognitive, Social, and Physiological Determinants of Emotional State," *Psychological Review*, 69 (September, 1962), 379-387, have recently reported a series of experiments where epinephrine-injected subjects defined their mood as euphoria or anger depending

From such examples as these, it seems likely that the degree of recognition and treatment of certain gynecological problems may be traced to the prevailing definition of what constitutes "the necessary part of the business of being a woman."[25] That such divergent definitions are still operative is shown by two recent studies. In the first, 78 mothers of lower socioeconomic status were required to keep health calendars over a four-week period. Despite the instruction to report *all* bodily states and dysfunctions, only 14 noted even the occurrence of menses or its accompaniments.[26] A second study done on a higher socioeconomic group yielded a different expression of the same phenomenon. Over a period of several years the author collected four-week health calendars from students. The women in the sample had at least a college education and virtually all were committed to careers in the behavioral sciences. Within this group there was little failure to report menses; very often medication was taken for the discomforts of dysmenorrhea. Moreover, this group was so psychologically sophisticated or self-conscious that they interpreted or questioned most physical signs or symptoms as attributable to some psychosocial stress. There was only one exception—dysmenorrhea. Thus, even in this "culturally advantaged" group, this seemed a sign of a bodily condition so ingrained in what one psychiatrist has called "the masochistic character of her sex" that the woman does not ordinarily subject it to analysis.

In the opening section of this paper, we presented evidence that a selective process might well be operating in what symptoms are brought to the doctor. We also noted that it might be this selective process and not an etiological one which accounts for the many unexplained or overexplained epidemiological differences observed between and within societies.[27] (There

---

on whether they spent time with a euphoric or angry stooge. Subjects without injections reported no such change in mood responding to these same social situations. This led them to the contention that the diversity of human emotional experiences stems from differential labeling of similar physical sensations.

25. A term used by Drs. R. Green and K. Dalton, as quoted in Hans Selye, *The Stress of Life* (New York: McGraw-Hill, 1956), p. 177.

26. John Kosa, Joel Alpert, M. Ruth Pickering, and Robert J. Haggerty, "Crisis and Family Life: A Re-Examination of Concepts," *The Wisconsin Sociologist*, 4 (Summer, 1965), 11-19.

27. For example, Saxon Graham, "Ethnic Background and Illness in a Pennsylvania County," *Social Problems*, 4 (July, 1956), 76-81, noted a significantly higher incidence of hernia among men whose backgrounds were Southern European (Italy or Greece) as compared with Eastern European (Austria, Czechoslavakia, Russia, or Poland). Analysis of the occupations engaged in by these groups revealed no evidence that the Southern Europeans in the sample were more engaged in strenuous physical labor than the Eastern Europeans. From what is known of tolerance to hernia, we suggest that, for large segments of the populations, there may be no differences in the actual incidence and prevalence of hernia but that in different groups different perceptions of the same physical signs may lead to dissimilar ways of handling them. Thus the Southern Europeans in Graham's sample may have been more concerned with problems in this area of the body, and have sought aid more readily (and therefore appear more frequently in the morbidity statistics). Perhaps the Southern Europeans are acting quite rationally and consistently while the

may even be no "real" differences in the prevalance rates of many deviations.[28] Such selective processes are probably present at all the stages through which an individual and his condition must pass before he ultimately gets counted as "ill." In this section we have focused on one of these stages, the perception of a particular bodily state as a symptom, and have delineated two possible ways in which the culture or social setting might influence the awareness of something as abnormal and thus its eventual tabulation in medical statistics.

Sample Selection and Methodology

The investigation to be reported here is not an attempt to prove that the foregoing body of reasoning is correct but rather to demonstrate the fruitfulness of the orientation in understanding the problems of health and illness. This study reports the existence of a selective process in what the patient "brings" to a doctor. The selectiveness is analyzed not in terms of differences in diseases but rather in terms of differences in responses to essentially similar disease entities.

Specifically, this paper is a documentation of the influence of "culture" (in this case ethnic-group membership) on "symptoms" (the complaints a patient presents to his physician.) The measure of "culture" was fairly straightforward. The importance of ethnic groups in Boston, where the study was done, has been repeatedly documented;[29] ethnicity seemed a reasonable urban counterpart of the cultures so often referred to in the previous pages. The sample was drawn from the outpatient clinics of the Massachusetts General Hospital and the Massachusetts Eye and Ear Infirmary; it was limited to those new patients of both sexes between 18 and 50 who were white, able to converse in English, and of either Irish Catholic, Italian Catholic, or Anglo-Saxon Protestant background.[30] These were the most

other groups are so threatened or ashamed that they tend to deny or mask such symptoms and thus keep themselves out of the morbidity statistics.

28. In studying the rates of peptic ulcer among African tribal groups Raper, *op. cit.*, first confirmed the stereotype that it was relatively infrequent among such groups and therefore that it was associated (as many had claimed) with the stresses and strains of modern living. Yet when he relied not on reported diagnosis but on autopsy data, he found that the scars of peptic ulcer were no less common than in Britain. He concluded: "There is no need to assume that in backward communities peptic ulcer does not develop; it is only more likely to go undetected because the conditions that might bring it to notice do not exist."

29. Oscar Handlin, *Race and Nationality in American Life* (Garden City, N.Y.: Doubleday, 1957); Oscar Handlin, *Boston's Immigrants* (Cambridge: Harvard University Press, 1959).

30. Ethnicity was ascertained by the responses to several questions: what the patients considered their nationality to be; the birthplaces of themselves, their parents, their maternal and paternal grandparents; and, if the answers to all of these were American, they were also asked whence their ancestors originated. For details, see Irving Kenneth Zola, *Sociocultural Factors in the Seeking of Medical Aid*, unpublished doctoral dissertation, Harvard University, Department of Social Relations, 1962.

numerous ethnic groups in the clinics; together they constituted approximately 50 percent of all patients. The actual interviewing took place at the three clinics to which these patients were most frequently assigned (the three largest outpatient clinics): the Eye Clinic, the Ear, Nose and Throat Clinic, and the Medical Clinic.

In previous research the specific method of measuring and studying symptoms has varied among case record analysis, symptom checklists, and interviews. The data have been either retrospective or projective, that is, requesting the subject either to recall symptoms experienced during a specific time period or to choose symptoms which would bother him sufficiently to seek medical aid.[31] Such procedures do not provide data on the complaints which people actually bring to a doctor, a fact of particular importance in light of the many investigations pointing to the lack of, and distortions in, recall of sickness episodes.[32] An equally serious problem is the effect of what the doctor, medicine-man, or health expert may tell the patient on the latter's subsequent perceptions of and recall about his ailment.[33] We resolved these problems by restricting the sample to new patients on their first medical visit to the clinics and by interviewing them during the waiting period *before* they were seen by a physician.[34]

The primary method of data collection was a focused open-ended interview dealing with the patient's own or family's responses to his presenting

31. The range of methods includes case research analysis—Berta Fantl and Joseph Schiro, "Cultural Variables in the Behavior Patterns and Symptom Formation of 15 Irish and 15 Italian Female Schizophrenics," *International Journal of Social Psychiatry*, 4 (Spring, 1959) 245-253; checklists—Cornerly and Bigman, *op. cit.;* standardized questionnaires—Sidney H. Croog, "Ethnic Origins and Responses to Health Questionnaires," *Human Organization*, 20 (Summer, 1961), 65-69; commitment papers—John B. Enright and Walter R. Jaeckle, "Psychiatric Symptoms and Diagnosis in Two Subcultures," *International Journal of Social Psychiatry*, 9 (Winter, 1963), 12-17; interview and questionnaire—Graham, *op. cit.;* Mark Zborowski, "Cultural Components in Response to Pain," *Journal of Social Issues*, 8 (Fall, 1952), 16-30; interview and psychological tests—Marvin K. Opler and Jerome L. Singer, "Ethnic Differences in Behavior and Psychopathology: Italian and Irish," *International Journal of Social Psychiatry*, 2 (Summer, 1956), 11-12; observation—Clark, *op. cit.;* and Lyle Saunders, *op. cit.*

32. See Jacob J. Feldman, "The Household Interview Survey as a Technique for the Collection of Morbidity Data," *Journal of Chronic Diseases*, 11 (May, 1960), 535-557; Theodore D. Woolsey, "The Health Survey," presented at the session, "The Contributions of Research in the Field of Health," 1959 AAPOR Conference, May, 1959, Lake George, New York.

33. Charles Kadushin, "The Meaning of Presenting Problems: A Sociology of Defense," paper read at the 1962 annual meeting of the American Sociological Association.

34. This particular methodological choice was also determined by the nature of the larger study, that is, how patients decided to seek medical aid, where the above-mentioned problems loom even larger. While only new admissions were studied, a number of patients had been referred by another medical person. Subsequent statistical analysis revealed no important differences between this group and those for whom the Massachusetts General Hospital or the Massachusetts Eye and Ear Infirmary was the initial source of help.

complaints. Interspersed throughout the interview were a number of more objective measures of the patient's responses—checklists, forced-choice comparisons, attitudinal items, and scales. Other information included a demographic background questionnaire, a review of the medical record, and a series of ratings by each patient's examining physician as to the primary diagnosis, the secondary diagnosis, the potential seriousness, and the degree of clinical urgency (i.e., the necessity that the patient be seen immediately) of the patient's presenting complaint.

The Patient and His Illness

The data are based on a comparison between 63 Italians (34 female, 29 male) and 81 Irish (42 female, 39 male), who were new admissions to the Eye, the Ear, Nose, and Throat, and the Medical Clinics of the Massachusetts General Hospital and the Massachusetts Eye and Ear Infirmary, seen between July, 1960, and February 1961.[35] The mean age of each ethnic group (male and female computed separately) was approximately thirty-three. While most patients were married, there was, in the sample, a higher proportion of single Irish men—a finding of other studies involving the Irish[36] and not unexpected from our knowledge of Irish family structure.[37] Most respondents had between 10 and 12 years of schooling, but only about 30 percent of the males claimed to have graduated from high school as compared with nearly 60 percent of the females. There were no significant differences on standard measures of social class, though in education, social class, occupation of the breadwinner in the patient's family, and the occupation of the patient's father, the Irish ranked slightly higher.[38] The Italians were overwhelmingly American-born children of foreign parents: about 80 percent were second generation while 20 percent were third. Among the Irish about 40 percent were second generation, 30 percent third, and 30 percent fourth.

With regard to general medical coverage, there were no apparent differences between the ethnic groups. Approximately 62 percent of the sample had health insurance, a figure similar to the comparable economic group

35. Forty-three Anglo-Saxons were also interviewed but are not considered in this analysis. They were dropped from this report because they differed from the Irish and Italians in various respects other than ethnicity: they included more students, more divorced and separated, more people living away from home, and more downwardly mobile; they were of higher socioeconomic and educational level, and a majority were fourth generation and beyond.

36. Opler and Singer, *op. cit.*

37. Conrad M. Arensberg and Solon T. Kimball, *Family and Community in Ireland* (Cambridge: Harvard University Press, 1948).

38. In Warner's terms (W. Lloyd Warner, *Social Class in America*, Chicago: Science Research Associates, 1949), the greatest number of patients was in Class V. Only a small proportion of new Irish and Italian patients were what might be traditionally labeled as charity cases, although by some criteria they were perhaps "medically indigent."

in the Rosenfeld survey of Metropolitan Boston.[39] Sixty percent had physicians whom they would call family doctors. The Irish tended more than
the Italians to perceive themselves as having poor health, claiming more
often they had been seriously ill in the past. This was consistent with their
reporting of the most recent visit to a doctor: nine of the Irish but none of
the Italians claimed to have had a recent major operation (e.g., appen-
dectomy) or illness (e.g., pneumonia). Although there were no differences
in the actual seriousness of their present disorders (according to the doctor's
ratings) there was a tendency for the examining physician to consider the
Irish as being in more urgent need of treatment. It was apparent that the
patients were not in the throes of an acute illness, although they may have
been experiencing an acute episode. There was a slight tendency for the
Irish, as a group, to have had their complaints longer. More significantly,
the women of both groups claimed to have borne their symptoms for a
longer time than the men.

In confining the study to three clinics, we were trying not only to econo-
mize but also to limit the range of illnesses. The latter was necessary for
investigating differential responses to essentially similar conditions.[40] Yet at
best this is only an approximate control. To resolve this difficulty, after all
initial comparisons were made between the ethnic groups as a whole, the
data were examined for a selected subsample with a specific control for
diagnosis. This subsample consisted of matched pairs of one Irish and one
Italian of the same sex, who had the same primary diagnosis, and whose
disorder was of approximately the same duration and was rated by the examining physician as similar in degree of "seriousness." Where numbers
made it feasible, there was a further matching on age, marital status, and
education. In all, thirty-seven diagnostically matched pairs (18 female
and 19 male) were created; these constituted the final test of any finding of
the differential response to illness.[41]

*Table 25.1.   Distribution of Irish and Italian clinic
admissions by location of chief complaint*

Location of Complaint	Italian	Irish[a]
Eye, ear, nose, or throat	34	61
Other parts of the body	29	17
Total	63	78

Note: $X^2 = 9.31$, $p < .01$.
[a]Since 3 Irish patients (two women, one man) claimed to be asymptomatic, no
location could be determined from their viewpoint.

39. Rosenfeld, *op. cit.*
40. This is similar to Zborowski's method, in his study of pain reactions, of confining his investigation to patients on certain specified wards. *Op. cit.*
41. These pairs included some eighteen distinct diagnoses: conjunctivitis; eyelid disease (e.g., blepharitis); mypopia; hyperopia; vitreous opacities; impacted cerumen;
external otitis; otitis media; otosclerosis; deviated septum; sinusitis; nasopharyngitis;

LOCATION AND QUALITY OF PRESENTING COMPLAINTS

In the folklore of medical practice, the supposed opening question is, "Where does it hurt?" This query provides the starting point of our analysis —the perceived location of the patient's troubles. Our first finding is that more Irish than Italians tended to locate their chief problem in either the eye, the ear, the nose, or the throat (and more so for females than for males). The same tendency was evident when all patients were asked what they considered to be the most important part of their body and the one with which they would be most concerned if something went wrong. Here, too, significantly more Irish emphasized difficulties of the eye, the ear, the nose, or the throat. That this reflected merely a difference in the conditions for which they were seeking aid is doubtful since the two other parts of the

Table 25.2   *Distribution of Irish and Italian clinic admissions by part of the body considered most important*

Most Important Part of the Body	Italian	Irish
Eye, ear, nose, or throat	6	26
Other parts of the body	57	55
Total	63	81

Note: $X^2 = 10.50$, $p < .01$.

body most frequently referred to were heart and "mind" locations, and these represent only 3 percent of the primary diagnoses of the entire sample. In the retesting of these findings on diagnostically matched pairs, while there were a great many ties, the general directions were still consistent.[42] Thus even when Italians had a diagnosed eye or ear disorder, they did not locate their chief complaints there, nor did they focus their future concern on these locations.

---

allergy; thyroid; obesity; functional complaints; no pathology; psychological problems.

To give some indication of the statistical significance of these comparisons, a sign test was used. For the sign test, a "tie" occurs when it is not possible to discriminate between a matched pair on the variable under study, or when the two scores earned by any pair are equal. All tied cases were dropped from the analysis, and the probabilities were computed only on the total N's excluding ties. In our study there were many ties. In the nature of our hypotheses, as will appear subsequently, a tie means that at least one member of the pair was in the predicted direction. Despite the problem, the idea of a diagnostically matched pair was retained because it seemed to convey the best available test of our data. Because there were specific predictions as to the direction of differences the probabilities were computed on the basis of a one-tailed sign test. This was used to retest the findings of Tables 25.1-25.6. See Sidney Siegel, *Non-Parametric Statistics for the Behavioral Sciences* (New York: McGraw-Hill, 1956), pp. 68-75.

42. For the prediction that the Irish would locate their chief complaint in eye, ear, nose or throat, and the Italians in some other part, 8 matched diagnostic pairs were in favor of the hypothesis, 1 against, 28 ties (p=.02); for the same with respect to most important part of the body there were 12 in favor of the hypothesis, 2 against, 23 ties (p=.006).

Pain, the commonest accompaniment of illness, was the dimension of patients' symptoms to which we next turned. Pain is an especially interesting phenomenon since there is considerable evidence that its tolerance and perception are not purely physiological responses and do not necessarily reflect the degree of objective discomfort induced by a particular disorder or experimental procedure.[43] In our study not only did the Irish more often than the Italians deny that pain was a feature of their illness but this difference held even for those patients with the same disorder.[44] When the Irish

Table 25.3.   *Distribution of Irish and Italian clinic admissions by presence of pain in their current illness*

Presence of Pain	Italian	Irish
No	27	54
Yes	36	27
Total	63	81

Note: $X^2 = 10.26$, p < .01.

were asked directly about the presence of pain, some hedged their replies with qualifications. ("It was more a throbbing than a pain . . . not really pain, it feels more like sand in my eye.") Such comments indicated that the patients were reflecting something more than an objective reaction to their physical conditions.

While there were no marked differences in the length, frequency, or noticeability of their symptoms, a difference did emerge in the ways in which they described the quality of the physical difficulty embodied in their chief complaint. Two types of difficulty were distinguished: one was of a more limited nature and emphasized a circumscribed and specific dysfunctioning; the second emphasized a difficulty of a grosser and more diffuse quality.[45] When the patients' complaints were analyzed according to these two types, proportionately more Irish described their chief problem in terms of specific dysfunction while proportionately more Italians spoke of a diffuse difficulty.

43. William P. Chapman and Chester M. Jones, "Variations in Cutaneous and Visceral Pain Sensitivity in Normal Subjects," *Journal of Clinical Investigation*, 23 (January, 1944), 81-91; James D. Hardy, Harold G. Wolff, and Helen Goodell, *Pain Sensations and Reactions* (Baltimore: Williams and Wilkins, 1952); Ronald Melzack, "The Perception of Pain," *Scientific American*, 204 (February, 1961), 41-49; Harry S. Olin and Thomas P. Hackett, "The Denial of Chest Pain in 32 Patients with Acute Myocardial Infection," *Journal of the American Medical Association*, 190 (December, 1964), 977-981; Zborowski, *op. cit.*

44. For the prediction that Italians would admit the presence of pain and the Irish would deny it, 16 matched diagnostic pairs were in favor of the hypothesis, 0 against, 21 ties (p=.001)

45. Complaints of the first type emphasized a somewhat limited difficulty and dysfunction best exemplified by something specific, e.g., an organ having gone wrong in a particular way. The second type seemed to involve a more attenuated kind of problem whose location and scope were less determinate, and whose description was finally more qualitative and less measurable.

Once again, the findings for diagnostically matched pairs were in the predicted directions.[46]

DIFFUSE VERSUS SPECIFIC REACTIONS

What seems to emerge from the above is a picture of the Irish limiting

*Table 25.4.   Distribution of Irish and Italian clinic admissions by
quality of physical difficulty embodied in chief complaint*

Quality of Physical Difficulty	Italian	Irish[a]
Problems of a diffuse nature	43	33
Problems of a specific nature	20	45
Total	63	78

Note: $X^2 = 9.44$, $p < .01$.

[a]Since 3 Irish patients (two women, one man) claimed to be asymptomatic, no rating of the quality of physical difficulty could be determined from their viewpoint.

and understating their difficulties and the Italians spreading and generalizing theirs. Two other pieces of information were consistent with this interpretation: first, an enumeration of the symptoms an individual presented—a phenomenon which might reflect how diffusely the complaint was perceived; second, the degree to which each patient felt his illness affected aspects of life other than purely physical behavior.

The first measure of this specific-diffuse dimension—number of distinguishable symptoms[47]—was examined in three ways: (1) the total number presented by each patient; (2) the total number of different bodily areas in which the patient indicated he had complaints, e.g., back, stomach, legs; (3) the total number of different qualities of physical difficulty embodied in the patient's presenting complaints.[48] The ethnic differences were consistent with the previous findings. Compared to the Irish, the Italians presented significantly more symptoms, had symptoms in significantly more bodily locations, and noted significantly more types of bodily dysfunction.[49]

The second analysis, the degree to which a patient felt his illness affected his more general well-being, was derived from replies to three questions: (1) Do you think your symptoms affected how you got along with your family? (2) Did you become more irritable? (3) What would you say has

46. For the prediction that the Italians would emphasize a diffuse difficulty and the Irish a specific one; there were 10 diagnostically matched pairs in favor, 0 against, 27 ties, (p = .001).

47. This number could be zero, as in a situation where the patient denied the presence of *any* difficulty, but others around him disagreed and so made the appointment for him or "forced" him to see a doctor.

48. Qualities of physical difficulty were categorized under nine headings.

49. The distributions for these two tables closely resemble those of Table 25.5 (p = .018 for bodily locations; p = .003 for types of bodily dysfunctions).

*Table 25.5.   Distribution of Irish and Italian clinic
admissions by number of presenting complaints**

Number of Presenting Complaints	Italian	Irish
Zero	0	3
One	5	21
Two	15	22
Three	14	16
Four	10	7
Five	9	7
Six or more	10	5
Total	63	81

Note: $p < .001$.
*The Mann-Whitney U-test was used. Probabilities were computed for one-tailed tests. They are, however, slightly "conservative"; with a correction for ties, the probabilities or levels of significance would have been even lower. See Siegel, *op. cit.*, pp. 116-127.

bothered you most about your symptoms?[50] An admission-of-irritability scale was created by classifying an affirmative response to any of the three questions as an admission that the symptoms affected extraphysical performance. As seen in Table 25.6, the Irish were more likely than the Italians to state that their disorders had not affected them in this manner. Here again the asides by the Irish suggested that their larger number of negative responses reflected considerable denial rather than a straightforward appraisal of their situation.

To examine these conclusions in a more rigorous manner, we turned to our subsample of matched diagnostic pairs. In general, the pattern and direction of the hypotheses were upheld.[51] Thus, even for the same diagnosis, the Italians expressed and complained of more symptoms, more bodily areas affected, and more kinds of dysfunctions, than did the

*Table 25.6.   Distribution of Irish and Italian clinic admissions by
responses to three questions concerning admission of irritability
and effect of symptoms on interpersonal behavior*

Response Pattern	Italian	Irish
No on all three questions	22	47
Yes on at least one question	41	34
Total	63	81

Note: $X^2 = 7.62$, $p < .01$.

Irish, and more often felt that their symptoms affected their interpersonal behavior.

50. For the latter question, the patient was presented with a card on which were listed eight aspects of illness and/or symptoms which might bother him. One of these statements was, "That it made you irritable and difficult to get along with."

51. For the prediction that the Italians would have more symptoms in all instances

The following composite offers a final illustration of how differently these patients reacted to and perceived their illnesses. Each set of responses was

Diagnosis	Question	Irish Patient	Italian Patient
1. Presbyopia and hyperopia	What seems to be the trouble?	I can't see to thread a needle or read a paper.	I have a constant headache and my eyes seem to get red and burny.
	Anything else?	No, I can't recall any.	No, just that it lasts all day long and I even wake up with it sometimes.
2. Myopia	What seems to be the trouble?	I can't see across the street.	My eyes seem very burny, especially the right eye ...Two or three months ago I woke up with my eyes swollen. I bathed it and it did go away but there was still the burny sensation.
	Anything else?	I had been experiencing headaches, but it may be that I'm in early menopause.	Yes there always seems to be a red spot beneath this eye. . . .
	Anything else?	No.	Well, my eyes feel very heavy...at night they bother me most.
3. Otitis externa A.D.	Is there any pain?	There's a congestion...but it's a pressure, not really a pain.	Yes....If I rub it, it disappears....I had a pain from my shoulder up to my to my neck and though it .might be a cold.
4. Pharyngitis	Is there any pain?	No, maybe a slight headache but nothing that lasts.	Yes, I have had a headache a few days. Oh, yes, every time I swallow it's annoying.
5. Presbyopia and hyperopia	Do you think the symptoms affected how you got along with your family? your friends?	No, I have had loads of trouble. I can't imagine this bothering me.	Yes, when I have a headache, I'm very irritable, very tense, very short-tempered.
6. Deafness, hearing loss	Did you become more irritable?	No, not me...maybe everybody else but not me.	Oh, yes...the least little thing aggravates me... and I take it out on the children.

there were for total number, 24 matched diagnostic pairs in favor of hypothesis, 7 against, 6 ties (p=.005); for number of different locations, 16 in favor, 5 against, 16 ties (p=.013); for number of different qualities of physical difficulties, 22 in favor, 9 against, 6 ties, (p=.025). For the prediction that Italians would admit irritability and Irish would deny it, there were 17 in favor, 6 against, 14 ties (p=.017).

given by an Italian and an Irish patient of similar age and sex with a disorder of approximately the same duration and with the same primary and secondary diagnosis (if there was one). In the first two cases, the Irish patient focused on a specific malfunctioning as the main concern while the Italian did not even mention this aspect of the problem but went on to mention more diffuse qualities of his condition. The last four responses contrast the Italian and Irish response to questions of pain and interpersonal relations.

Sociocultural Communication

What has so far been demonstrated is the systematic variability with which bodily conditions may be perceived and communicated. Until now the empirical findings have been presented without interpretation. Most of the data are quite consistent with those reported by other observers.[52] Although no data were collected in our investigation on the specific mechanics of the interplay between being a member of a specific subculture and the communication of "symptoms," some speculation on this seems warranted.

In theorizing about the interplay of culture and symptoms particular emphasis was given to the "fit" of certain bodily states with dominant value orientations. The empirical examples for the latter were drawn primarily from data on social roles. Of course, values are evident on even more general levels, such as formal and informal societal sanctions and the culture's orientation to life's basic problems. With an orientation to problems usually goes a preferred solution or way of handling them.[53] Thus a society's values may also be reflected in such preferred solutions. One behavioral manifestation of this is defense mechanisms—a part of the everyday way

52. The whole specific-diffuse pattern and the generalizing-withholding illness behavior dovetails neatly with the empirical findings of Opler and Singer, *op. cit.*, Fantl and Schiro, *op. cit.*, and Paul Barrabee and Otto von Mering, "Ethnic Variations in Mental Stress in Families with Psychotic Children," *Social Problems*, 1 (October, 1953), 48-53. The specific emphasis on expressiveness has been detailed especially by Zborowski, *op. cit.*, and the several studies of Italian mental patients done by Anne Parsons, "Some Comparative Observations on Ward Social Structure: Southern Italy, England, and the United States," *Tipografia dell'Ospedale Psichiatrico*, Napoli, April, 1959; "Family Dynamics in Southern Italian Schizophrenics," *Archives of General Psychiatry*, 3 (November, 1960), 507-518; "Patriarchal and Matriarchal Authority in the Neapolitan Slum, *Psychiatry*, 24 (May, 1961), 109-121. The contrast on number of symptoms has been noted by Croog, *op. cit.*, and Graham, *op. cit.*

53. Florence R. Kluckhohn, "Dominant and Variant Value Orientations," in *Personality in Nature, Society, and Culture*, 2nd ed., Clyde Kluckhohn, Henry A. Murray, and David M. Schneider, eds. (New York: Knopf, 1956), pp. 342-357; Florence R. Kluckhohn and Fred L. Strodtbeck, *Variations in Value Orientations* (Evanston, Ill.: Row Peterson, 1961); John Spiegel, "Some Cultural Aspects of Transference and Counter-Transference," in *Individual and Family Dynamics*, Jules H. Hasserman, ed. (New York: Grune & Stratton, 1959), pp. 160-182; John P. Spiegel, "Conflicting Formal and Informal Roles in Newly Acculturated Families," in *Disorders of Communication*, 42 (Research Publications, Association for Research in Nervous and Mental Disease, 1964), pp. 307-316; John P. Spiegel and Florence R. Kluckhohn, "The

individuals have of dealing with their everyday stresses and strains.[54] We contend that illness and its treatment (from taking medicine to seeing a physician) is one of these everyday stresses and strains, an anxiety-laden situation which calls forth coping or defense mechanisms.[55] From this general reasoning, we would thus speculate that Italian and Irish ways of communicating illness may reflect major values and preferred ways of handling problems within the culture itself.[56]

For the Italians, the large number of symptoms and the spread of the complaints, not only throughout the body but into other aspects of life, may be understood in terms of their expressiveness and expansiveness so often seen in sociological, historical, and fictional writing.[57] Yet their illness behavior seems to reflect something more than lack of inhibition, and valuation of spontaneity. There is something more than real in their behavior, a "well-seasoned, dramatic emphasis to their lives." In fact, clinicians have noted that this openness is deceptive. It only goes so far and then. . . .Thus this Italian overstatement of "symptoms" is not merely an expressive quality but perhaps a more general mechanism, their special way of handling problems—a defense mechanism we call dramatization. Dynamically, dramatization seems to cope with anxiety by repeatedly overexpressing it and thereby dissipating it. Anne Parsons delineates this process in a case study of a schizophrenic woman. Through a process of repetition and exaggeration she was able to isolate and defend herself from the destructive consequences of her own psychotic breakdown. Thus Anne Parsons concludes:

> rather than appearing as evidence for the greater acceptance of id impulses the greater dramatic expression of Southern Italian culture might be given a particular place among the ego mechanisms, different from but in this respect fulfilling the same function as the emphasis on rational mastery of the objective or subjective world which characterizes our own culture (U.S.A.).[58]

Influence of the Family and Cultural Values on the Mental Health and Illness of the Individual," unpublished Progress Report of Grant M-971, U. S. Public Health Service.

54. Anna Freud, *The Ego and the Mechanisms of Defense* (London: Hogarth, 1954).

55. That illness is almost an everyday problem is shown by the data in our opening section on the prevalence of illness. That illness and its concomitants are anxiety-laden is suggested by the findings of many studies on patient delay. Barbara Blackwell, "The Literature of Delay in Seeking Medical Care for Chronic Illnesses," *Health Education Monographs,* 16 (1963), 3-32; Bernard Kutner, Henry B. Malcover, and Abraham Oppenheim, "Delay in the Diagnosis and Treatment of Cancer," *Journal of Chronic Diseases,* 7 (January, 1958), 95-120; *Journal of Health and Human Behavior,* 2 (Fall, 1961), 171-178.

56. Speculation as to why the Italians and the Irish, with similar problems of hardship and poverty, should develop dissimilar ways of handling such problems is beyond the scope of this paper.

57. In addition to the references cited in footnotes 52 and 53, we have drawn our picture from many sociological, literary, and historical works. A complete bibliography is available on request. For the compilation and annotation of many of these references I am particularly indebted to Mrs. Marlene Hindley.

58. Anne Parsons, *Psychiatry, op. cit.,* p. 26.

While other social historians have noted the Italian flair for show and spectacle, Barzini has most explicitly related this phenomenon to the covering up of omnipresent tragedy and poverty, a way of making their daily lives bearable, the satisfactory *ersatz* for the many things they lack.

> The most easily identifiable reasons why the Italians love their own show.
> . . .First of all they do it to tame and prettify savage nature, to make life
> bearable, dignified, significant, and pleasant for others, and themselves. They
> do it then for their own private ends; a good show makes a man *simpatico*
> to powerful people, helps him get on in the world and obtain what he wants,
> solves many problems, lubricates the wheels of society, protects him from the
> envy of his enemies and the arrogance of the mighty—they do it to avenge
> themselves on unjust fate.[59]

Through many works on the Southern Italian there seems to run a thread—a valued and preferred way of handling problems shown in the tendency toward dramatization. The experience of illness provides but another stage.

But if the Italian view of life is expressed through its fiestas, for the Irish it is expressed through its fasts.[60] Their life has been depicted as one of long periods of plodding routine followed by episodes of wild adventure, of lengthy postponement of gratification of sex and marriage, interspersed with brief immediate satisfactions like fighting and carousing. Perhaps in recognition of the expected and limited nature of such outbursts that the most common Irish outlet, alcoholism, is often referred to as "a good man's weakness." Life was black and long-suffering, and the less said the better.[61]

It is the last statement which best reflects the Irish handling of illness. While in other contexts the ignoring of bodily complaints is merely descriptive of what is going on, in Irish culture it seems to be the culturally prescribed and supported defense mechanism—singularly most appropriate for their psychological and physical survival.[62] When speaking of the

59. Luigi Barzini, *The Italians* (New York: Bantam, 1965), p. 104.
60. In addition to the papers in footnote 52, Arensberg and Kimball, *op. cit.*, remains the classic reference work.
61. The ubiquitous comic spirit, humor, and wit for which the Irish are famous can be regarded in part as a functional equivalent of the dramatization by Italians. It is a cover, a way of isolating life's hardships, and at the same time a preventive of deeper examination and probing. Also, while their daily life was endowed with great restrictions, their fantasy life was replete with great richness (tales of the "wee folk").
62. Spiegel and Kluckhohn, *op. cit.*, state that the Irishman's major avenue of relief from his oppressive sense of guilt lies in his almost unlimited capacity for denial. This capacity they claim is fostered by the perception in the rural Irish of a harmonic blending between man and nature. Such harmonizing of man and nature is further interpreted as blurring the elements of causality, thus allowing for continually shifting the responsibility for events from one person to another, and even from a person to animistically conceived forces. Thus denial becomes not only a preferred avenue of relief but also one supported and perhaps elicited by their perception of their environment.

discomfort caused by her illness, one stated, "I ignore it like I do most things." In terms of presenting complaints this understatement and restraint was even more evident. It could thus be seen in their seeming reluctance to admit they have any symptoms at all, in their limiting their symptoms to the specific location in which they arose, and finally in their contention that their physical problems affected nothing of their life but the most minute physical functioning. The consistency of the Irish illness behavior with their general view of life is shown in two other contexts. First it helped perpetuate a self-fulfilling prophecy. Thus their way of communicating complaints, while doing little to make treatment easy, did assure some degree of continual suffering and thus further proof that life is painful and hard (that is, "full of fasts").[63] Secondly, their illness behavior can be linked to the sin and guilt ideology which seems to pervade so much of Irish society. For, in a culture where restraint is the *modus operandi*, temptation is ever-present and must be guarded against. Since the flesh is weak, there is a concomitant expectation that sin is likely. Thus, when unexpected or unpleasant events take place, there is a search for what they did or must have done wrong. Perhaps their three most favored locations of symptoms (the eyes, ears, and throat) might be understood as symbolic reflections of the more immediate source of their sin and guilt—what they should not have seen; what they should not have heard; and what they should not have said.

In these few paragraphs, we have tried to provide a theoretical link between membership in a cultural group and the communication of bodily complaints. The illness behavior of the Irish and the Italians has been explained in terms of two of the more generally prescribed defense mechanisms of their respective cultures—with the Irish handling their troubles by denial and the Italians theirs by dramatization.[64]

Qualifications and Implications

The very fact that we speak of trends and statistical significance indicates the tentativeness of this study. In particular, the nature of sample selection affected the analysis of certain demographic variables since the lack of significant differences in some cases may be due to the small range available for comparison. Thus, there were no Italians beyond the third generation and few in the total sample who had gone to college. When comparisons were made within this small range (for example, only within the second

63. Their "fantasying" and their "fasting" might be reflected in the serious illness they claim to have had in the past, and the dire consequences they forecast for their future. We do not know for a fact that the Irish *had* more serious illnesses than the Italians, but merely that they claimed to. The Italians might well have had similar conditions but did not necessarily consider them serious.
64. The Anglo-Saxons complete the circle with an emphasis on neutralizing their anxiety.

generation or only within the high school group) there were, with but one exception, no significant differences from previously reported findings.[65] Despite the limitations cited, it can be stated with some confidence that, of the variables capable of analysis, sociocultural ones were the most significant. When a correlational analysis (and within this, a cluster analysis) was performed on all the codable and quantifiable material (including the demographic data, the health behaviors, and attitude scales) the variable which consistently correlated most highly with the "illness behaviors" reported in this study was ethnic group membership.

There is one final remark about our sample selection which has ramifications, not for our data analysis, but rather for our interpretation. We are dealing here with a population who had decided to seek or were referred for medical aid at three clinics. Thus we can make no claim that in a random selection of Irish, they will be suffering primarily from eye, ear, nose, and throat disorders or even locate their chief symptoms there. What we are claiming is that there are significant differences in the way people present and react to their complaints, *not* that the specific complaints and mechanisms we have cited are necessarily the most common ones. (We would, of course, be surprised if the pattern reported here did not constitute one of the major ones.) Another difficulty in dealing with this population is the duration of the patients' disorders. Since the majority of these patients have had their conditions for some time, one may wonder if similar differences in perception would exist for more acute episodes, or whether the very length of time which the people have borne their problems has allowed for coloration by sociocultural factors. As a result of this we can only raise the issues as to whether the differences reported here between members of a cultural group exist only at a particular stage of their illness, or reflect more underlying and enduring cultural concerns and values.[66]

While there has long been recognition of the subjectivity and variability of a patient's reporting of his symptoms, there has been little attention to the fact that this reporting may be influenced by systematic social factors

65. The previously reported ethnic differences with respect to presenting complaints did begin to blur. The Italian and the Irish males tended to "move" toward the "middle position" of the Anglo-Saxon Protestant group. In many of the major comparisons of this study, the Anglo-Saxon group occupied a position midway between the responses of the two other ethnic groups, though generally closer to the Irish. For example, when asked about the presence of pain some 70 percent of the Irish males denied it, as compared to almost 60 percent of the Anglo-Saxon males, and 40 percent of the Italian males.

66. Such a problem was explicitly stated and investigated by Ellen Silver, "The Influence of Culture on Personality: A Comparison of the Irish and Italians with Emphasis on Fantasy Behavior," mimeographed, Harvard University, 1958, in her attempted replication of the Opler and Singer work, *op. cit.*, and was emphasized by the somewhat ambiguous findings of Rena S. Grossman, "Ethnic Differences in the Apperception of Pain," unpublished undergraduate honors thesis, Department of Social Relations, Radcliffe College, 1964, in her replication of Zborowski's findings, *op. cit.*, on a nonhospitalized population.

like ethnicity. Awareness of the influence of this and similar factors can be of considerable aid in the practical problems of diagnosis and treatment of many diseases, particularly where the diagnosis is dependent to a large extent on what the patient is able and willing, or thinks important enough, to tell the doctor.[67] The physician who is unaware of how the patient's background may lead him to respond in certain ways, may, by not probing sufficiently, miss important diagnostic cues, or respond inappropriately to others.[68]

The documentation of sociocultural differences in the perception of and concern with certain types of "symptoms" has further implications for work in preventive medicine and public health. It has been found in mental health research that there is an enormous gulf between lay and professional opinion as to when mental illness is present, as well as when and what kind of help is needed.[69] If our theorizing is correct, such differences reflect not merely something inadequately learned (that is, wrong medical knowledge) but also a solidly embedded value system.[70] Such different frames

67. Several examples are more fully delineated in Irving Kenneth Zola, "Illness Behavior of the Working Class: Implications and Recommendations," in Arthur B. Shostak and William Gomberg, eds. *Blue Collar World* (Englewood Cliffs, N.J.: Prentice-Hall, 1964), pp. 350-361.

68. This may be done to such an extreme that it is the physician's response which creates epidemiological differences. Such a potential situation was noted using data from the present study and is detailed in Irving Kenneth Zola, "Problems of Communications, Diagnosis, and Patient Care: The Interplay of Patient, Physician, and Clinic Organization," *Journal of Medical Education,* 38 (October, 1963), 829-838.

69. The explanations for such differences have, however, more often emphasized negative aspects of the respondents' background—their lower education, lower socioeconomic status, lesser psychological sophistication, and greater resistance and antipathy—by virtue of their membership in certain racial and cultural minorities. See Bernard Bergen, "Social Class, Symptoms, and Sensitivity to Descriptions of Mental Illness—Implications for Programs of Preventive Psychiatry," unpublished doctoral dissertation, Harvard University, 1962; Elaine Cumming and John Cumming, *Closed Ranks: An Experiment in Mental Health Education* (Cambridge: Harvard University Press, 1957); Howard E. Freeman and Gene G. Kassebaum, "Relationship of Education and Knowledge to Opinions about Mental Illness," *Mental Hygiene,* 44 (January, 1960), 43-47; Gerald Gurin, Joseph Veroff, and Sheila Feld, *Americans View Their Mental Health* (New York: Basic Books, 1960); Jum C. Nunnally, *Popular Conceptions of Mental Health* (New York: Holt, Rinehart & Winston, 1961); Glenn V. Ramsey and Melita Seipp, "Attitudes and Opinions Concerning Mental Illness," *Psychiatric Quarterly,* 22 (July, 1949), 1-17; Elmo Roper and Associates, *People's Attitudes Concerning Mental Health* (New York: Private Publication, 1950); Shirley Star, "The Public's Ideas about Mental Illness," paper presented to the Annual Meeting of the National Association for Mental Health, Indianapolis, 1955; Shirley Star, "The Place of Psychiatry in Popular Thinking," paper presented at the annual meeting of the American Association for Public Opinion Research, Washington, D.C., 1957; Julian L. Woodward, "Changing Ideas on Mental Illness and Its Treatment," *American Sociological Review,* 16 (August, 1951), 443-454.

70. This approach is evident in such works as Stanley King, *op. cit.;* Clyde Kluckhohn "Culture and Behavior," in Gardner Lindzey, *Handbook of Social Psychology,* Vol. 2 (Cambridge: Addison-Wesley, 1954), pp. 921-976; Walter B. Miller, "Lower Class Culture as a Generating Milieu of Gang Delinquency," *Journal of Social Issues,* 14 (July, 1958), 5-19; Marvin K. Opler, *Culture, Psychiatry, and Human Values*

of reference would certainly shed light on the failure of many symptom-based health campaigns. Often these campaigns seem based on the assumption that a symptom or sign is fairly objective and recognizable and that it evokes similar levels of awareness and reaction. Our study adds to the mounting evidence which contradicts this position by indicating, for example, the systematic variability in response to even the most minor aches and pains.

The discerning of reactions to minor problems harks back to a point mentioned in the early pages of this report. For, while sociologists, anthropologists, and mental health workers have usually considered sociocultural factors to be etiological factors in the creation of specfic problems, the interpretative emphasis in this study has been on how sociocultural background may lead to different definitions and responses to essentially the same experience. The strongest evidence in support of this argument is the different ethnic perceptions for essentially the same disease. While it is obvious that not all people react similarly to the same disease process, it is striking that the pattern of response can vary with the ethnic background of the patient. There is little known physiological difference between ethnic groups which would account for the differing reactions. In fact, the comparison of the matched diagnostic groups led us to believe that, should diagnosis be more precisely controlled, the differences would be even more striking.

The present report has attempted to demonstrate the fruitfulness of an approach which does not take the definition of abnormality for granted. Despite its limitations, our data seem sufficiently striking to provide further reason for reexamining our traditional and often rigid conceptions of health and illness, of normality and abnormality, of conformity and deviance. Symptoms, or physical aberrations, are so wide-spread that perhaps relatively few, and a biased selection at best, come to the attention of official treatment agencies like doctors, hospitals, and public health agencies. There may even be a sense in which they are part and parcel of the human condition. We have thus tried to present evidence showing that the very labeling and definition of a bodily state as a symptom or as a problem is, in itself, part of a social process. If there is a selection

(Springfield, Ill.: Charles C Thomas, 1956); Marvin K. Opler, *Culture and Mental Health* (New York: Macmillan, 1959); Benjamin D. Paul, *Health, Culture, and Community—Case Studies of Public Reactions to Health Programs* (New York: Russell Sage Foundation, 1955); Henry J. Wegroski, "A Critique of Cultural and Statistical Concepts of Abnormality," in Clyde Kluckhohn, Henry A. Murray, and David M. Schneider, *Personality in Nature, Society, and Culture*, rev. ed. (New York: Knopf, 1956), pp. 691-701.

and definitional process, then focusing solely on reasons for deviation (the study of etiology) and ignoring what constitutes a deviation in the eyes of the individual and his society may obscure important aspects of our understanding and eventually our philosophies of treatment and control of illness.[71]

71. This is spelled out from various points of view in such works as Samuel Butler, *Erewhon* (New York: Signet, 1961); Rene Dubos, *op. cit.,* Josephine D. Lohman (participant), "Juvenile Delinquency: Its Dimensions, Its Conditions, Techniques of Control, Proposals for Action," Subcommittee on Juvenile Delinquency of the Senate Committee on Labor and Public Welfare, 86th Congress, S. 765, S. 1090, S. 1314, Spring, 1959, p. 268; Talcott Parsons, "Social Change and Medical Organization in the United States: A Sociological Perspective," *Annals of the American Academy of Political and Social Science,* 346 (March, 1963), 21-34; Edwin M. Schur, *Crimes Without Victims—Deviant Behavior and Public Policy* (Englewood Cliffs, N.J.: Prentice-Hall, 1965); Thomas Szasz, *The Myth of Mental Illness* (New York: Hoeber-Harper, 1961); Thomas Szasz, *Law, Liberty, and Psychiatry* (New York: Macmillan, 1963); Irving Kenneth Zola, "Problems for Research—Some Effects of Assumptions Underlying Socio-Medical Investigations," in Gerald Gordon, ed., *Proceedings, Conference on Medical Sociology and Disease Control* (National Tuberculosis Association, 1966), pp. 9-17.

26

JUDITH LORBER

Deviance as Performance:
The Case of Illness

The labeling theory of deviance, proposed originally by Lemert in *Social Pathology*, and developed by him and a growing number of sociologists,[1] has shifted attention away from the individual attributes of the deviant and focused attention on societal reaction to those attributes. In this theory, deviance is seen not as a psychological or physical flaw, but as the outcome of a social process which involves conflicting values of social groups, a social language of labels, social reactions and expectations.

The emphasis on how and why and with what consequences certain groups come to label certain behaviors as wrong, abnormal, to be punished, treated, or controlled, has been an antidote to the clinical interpretation of deviance. The latter concentrates on the characteristics of the *deviant*. The labeling approach concentrates instead on the characteristics of the *controllers*—the formal and informal agents of social control who

Reprinted from *Social Problems*, 14, No. 3 (1967), pp. 302-310, by permission of the author and The Society for the Study of Social Problems.

This paper is a revision of my Master's thesis written under N.I.M.H. Grant No. 5 TI-MH-8126-02. I am indebted to Professor Eliot Freidson for his encouragement and criticism throughout the various stages of its preparation, and to my fellow members of the N.I.M.H. Training Program for their perceptive and helpful comments on an earlier version.

1. Edwin M. Lemert, *Social Pathology* (New York: McGraw-Hill, 1951); Edwin M. Lemert, "Social Structure, Social Control, and Deviation," in Marshall B. Clinard, ed. *Anomie and Deviant Behavior* (New York: The Free Press, 1964, pp. 57-97; Howard S. Becker, *Outsiders: Studies in the Sociology of Deviance* (New York: The Free Press, 1963); Howard S. Becker, ed., *The Other Side: Perspectives on Deviance* (New York: The Free Press, 1964); Edwin M. Schur, *Crimes without Victims: Deviant Behavior and Public Policy* (Englewood Cliffs, N.J.: Prentice-Hall, 1965); Jane R. Mercer, "Social System Perspective and Clinical Perspective: Frames of Reference for Understanding Career Patterns of Persons Labelled as Mentally Retarded," in this volume; Eliot Freidson, "Disability as Social Deviance," in this volume; Thomas J. Scheff, *Being Mentally Ill: A Sociological Theory* (Chicago, Ill.: Aldine, 1966).

ferret out, define, and do something about a certain kind of activity. The labeling approach tends to ignore the motives or intentions of the deviant.

This theoretical bias of the labeling approach has helped form a more purely sociological analysis of deviance and social control. Neglect of the deviant, however, while possibly justified operationally, creates large gaps in the study of deviance. Using as data the social labels only and omitting the activity, intentions, or self-view of the individual deviant make it impossible to distinguish between the falsely accused and the true deviant, and between the truly innocent and the hidden deviant. The argument of the situational theorists would be that the distinction is immaterial, that only the social label matters, not what the individual thinks or does—the mental patient in on a bum rap undergoes the same institutionalization as the genuine schizophrenic;[2] the hidden homosexual is not a social problem.[3] Only that behavior which *others* label as deviance is salient.

If the labeling theory is strictly applied, secret deviance must be excluded. As it is hidden, it is unlabeled, and as it is unlabeled, it is socially nonexistent. Nevertheless, Becker's analysis of marijuana users in *Outsiders* discusses secret deviance,[4] and other proponents of the labeling theory would no doubt regret the arbitrary omission of this category of deviance from sociological research.

The problem of combining the notion of secret deviance with the concept of deviance as something created by labeling can be solved by introducing the deviant into the social process of labeling. Hidden deviance implies that even though his social group assumes his innocence, the deviant either sees himself as doing wrong according to his own reference group, or, condoning his own behavior, he realizes that others will condemn his actions according to their standards. In either case, to avoid the consequences he feels will occur if his deviance comes out into the open (is socially labeled), he pretends to be conforming to the standards of the group in a position to condemn him for what he is doing secretly. In short, in response to his self-label of his behavior as apt to incur sanctioning, he acts in such a way as to achieve a social label of conformity. Like any other social actor who attempts to influence the response of others to him, *he puts on a performance.*[5]

Ironically, while an aware rule-breaker may be able to carry off a convincing impression of morality and so hide his deviance, someone who believes he is doing right but is unaware of possible public response may find himself accused of deviance. On the other hand, even the conformist may have to put on a deliberate show of sameness to achieve the label of

2. Erving Goffman, *Asylums* (Garden City, N.Y.: Anchor Books, 1961), pp. 127-169.
3. Schur, *op. cit.*, p. 107.
4. Becker, *Outsiders, op. cit.*, pp. 66-72.
5. See Erving Goffman, *The Presentation of Self in Everyday Life* (Garden City, N.Y.: Anchor Books, 1959), pp. 3-4.

social approval, and a conscious performance of rule-breaking may, in extraordinary circumstances, be required to socially validate immoral behavior. Of course, performances fail, and so a social label of deviant may be the price of an unsuccessful performance of conformity by either the conformist or the secret deviant.

As performances, deviance and conformity involve a presentation of self no different in arts and techniques from the everyday performances described by Goffman.[6] However, where Goffman's performers are by and large members of teams who must manage the definition of the situation so the action is not interrupted, the moral performer frequently works alone to achieve the application of a certain label—deviant or conformist.[7]

What's in a Label?

So far we have been talking too simply of the labels of conformity and deviance. As a social label, *conformity* can be applied to socially approved behavior, to deviance that is socially unimportant, and to secret deviance. In the case of conformity, the consequences of the social label are the same; it is the nature of the *self*-label that determines the kind of performance the individual may have to put on to achieve moral certification.

Deviance as a social label, however, has different consequences depending on the type of deviance implied by the label. One kind of social label of deviance imputes maliciousness or willfulness to the deviance, and carries consequences of punishment. A second kind defines the deviance as accidental, implying acquisition without the individual's wanting to be deviant. Some familiar kinds of deviance socially defined as accidental are illness, foreignness, crippling, or inherited defects.[8]

Deviance that is socially defied as accidental is usually treated more kindly than deviance that is socially defined as deliberate. In our society, mercy and mitigation of punishment are traditional for those who are considered to have fallen into sin or disgrace through no fault of their own. Today, we are more likely to give therapy to those who are defined as ill (accidental deviance) and punish those who are defined as criminal (deliberate deviance).[9] If he cannot achieve a level of conformity, it is to the deviant's advantage to have his behavior socially defined as accidental rather than de-

---

6. *Ibid.*, *passim*.

7. Actually, Goffman notes that most of us spend our lives merchandising our morality. Thus, he says, "the very obligation and profitability of appearing always in a steady moral light, of being a socialized character, forces one to be the sort of person who is practiced in the ways of the stage." *Ibid.*, p. 251.

8. Freidson, *op. cit.*, pp.338-339.

9. Cf. Vilhelm Aubert and Sheldon L. Messinger, "The Criminal and the Sick," in this volume. Thus, as Schur suggests, if abortion, homosexuality, and drug addiction are to be considered medical problems, they must be transformed into illnesses—the addict must be considered compulsively driven, the pregnant woman physically or

liberate. If his *self*-label is that his deviance is not his fault, he must convince his audience to believe him; if his self-label is that he acted deliberately, he still may attempt to show that he deserves merciful treatment by pretending he is not responsible for his behavior.

We might now present a typology which would chart these different kinds of conformity and deviance labels:

Table 26.1.   A typology of deviance

| Social Label | Self-Label | | |
	conformity	accidental deviance	deliberate deviance
conformity	Reasonable adherence to norms	Acceptable differences	Undetected violation of rules, norms, laws
accidental deviance	Culture and role conflicts	Illnesses, inherited defects, crippling	Crimes of passion, hunger, rage
deliberate deviance	Deliberate violation of laws or rules for political or religious reasons	"Nuremberg pleas" ("Could happen to anyone")[10]	"Professional" deviance

These abstract categories are entirely dependent for their content on the specific norms and values of the labelers and labeled. The definitions of conformity and deviance, and of accident and deliberateness, as well as the consequences of the labels, cannot be separated from time, place, and social situation. For this reason, performances to achieve any of the labels will vary as the categories of perception and evaluation vary.[11]

Two recent studies indicate how, in particular types of deviance, impressions may be varied to achieve different labels. In his study of suicide, Jack Douglas discusses the attempts of suicides to remove responsibility for their deed from themselves by placing the blame on what "drove them to it"—

mentally incapable of surviving childbirth, and the homosexual a victim of early childhood conditioning. *op. cit.*, pp. 178-179.

10. Essentially, a *rejected* plea in which the person being judged claims he was only following orders, didn't really know what he was doing, or was no different from anyone else in the same situation.

11. The typology can conceivably be used to analyze virtue as well as vice. Thus, a helping hand might be accidental virtue unremarked socially, and anonymous philanthropy would be secret virtue. Revolts against oppression, good samaritanism, and heorism under fire might fill in the second row across. In the third row, we might have martyrdom, denied saintliness (for example, Joan of Arc's plight after capture by the British), and missionary work.

loss of job, family trouble, illness, rejecting lover, and so on.[12] In our terms, the suicide is trying to create the impression that the deviance was not a willful act, but forced on him.

A study of county lunacy commission hearings gives another example of impression management to achieve a label with desired consequences.[13] The authors note that

> those persons who were able to approach the judge in a controlled manner, use proper eye contact, sentence structure, posture, etc., and who presented their stories without excessive emotional response or blandness and with proper demeanor, were able to obtain the decision they wanted—whether it was release or commitment—despite any "psychiatric symptomatology."[14]

The study also gives examples of failed performances. Some self-defined patients were not committed to the mental hospital because they could not hide their eagerness to be committed; that is, they were defined as chronic alcoholics and malingerers (deliberate deviants) who did not deserve the treatment reserved for the "truly" ill (accidental deviants).

Illness as a Performance of Innocence

Illness is commonly considered a type of accidental deviance—it is not felt that the individual deliberately or willfully chose to become ill. However, as Aubert and Messinger note, "any situation in which an individual stands to gain from withdrawal is such as to render suspect his claim to illness."[15] Absences from school and work, and going on sick call in the army, are cases in point. Aubert and Messinger also state:

> The reverse situation may be seen to obtain as well—that is, it is easier to be categorized as ill when the situation points to significant deprivation following validation of a claim to illness.[16]

Szasz suggests that the juxtaposition of motives and symptoms forms a continuum of types of imputation within the category of illness. If a person has no motive to be ill and has symptoms, he is clearly ill. If he has a motive and symptoms, his condition may be psychosomatic or hysterical. If he has a motive and questionable symptoms, he is open to the charge of malingering.[17]

12. Jack D. Douglas, "The Sociological Analysis of Social Meanings of Suicide," *Archives Européenes de Sociologie*, 1966.

13. Dorothy Miller and Michael Schwartz, "County Lunacy Commission Hearings: Some Observations of Commitments to a State Mental Hospital," *Social Problems*, 14 (Summer, 1966), 26-35.

14. *Ibid.*, p. 34.

15. Aubert and Messinger, *op. cit.*, p. 239

16. *Ibid.*, p. 294.

17. Thomas S. Szasz, "Malingering: 'Diagnosis' or Social Condemnation?" in this volume.

Table 26.2. *A typology of illness*

Social Label	Self-Label		
	conformity	*accidental deviance*	*deliberate deviance*
conformity	Health	Minor Illness	Concealed illness
accidental deviance	Illness discovered by doctor	Treated illness	Conversion hysteria
deliberate deviance	Refusal of treatment	"Parlayed" compensation case	Malingering

As a form of deviance in itself, illness may be fitted into the abstract typology presented above. The self-labeler is the patient; the social labelers are the medical profession.[18] Of course, as will be seen from the following discussion, this typology is still too abstract, as doctors vary in their categorization of different symptoms, and patients also have greatly varied views of illness. However, a discussion of impression management in illness, based on the typology given, may illustrate the usefulness of the performance concept in the analysis of deviance.

In the first column, the actor feels that he is healthy—that his physical state is "normal." Presumably, unless he has some peculiar physical quirks which he knows do not affect his capacities, but which the physician has to check out for himself, there is no real need for a performance to convince a physician that he is healthy as long as his physical aspects fall into the medical boundaries of normality.[19] If an individual does have a medical abnormality that the doctor discovers, he is, despite his self-label of health, categorized as ill, or accidentally deviant. If he accepts the diagnosis and consents to treatment, he moves into the middle cell, treated illness. If he does not accept the doctor's label, insists that he is healthy, and refuses treatment, he may be categorized as a deliberate deviant by the doctor. He is now considered responsible for his deviance (or at least for permitting himself to get worse). Those who are diagnosed as ill have, in a sense, "failed" in their performances of health.

In the second column, the label desired by the deviant is one of "true" illness, that is accidental deviance. Of course, he must in the first place define

18. Somewhat different categories would have to be inserted into the typology were the social labelers other laymen. For example, venereal disease might be considered deliberate deviance. The question of stigmatization, which arises when the audience is primarily composed of laymen, is discussed by Freidson, *op. cit.*, pp. 337-338.

19. In checking out a physical peculiarity, the physician may "create" a *non*-illness, verifying that an individual does *not* have such-and-so, which in itself is a defined state. See Clifton K. Meador, "The Art and Science of Nondisease," in this volume.

his symptoms as adding up to illness to give *himself* the label. For instance, a study of office workers with colds found that some employees would stay home from work only if they had severe colds with fever—conditions they defined as true illness.[20] Unless their colds were severe, they did not feel they had a warrant to stay home from work. In this instance, the self-label alone operated, for these employees did not feel they had to convince others that they were ill in order to get permission to stay out of work. In other instances, the person who feels he is ill through no fault of his own must manage to convince others that he neglects his obligations only because he is incapacitated, not because he wants to get out of his duties. In such cases, in order to get clear title to the label of illness, he may need the validation of a physician, which puts him into the category of treated illness.[21]

The compensation case in which the physical state is milked for financial gain is an illustration of a performance designed to achieve a label of accidental deviance which may ultimately be refused. Interestingly enough, there is even some evidence that the industrial accident which led to the compensation itself may have been engineered.

Hirschfeld and Behan, in their review of about 300 cases of industrial accidents and injuries, found a prevalent pattern of feuding with management, almost deliberate infraction of previously followed safety rules, and an increased frequency of sick calls in the period just before the accident.[22] As psychiatrists, these authors explain the accident as an unconscious solution to an otherwise insoluble psychological conflict in the worker's life, such as inability to handle heavy physical work because of advanced age. An accident, however, might just as validly be seen as the "planned" solution to a socially imposed problem, for there is no more legitimate escape from the obligations of work in our society for a man of technical working age than through physical disability. When legal compensation for disability enters the picture, the managed aspects of accidents are thrown even more clearly into focus. Hirschfeld and Behan themselves note:

> it is our conclusion that, in most cases in which legal problems contribute to chronicity, the patient's reaction is not unconscious. These people are usually aware of what they are doing. . . . It is difficult to listen to descriptions of how the

20. Judith Lorber, "Management of the Common Cold in Office Workers," unpublished Master's thesis, New York University, New York, 1966.

21. A label of incapacity may also depend on the requirements of the ill individual's working group—its need for manpower, and its assessment of the relative value to the group of the individual's continuing to work. Cf. David Mechanic, "Illness and Social Disability: Some Problems in Analysis," *Pacific Sociological Review*, 2 (Spring, 1959), 37-41. Parsons also notes that "incapacity" is a socially determined label dependent on institutionalized expectations of standards of "adequate" performance. See Talcott Parsons, "Definitions of Health and Illness in the Light of American Values and Social Structure," in *Social Structure and Personality* (New York: The Free Press, 1964), p. 265.

Of course, just as the individual's importance to the group may make it difficult for him to get labeled ill, his position may subject him to label of illness for every minor symptom: the President of the United States goes to the hospital with a cold.

patient has come to regard his injury as a means of financing his future without believing that an ordinarily intelligent man knows what he is saying.[23]

Even if the social labelers feel an accident is not accidental, they must confer a label of illness since there is a palpable injury. If a state is medically defined as illness, it must be treated; if punishment is to take place for deliberate self-injury, it can only be done when the patient is symptom-free. Then he gets a kind of retrospective label of malingering.

Ill individuals who want to *avoid* the label of illness may insist that their physical symptoms are not disabling. If they are chronically ill and wish to lead as normal a life as possible, they will try to convey the impression that they are healthy. They are, in their way, secret deviants, and therefore belong in the first cell of the third column.

In the case of conversion reactions (the hysterical enactment of an illness), where there seems to be a definite gain from the label of illness, the management of the performance to achieve a label of accidental rather than deliberate deviance must be particularly delicate. According to Ziegler and his co-workers, hysterical symptoms are chosen for their symbolic communication of emotional distress, yet to be accepted as physical and not emotional illness they must grossly coincide with medical conceptions.[24] These authors feel that this type of enactment of the sick role is an unconscious mechanism of psychological avoidance, because the patients are convinced of the somatic origin of their symptoms. The authors also suspect, however, "that their environmental circumstances strongly support this rather manipulative emotional pattern. . . ."[25] Thus, women are more likely to utilize conversion reactions, because dependency is acceptable in the female role. In men, complicated conversion reactions involving many symptoms over a long period of time are usually found in settings permitting compensation for illness, such as veterans' hospitals. Conversion reactions can also be "unreasonable exaggerations of genuine physical problems."[26] The performance may not fool a psychiatrist or a psychiatrically minded physician, but by judicious "shopping around," the conversion reactor may achieve the label of legitimate illness and the secondary gains of sympathy and support. If he does not achieve the label of accidental deviance by being treated for his symptoms, the hysteric may get the stigmatizing label "malingerer."

The treatment the hysteric gets may be psychiatric rather than physical. The difficulty doctors have in distinguishing hysteria and malingering have

22. Alexander H. Hirschfeld and Robert C. Behan, "The Accident Process, I. Etiological Considerations of Industrial Injuries," *Journal of the American Medical Association,* 186 (October 19, 1963), 114-115.
23. *Ibid.,* p. 118.
24. Frederick J. Ziegler, John B. Imboden, and Eugene Meyer, "Contemporary Conversion Reactions: A Clinical Study," *American Journal of Psychiatry,* 116 (April, 1960), 901-909; Frederick J. Ziegler, John B. Imboden, and David A. Rodgers, "Contemporary Conversion Reactions: Diagnostic Considerations," *Journal of the American Medical Association,* 186 (October 26, 1963), 307-311.
25. Ziegler, Imboden, and Rodgers, *op. cit.,* p. 308.
26. *Ibid.,* p. 309.

led some of them to turn the whole problem over to the psychiatrist. The following discussion by a doctor is an excellent summation of the self- and social labeling process and the possible ultimate disposition of these kinds of deviants:

> Hysterical patients have no organic basis for their symptoms and findings so that in a sense, they are "faking" their disease. The important point is that this faking is on a subconscious level and the patient is perfectly sincere in the belief that his symptoms and findings are bona fide. The malingerer is also a faker but his dissimulation is on a conscious level and he knows perfectly well that he is "putting it on" for a purpose. The only difference between hysteria and malingering is the presence or absence of awareness by the patient that he is faking. This awareness is extremely difficult to prove unless the patient will confess. The borderline between hysteria and malingering is indeed a thin one because fakers may convince themselves of their illness and develop an hysterical overlay while hysterics may come to see the benefits of their illness and consciously embellish it with ornamental additions. For these reasons, recognition of the malingerer is unusual, the true malingerer actually is quite rare, probably most such patients have abnormal personality traits anyway and most often they end up with a psychiatric diagnosis of some sort.[27]

A *psychiatric* label of illness resolves the problem of distinguishing between accidental and deliberate deviance from the doctor's point of view by keeping it a "true" illness (not the deviant's doing, but due to abnormal personality traits).

As long as he incurs no stigmatization for undergoing psychiatric treatment, the malingerer may not find it disadvantageous to be labeled an abnormal personality. Even if he doesn't get "well," professional ideology prevents punishment of his deviance. Without this shift to the area of psychological deviance, the label of malingerer represents the failure of all performances of "innocence."

None of the types of illness discussed is stable or permanent; self-labels and social labels change, depending on the development of physical symptoms, shifting perceptions and evaluations, contacts with the medical profession, and consistency of performance. The compensation case may be denied further compensation, malingering may be transformed into mental illness, hidden illness may be discovered and treated, minor illness may get worse and be treated, and then may be exaggerated into hysteria.[28] Like other social situations, illness is a combination of physical reality and social evaluation and response. It is an interactive process with elements of conflict. The deviant struggles to achieve the kind of label he desires, using his

27. Warner F. Bowers, *Interpersonal Relationships in the Hospital* (Springfield, Ill.: Charles C Thomas, 1960), pp. 65-66.

28. If the illness results in a permanent disability, the person enters into a different area of deviance, with its own labels and performances. See Fred Davis, "Deviance Disavowal: The Management of Strained Interaction by the Visibly Handicapped," *Social Problems*, 9 (Fall, 1961), 120-132; and Erving Goffman, *Stigma: Notes on the Management of Spoiled Identity* (Englewood Cliffs, N.J., Prentice-Hall, 1963).

physical state and his performing arts to build up an impression that will convince his social audience "to act voluntarily in accordance with his own plan."[29]

Summary

Although the basic theoretical vocabulary of the labeling concept of deviance is that of symbolic interaction (it assumes the far-reaching effect of a linguistic symbol and self-identification as a result of social identification), the most recent emphasis has been on the *other,* on the responder. The self, the initiator of the action, has been neglected. The emphasis on the labeler has made him the initiator of action, and the deviant the responder, which ignores the fact that deviance is a reciprocal interaction process in which deviant and labeler take turns acting and responding.[30]

This paper has suggested that the deviant often more or less deliberately conveys an impression which he hopes will lead to the imposition of a certain label by his audience. The impression or performance he gives, it was further suggested, depends on his view of himself (his self-label) and his ability to determine possible social response to his behavior. The interaction sequence in deviance should follow the pattern of social interaction described by Mead: intent, recognition of the response of the other, action, actual response, revised intent, revised behavior, response, and so on.[31] Or, using the language of labeling theory: self-label, awareness of societal reaction, performance, social label, revision of self-label, performance in the role implied by the social label. In short, the sequence of interaction in deviance should be no different from that in other social situations, where roles are built up through a dialectic of self and other.

In this paper, both self-labels and social labels were broken down into conformity, accidental deviance, and deliberate deviance, and a ninefold typology of deviance was offered. Illness as a type of deviance usually defined as accidental was analyzed for its labeling and performance aspects, as an illustration of the uses of the approach.

Restoring the deviant individual to the analysis of deviance permits the use of the labeling theory in the study of all forms of deviance, hidden as well as socially labeled. Besides correcting a limiting theoretical bias, a fully interactive conceptualization of deviance also avoids an unfortunate *moral* bias. A concentration on social responses, and a neglect of the interaction processes that culminate in those responses, "sentimentalizes"

29. Goffman, *The Presentation of Self, op. cit.,* p. 4.

30. Albert K. Cohen makes a similar point in "The Sociology of the Deviant Act: Anomic Theory and Beyond," *American Sociological Review,* 30 (February, 1965), 5-14. The point is made on pp. 9-10.

31. George Herbert Mead, *Mind, Self and Society* (Chicago, Ill.: The University of Chicago Press, 1934), pp. 135-226.

the deviant by making him a put-upon victim, with the social control agents the villains of the piece.[32] An interaction approach admits the possibility that the deviant individual is very much aware that he is breaking rules, that he is choosing to do so, and that, with this awareness, he can attempt to manipulate those in a position to label. Thus, he may get what he wants within the limitations of the social structure that encompasses him.

32. A warning about sentimentalizing the subjects with whom the researcher feels in sympathy is attributed to Freidson by Becker in the introduction to *The Other Side*. Becker makes the distinction between *conventional* sentimentality, or sympathy with the establishment, and *unconventional* sentimentality, or sympathy with deviants. He cautions against both kinds of sentimentality, but feels the latter is the lesser evil. *Op. cit.*, pp. 4-6.

27

JANE R. MERCER

Career Patterns of Persons Labeled as Mentally Retarded

A growing body of sociological literature is diverging from the tradi-tional treatment of deviance. This new approach, which we are calling the "social system perspective," views deviance as a label emerging from an interpersonal process in which one individual or group of individuals defines the behavior or physical attributes of another individual or group as "different," "strange," or beyond tolerable limits.[1,2,3] The social sys-tem perspective contrasts sharply with the more conventional view of de-viance as an attribute of the deviant, a perspective we will call the "clini-cal perspective." Both perspectives are useful in certain contexts; however, it is essential that an investigator be aware of the perspective which he is adopting in any given analysis. After defining more specifically what is meant by each of these concepts, we will attempt to illustrate how the use of the social system perspective can assist in understanding processes in the career patterns of persons who have been labeled mentally retard-ed.[4]

Reprinted from *Social Problems*, 13, No. 1 (1965), pp. 18-34, by permission of the author and The Society for the Study of Social Problems.

Supported in part by the National Institute of Mental Health, Grant No. 3M-9130: Population Movement of Mental Defectives and Related Physical, Behavioral, Social, and Cultural Factors; and Grant No. MH-5687: Mental Retardation in a Community, Pacific State Hospital, Pomona, California. Appreciation for assistance is expressed to the Western Data Processing Center, Division of the Graduate School of Business Administration, University of California, Los Angeles.

1. Howard S. Becker, *Outsiders: Studies in the Sociology of Deviance* (Glencoe, Ill.: The Free Press, 1963).

2. Howard S. Becker, ed., *The Other Side: Perspectives on Deviance* (Glencoe, Ill.: The Free Press, 1964).

3. John I. Kitsuse, "Societal Reaction to Deviant Behavior: Problems of Theory and Method," *Social Problems*, 9 (Winter, 1962), 247-257.

4. The author wishes to express appreciation to Harvey F. Dingman, Ph.D., and Lindsey C. Churchill, Ph.D., for helpful suggestions and observations made in the preparation of this manuscript.

The clinical perspective is the frame of reference most commonly adopted in studies of mental deficiency, mental illness, drug addiction, and other areas which the students of deviance choose to investigate.[5,6] This viewpoint is readily identified by several distinguishing characteristics.

First, the investigator accepts as the focus for study those individuals who have been labeled deviant. In so doing, he adopts the values of whatever social system has defined the person as deviant and assumes that its judgments are the valid measure of deviance. The evaluations which have produced the definition "mental retardate," "drug addict," or "alcoholic" are taken as given, and the individual is perceived within the frame of reference of the evaluating group. Groups in the social structure sharing the values of the core culture tend to accept the labels attached as a consequence of the application of these values without serious questioning. For example, it seems obvious to a member of a middle-class American family that there is something seriously wrong with any adult who cannot read or write. This opinion would be widely shared by other persons in the core groups, but not nearly so widely shared by persons in more peripheral social systems.

This acceptance of the core group definition of deviance as a starting point for investigation results in a second distinguishing characteristic of the clinical perspective: a tendency to perceive deviance as an attribute of the person, as a meaning inherent in his behavior, appearance, or performance. Mental retardation, for example, is viewed as a characteristic of the person, a lack to be explained. This viewpoint results in a quest for etiology. Thus, the clinical perspective is essentially a medical frame of reference, for it sees deviance as individual pathology requiring diagnostic classification and etiological analysis for the purpose of determining proper treatment procedures and probable prognosis.

The perceived necessity for accurate diagnosis leads to three additional characteristics of the clinical perspective: the development of a diagnostic nomenclature, the creation of diagnostic instruments, and the professionalization of the diagnostic function. In areas of deviance with a long social history, extensive effort has been expended in elaborating diagnostic nomenclatures, and a corps of professional diagnosticians has evolved with official sanction to label deviants by using complex instruments which require special training and skill to administer. This professional group acquires a position as the legitimate "labelers." The development of special labeling devices and measurements results in the formal codification of what is officially considered "normal," and written norms are created, on the basis of which individuals are labeled as deviant or nondeviant and assigned to subcategories within the larger area of deviance.

5. August B. Hollingshead and Fredrick C. Redlich, *Social Class and Mental Illness* (New York: John Wiley, 1958), chap. 11.

6. H. E. Freeman and O. G. Simmons, "Social Class and Posthospital Performance Levels," *American Sociological Review*, 2 (June, 1959), 348.

The more formal the norms and the more elaborate the measuring devices, the stronger the tendency to professionalize the diagnostic function and to adopt a clinical perspective. This is very evident in the highly formalized and professionalized processes which operate in the labeling of the mental retardate. Low performance on carefully normed intelligence measures administered by duly trained and licensed professionals is the recognized criterion for placing persons in special education classes, hospitals for the retarded, or on categorical aid programs for the totally disabled. In areas where norms are still fluid and the diagnostic function less highly professionalized, as in definitions of juvenile delinquency, the tendency to see deviance as a trait of the individual is somewhat less pronounced.

When the investigator begins his research with the diagnostic designations assigned by official defining agents, he tends to assume that all individuals placed in a given category are essentially equivalent in respect to their deviance. If there are significant differences in the life careers of persons in the same category, such as difference in rates for admission or release from social institutions, the explanation for these differences is sought in some other attribute of the individual, i.e., his age, sex, body structure, or degree of physical handicap. Research design frequently follows a typical pattern. Individuals assigned to different categories of deviance are compared with each other or with a "normal" population consisting of persons who, for whatever reason, have escaped being labeled. The focus is on the individual.

Another characteristic of the clinical perspective is its assumption that the official definition is somehow the "right" definition. If persons in other social systems, especially the family, do not concur with official findings and refuse to define a member as "retarded," "delinquent," or "mentally ill," the clinical perspective assumes that they are either unenlightened or are evidencing psychological denial. It follows, then, that they need to be educated to understand the "real" situation or, if resistance is intense, need therapy to help them gain insight into the psychological roots of their denial.

Finally, when deviance is perceived as individual pathology, social action tends to center upon changing the individual or, that failing, removing him from participation in society. Prevention and cure become the primary social goals. Seldom considered are the alternative possibilities of redefining his behavior by modifying the norms of the social system or of attempting to locate the individual in the structure of social systems which will not perceive his behavior as pathological.

Uncritical acceptance of the frame of reference of the official defining group, whether it be psychiatrists labeling persons as mentally ill, criminal courts labeling persons as criminal, or psychometrists labeling persons as "gifted," "average," or "retarded," obviates the possibility of investigating the labeling process itself. It also rules out exploration of the possibility that different definitions of the individual's behavior may have been made by other social systems—for example, his family or friendship group—and that these alternative definitions may be even more significant in influencing his future career than the official definition. By ignoring the values of social systems other than the recognized defining agencies, we exclude from review many facets of the nature of deviance.

The social system perspective, on the other hand, attempts to see the definition of an individual's behavior as a function of the values of the social system within which he is being evaluated. The professional definers are studied as one of the most important of the evaluating social systems but within the context of other social systems which may or may not concur with official definitions.

Defining an individual as mentally ill, delinquent, or mentally retarded is viewed as an interpersonal process in which the definer makes a value judgment about the behavior of the persons being defined. Depending upon the role expectations current in the social system for the roles which the defined is playing, his behavior will be judged normal, subnormal, or superior. Role expectations vary from system to system according to the performance of persons playing roles. For example, if a sizable percentage of the persons playing adult roles in a defining social system has little or no formal education and is unemployed and living on welfare, these persons are unlikely to regard such behavior as deviant, regardless of what labels may be attached to it by official agencies. Thus, the extent of deviation depends not only on the behavior of the individual, but also on the framework of norms within which the definer operates in making his judgments. Deviation is not seen as a characteristic of the individual or as a meaning inherent in his behavior, but as a socially derived label which may be attached to his behavior by some social systems and not by others.[7]

In order to understand what is meant by the label "mentally retarded," from this viewpoint, it then becomes essential to know who is defined by whom as retarded, and what impact the labeling has upon the career of the individual.

Customarily, research in mental retardation has proceeded under the assumptions of the clinical perspective. However, the second approach, which sees mental retardation as bound to a particular social system, has considerable value. If it is postulated that the label "mentally subnormal" is an evaluation of an individual made within a particular social system and based on the norms of that system, then it becomes clear that the label may not be applied to the person when he is evaluated by the norms of a different social system. Thus, it follows that a person may be mentally retarded in one system and not mentally retarded in another. He may

7. Becker, 1964, *op. cit.*

change his label by changing his social group. This viewpoint frees us from the necessity of seeing the person as permanently stigmatized by a deviant label and makes it possible to understand otherwise obscure patterns in the life careers of individuals. It turns attention from questions directed at determining whether the individual is "really" retarded and from discussions of "proper" diagnosis to such questions as: "Who sees whom as retarded?" "What are the characteristics of the social systems which attach different labels to the same individual?" and "What impact does differential labeling have on the life career of the person?"

The research reported in this paper attempts to answer these questions about a group of persons who shared the common experience of having been labeled retarded by official defining agencies and placed in a public institution for the retarded. The sample was selected to include two groups whose life careers took different courses at a critical juncture. One group was released to their families after a period of institutionalization, while the other group, after an equivalent period of institutionalization, remained residents of the institution.

The specific question which this study seeks to investigate within the above framework is: "Why do the families of some individuals take them back home after a period of institutionalization in a hospital for the retarded while other families do not, when, according to official evaluations, these individuals show similar degrees of deviance, that is, have comparable intelligence test scores, and are of equivalent age, sex, ethnic status, and length of hospitalization?"

In trying to answer this question we used a social system perspective. We anticipated that those patients who were released would tend to come from family social systems which were most distant, structurally, from societal core groups and which evidenced a style of life contrary to many middle-class values. In such a social system the nonachieving, dependent person with a low intelligence score would be closer to group norms than in a high achieving, independent, upper-status milieu.

The literature on the value systems of different classes in American society supports this as a plausible hypothesis. For example, Hyman, in a secondary analysis of several studies using national samples and spaced over a period of years, concluded that lower-class persons place a lower evaluation on education achievement than middle-class persons. In addition, they more frequently show a preference for a low-paying job, if it is secure, than a high-paying job involving risk, and consistently show a pattern of limited expectations and striving.[8] Hollingshead and Redlich, in their study of mental illness, found that lower-status families are less likely to define the behavioral manifestations associated with emotional

8. Herbert H. Hyman, "The Value Systems of Different Classes: A Social Psychological Contribution to the Analysis of Stratification," *Class, Status and Power,* Reinhard Bendix and Seymour M. Lipset, eds. (Glencoe, Ill.: The Free Press, 1953).

disturbance as a symptom of mental illness.[9] This finding for mental patients has been confirmed by other investigators.[10][11] Freeman and Simmons found that middle-class families were less tolerant of the ex-mental patient's behavior and were more likely to exclude him, following release, than lower-class families.[12] Downey reports that more educated families demonstrate less interest in their children after placing them in a hospital for the retarded because they tend to view them in terms of their ability to be educated and anticipate they will be unable to conform to the family's career expectations.[13]

These differences in group norms should be evident not only in a different style of life but should be apparent in divergent definitions of the patient. If our reasoning is correct, the higher-status family, because it is closer to core cultural values and thus closer to the values of the social defining agencies, should more frequently concur in the definition of the patient as "retarded," more frequently see the patient's condition as unchangeable, and have fewer expectations that he will ever be able to fill adult roles, since adult roles carry more demanding role expectations in higher-status levels than lower-status levels. This would also lead us to believe that there should be significant differences in the processes by which the patient was first labeled "retarded," differences that would somehow be congruent with the divergent definitions held by the families.

Method

Two groups of labeled retardates were studied. One group consisted of patients who had been released to their families from a state hospital for the retarded and the other group consisted of a matched group of patients still resident in the hospital at the time of the study.[14]

Specifically, the released group was made up of all patients released to their families during a three-year period (1957-59), who had not been readmitted to another institution for the retarded at the time of the study, and who were reported to be living within a one-hundred-mile radius of the hospital. Only those cases in which the family had assumed responsibility for the patient were included. Of the 76 patients who met these qualifications, it was possible to complete interviews with 63 of the families. Six families refused to be interviewed and seven could not be located.

9. Hollingshead and Redlich, *op. cit.*, Chap. 11.

10. E. H. Hare, "Mental Illness and Social Class in Bristol," *British Journal of Preventative and Social Medicine,* 9 (October, 1955), 191-195.

11. Bertram Mandelbrote and Steven Folkard, "The Outcome of Schizophrenia in Relation to a Developing Community Psychiatric Service," *Mental Hygiene,* 47 (January, 1964), 43-56.

12. Freeman and Simmons, *op. cit.*, p. 348.

13. Kenneth J. Downey, "Parental Interest in the Institutionalized Severely Mentally Retarded Child," *Social Problems,* 11 (Fall, 1963), 186-193.

14. Pacific State Hospital, Pomona, California, is a state-supported hospital for the mentally retarded with a population of approximately 3,000 patients.

Since we wished to focus this study on variables in the social systems from which these persons came, it was essential to match individual characteristics known to influence rate of release; consequently, the resident group was selected to match the released group in intelligence quotient, age, sex, ethnic status, and year of admission, other studies having demonstrated that these factors are related to the probability of release.[15]

The matched group of resident patients was selected in the following manner: all patients on the hospital rolls were sorted into two groups by sex, two groups by age, three groups by ethnic status, three groups by intelligence quotient, and two groups by year of admission. All released patients were likewise assigned to the proper category. Resident patients were then chosen at random from within each cell in sufficient numbers to correspond to the number of discharged patients also falling in that cell. Each resident case was required to have a family living within a one-hundred-mile radius of the hospital. If a case did not meet this requirement, another case was drawn randomly from the appropriate cell until there were an equal number of discharged and resident cases in each cell. Sex distribution in each group was 53 males and 23 females; ethnic distribution, 47 Caucasians, 20 Mexicans, and 9 Negroes.

Statistical tests comparing age, intelligence quotient, and year of admission for the patients in the two groups were made to determine if the matching process had indeed controlled for these factors. Table 27.1 presents the distribution of intelligence quotients, birth years, and years of admission for the interviewed cases. Of the 76 resident cases, interviews were completed with 70 families. Two refused to be interviewed and four families could not be located. Using a Kolmogornov-Smirnov Test of two independent samples, we found that all differences between the interviewed groups could be accounted for by chance.

When the 19 noninterviewed cases were compared with the 133 interviewed cases, no significant differences were found in the sex, age, I.Q., or ethnic status of the patients, or the socioeconomic level of the families. We concluded that no significant bias was introduced by inability to contact 19 of the families originally selected for study.

The hospital file for each patient selected for study was searched for relevant data and an interview was held with a family member. In 75 percent of the cases the mother was interviewed; in 8 percent the father was interviewed; and in the remaining cases some other relative served as informant. All but two of the interviews were held in the home of the respondent. Four graduate students in the behavioral sciences and the author served as interviewers. A letter from the hospital first explained that the research department was interested in learning more about its

15. G. Tarjan, S. W. Wright, M. Kramer, P. H. Person, Jr., and R. Morgan, "The Natural History of Mental Deficiency in a State Hospital. I: Probabilities of Release and Death by Age, Intelligence Quotients, and Diagnosis," *AMA Journal of Disturbed Children,* 96 (1958), 64-70.

patients and their families, and an appointment for an interview was then made by telephone. In those cases in which the family had no phone, initial contacts were made without appointment.

Table 27.1.   *Comparison of interviewed cases by birth year,*
intelligence quotient, and year of admission.

Matched Variable	Released (63)	Resident (70)	Significance Level
Birth Year			
Before 1920	4	5	
1921-1930	13	12	
1931-1940	33	34	> .05 [a]
1941-1950	12	17	
1951-1960	1	2	
Intelligence Quotient			
0-9	2	4	
10-19	2	1	
20-29	4	3	
30-39	6	4	> .05 [a]
40-49	13	15	
50-59	14	18	
60-69	19	19	
70 +	3	6	
Year of Admission			
Before 1945	5	9	
1945-1950	20	14	
1951-1956	33	31	> .05 [a]
1957 and later	5	16	

[a] The Kolmogornov-Smirnov Test of two independent samples was used.

Since this study focuses on factors in release, it is useful at this point to examine briefly the process by which a patient may be discharged to his family. In the hospital studied, a patient's release to his family may be initiated either by the family or as the result of a suggestion from a hospital staff member. In the latter case, release is contingent upon the family's willingness to reaccept the patient. Families offered the choice frequently reject the hospital's promptings.

To clarify the circumstances under which the released group returned to their families, the respondent was asked two questions: "Who was the most important person in getting you to take —— out of the hospital?" and "What were the main reasons you decided to have —— discharged from the hospital?"

In 12 cases the parents reported that someone in the hospital, i.e., a social worker, family care mother, or a ward technician, had first suggested that the patient could be released to the family. In the 51 remaining cases the families were the active agents in release. Reasons given by the families for seeking a discharge are described in Table 27.2.

Table 27.2   The release process as reported by the families of
released patients

	f	%
Hospital-initiated releases	12	19
Family-initiated releases		
Family opposed to placement from beginning	9	14
Parents lonely without patient or need him for some practical reason, e.g., to help with younger children, earn money, etc.	8	13
Patient was unhappy in the hospital. Hospital failure: mistreated patient, made him work too hard, etc.	6	9
Hospital success: Patient improved enough to come home.	9	14
Home conditions changed to permit return, e.g., found patient a job, mother's health better, etc.	10	16
Total release cases	63	

It is clear from this table that most of the patients who returned to their families returned because the family made an effort to secure their release. Some families had been opposed to placement from the beginning while others, initially favorable to placement, had become disillusioned with hospital care because the patient was unhappy or because they felt he was mistreated. Others, expressing a more positive note, sought the patient's return because they missed him, because home conditions had changed to permit his return, or because his behavior had improved sufficiently to make them willing to reaccept him. Whatever their stated reason, however, the critical point for the present discussion is that most of these families actively wanted the patient at home.

Findings

SOCIAL STATUS OF RELEASED PATIENTS

Several indices were used to measure the socioeconomic level of the family of each retardate. A socioeconomic index score based on the occupation and education of the head of the household, weighted according to Hollingshead's system, was used as the basic measure. In addition, the interviewer rated the economic status of the street on which the patient's home was located, rated the physical condition of the housing unit, and completed a checklist of equipment present in the household. As can be seen in Table 27.3, the families of the released patients rated significantly lower than the families of the resident patients on every measure. The heads of the households in the families of released patients had less education and lower-level jobs, the family residence was located among less affluent dwellings, the housing unit was in a poorer state of repair, and the dwelling was less elaborately furnished and equipped. Contrary to the pattern found in studies of those placed as mentally ill,[16] it is the "retardate" from lower socioeconomic background who is most likely to be released to

16. Hollingshead and Redlich, 1958, *op. cit.*, chap. 11.

*Table 27.3.   Socioeconomic differences between patients released to their
families and those still resident in the state hospital*

Socioeconomic Measure		Released Living at Home (63%)	Resident in State Hospital (70%)	significance level
Socioeconomic index score of head of household	Above median	36.5	61.4	
	Below median	61.9	38.6	<.01 [c]
	Unknown	1.6	0.0	
Economic status of street [a]	Housing value $10,000 and above	29.0	55.1	<.05 [c]
	Housing value less than $10,000	71.0	44.9	
Condition of housing unit [a]	Run-down	48.4	23.2	
	Average	46.8	57.2	<.05 [c]
	Above average	4.8	18.8	
Household equipment scale [a]	0-2	19.0	11.9	
	3-5	27.6	20.9	<.05 [b]
	6-8	43.1	.41.8	
	9-11	10.3	25.4	

[a] Some cases are not included because data were not available.
[b] Test of significance of difference between unrelated means was used.
[c] Chi Square Test was used.

his family while higher-status "retardates" are more likely to remain in the hospital.

From the clinical perspective, several explanations may be proposed for these differences. It has been found in hospital populations that patients with an I.Q. below 50 are more likely to come from families which represent a cross-section of social levels, while those with an I.Q. between 50 and 70 are more likely to come from low-status families.[17] Since persons with higher I.Q.'s have a higher probability of release, this could account for higher rates of release for low-status persons. However, in the present study, the tested level of intelligence was equal for both groups, and this hypothesis cannot be used as an explanation.

A second possible explanation from a clinical perspective might be based on the fact that persons who have more physical handicaps tend to be institutionalized for longer periods of time than persons with few handicaps.[18] Should it be found that high-status patients have more physical

17. Georges Sabagh, Harvey F. Dingman, George Tarjan, and Stanley W. Wright, "Social Class and Ethnic Status of Patients Admitted to a State Hospital for the Retarded," *Pacific Sociological Review*, 2 (Fall, 1959), 76-80.
18. Tarjan, Wright, Kramer, Person, Jr., and Morgan, *op. cit.*, pp. 64-70.

handicaps than low-status patients, then this could account for the latter's shorter hospitalization. Data from the present sample were analyzed to determine whether there was a significant relationship between physical handicap and social status. Although released patients tended to have fewer physical handicaps than resident patients, this was irrespective of social status. When high-status patients were compared with low-status patients, 50 percent of the high-status and 56 percent of the low-status patients had no physical handicaps. A chi square of 1.9 indicates these differences could be accounted for by chance variation.

A third explanation from the clinical perspective may hinge on differences in the diagnostic categories to which retardates of different social status were assigned. In addition to categorizing persons according to intelligence level as measured by tests, professional evaluators also assign them to categories according to the physical symptomotology and supposed etiology of their retardation.[19] Without going into an extensive discussion of this professional nomenclature, we can say that diagnostic labels give a rough measure of the extent of physical deformity which accompanies low intellectual performance. A diagnostic label of "familial" or "undifferentiated" ordinarily indicates that the individual has few or no physical stigmata and is essentially normal in body structure. All other categories ordinarily indicate that he has some type of physical symptomotology. Although released patients were more likely to be diagnosed as familial or undifferentiated than resident patients $X^2=7.08$, p$<$.01, this, like physical handicap, was irrespective of social status. Fifty-seven percent of the high-status retardates, and 69 percent of the low-status retardates were classified as either undifferentiated or familial, a difference which could be accounted for by chance.

Since differences in the release rates of different status level patients to their families cannot be explained within the clinical perspective as due to differences in the individual characteristics of patients from high and low-status families, we turn to an exploration of differences in the social systems from which the patients came for a possible explanation of the dissimilarity of their life careers.

DIVERGENT DEFINITIONS

In analyzing social status, four types of situations were identified. The modal category for resident patients were high social status with a smaller number of released patients coming from higher-status families. If we are correct in our hypothesis (that higher release rates for low-status patients are related to the fact that the family social system is structurally more distant from the core culture and that its style of life, values, and definitions of the patient are more divergent from official definitions than that of

19. National Committee for Mental Hygiene, *Statistical Manual for the Use of Institutions for Mental Defectives* (New York: NCMH, 1946).

high-status families), we would expect the largest differences to occur when high-status resident families are compared to low-status released families. The two nonmodal categories would be expected to fall at some intermediate point. For this reason, the analysis of all subsequent variables has retained these four basic classifications.

Table 27.4 presents the responses made to three questions asked to determine the extent to which the family concurred in the official label of "retardation," the extent to which they believed the patient's condition amenable to change, and the extent to which they anticipated that the individual could live outside the hospital and, perhaps, fill adult roles. The patterns of the divergent definitions of the situation which emerged for each group are illuminating.

When asked whether *he* believed the patient to be retarded, the high-status parent more frequently concurred with the definitions of the official defining agencies while the low-status parent was more prone to disagree outright or to be uncertain. This tendency is especially marked when the two modal categories are compared. While 33.3 percent of the parents of the low-status released patients stated that they did not think the patient was retarded and 25.6 percent were uncertain whether he was retarded, only 4.6 percent of the parents of high-status resident patients felt he was not retarded and 20.9 percent were uncertain.

When parents were asked whether they believed anything could change the patient's condition, the differences between all groups were significant at the .02 level or beyond. The high-status parent was most likely to believe that nothing could change his child's condition, and this was significantly more characteristic of parents whose children were still in the hospital than those who had taken their child from the hospital on both status levels.

When asked what they saw in the future for their child, all groups again differed significantly in the expected direction. The modal, high-status group was least optimistic and the modal, low-status group, most optimistic about the future. Fully 46 percent of the parents of the latter group expressed the expectation that their child would get a job, marry, and fulfill the usual adult roles while only 6.9 percent of the modal high-status group responded in this fashion. High-status parents, as a group, more frequently see their child playing dependent roles. It is interesting to note that, although a large percentage of parents of released patients believe the patient will be less dependent, they demonstrate their willingness to accept responsibility for the retarded child themselves by their responding that they foresee him having a future in which he is dependent at home. Only 9.3 percent of the high-status and 22.2 percent of the low-status parents of the resident patients see this as a future prospect. Release to the family clearly appears to be contingent upon the willingness of the family to accept the patient's dependency, if they do not foresee him assuming independent adult roles.

Table 27.4 Patterns of divergent definitions

Question	Response Categories	High Status resident (43) %	High Status released (23) %	Low Status resident (27) %	Low Status released (39) %	high status / low status	high status resident / low status released	high status resident / high status released	low status resident / low status released
1. We know that many people have told you ___ is retarded but we want to know what you think. Do you think he/she is retarded?	Yes	74.4	47.8	66.6	41.0				
	Uncertain	20.9	39.1	14.8	25.6	< .02 [a]	< .02 [a]	NS [a]	NS [a]
	No	4.6	13.0	18.5	33.3				
2. Do you believe anything can change ___'s condition?	Nothing	74.3	39.0	66.6	33.3				
	Uncertain	2.3	17.3	11.1	38.4	< 02 [b]	< .001 [b]	< .01 [b]	< .01 [b]
	Training, medical care, etc.	23.2	43.4	22.2	28.2				
3. What do you see in the future for ___?	Dependent in institution	83.7	13.0	74.0	2.5				
	Dependent at home	9.3	60.8	22.2	48.7	< .02 [b]	< .001 [b]	< .001 [b]	< .001 [b]
	Normal adult roles	6.9	26.0	3.7	46.1				

[a] The Kolmogornov-Smirnov Test of two independent samples was used.
[b] The Log-Likelihood Ratio Test was used. (Barnett, Wolf, "The Log-Likelihood Ratio Test [The G-Test]: Methods and Tables for a Test of Heterogeneity in Contingency Tables," *Annals of Human Genetics*, 21:4 [June, 1957], 397-409.)

FACTORS IN THE LABELING PROCESS

From the social system perspective, retardation is viewed as a label placed upon an individual after someone has evaluated his behavior within a specific set of norms. Retardation is not a meaning necessarily inherent in the behavior of the individual. We have seen that the parents of low-status, released patients tend to reject the label of retardation and to be optimistic about the future. We surmised that this divergent definition could well be related to factors in the process by which the child was first categorized as subnormal, such as his age at the time, the type of behavior which was used as a basis for making the evaluation, and the persons doing the labeling. Consequently, parents were asked specifically about these factors. Table 27.5 records their responses.

Children from lower-status families were labeled as mentally subnormal at a significant later age than children from high-status families. Seventy-nine percent of the patients at the high-status, modal group were classified as retarded by the age of six while only 36.1 percent of those in the low-status, modal group were identified at such an early age. The largest percentage of low-status retardates were first classified after they reached public school age. This indicates that relatives and friends, who are the individuals most likely to observe and evaluate the behavior of young children, seldom saw anything deviant in the early development of lower-status children later labeled retarded, but that the primary groups of higher-status children did perceive early deviation.

This is related to the responses made when parents were asked what first prompted someone to believe the patient retarded. The modal, high-status group reported slow development in 48.8 percent of the cases and various types of physical symptoms in an additional 20.9 percent, while only 14.7 percent and 11.8 percent of the modal, low-status parents gave these responses. On the other hand, 55.9 percent of the modal, low-status group were first labeled because they had problems learning in school, while this was true of only 9.3 percent of the modal high-status group.

When parents were asked who was the most important person influencing them in placing the child in the hospital, a parallel pattern emerged. Medical persons are the most important single group for the modal high-status persons while the police and welfare agencies loom as very significant in 64.1 percent of the cases in the modal, low-status group. These findings are similar to those of Hollingshead and Redlich in their study of paths to the hospital for the mentally ill.[20] Of additional interest is the fact that the person important in placement differentiates the low-status released from the low-status resident patient at the .01 level. The resident low-status patient's path to the hospital is similar to that of the high-status patient and markedly different from released low-status persons. When authoritative figures

20. Hollingshead and Redlich, *op. cit.*, chap. 11.

Table 25.5. Factors in the labeling process

Question	Response Categories	High Status resident (43) %	High Status released (23) %	Low Status resident (27) %	Low Status released (39) %	high status / low status	resident high / released low	resident high / released high	resident low / released low
1. How old was ___ when someone first said he was retarded?	1-2 years	44.1	18.1	23.2	16.7	<.001 [a]	<.02 [a]	NS [a]	NS [a]
	3-6 years	34.8	50.0	30.2	19.4				
	7-10 years	9.3	22.7	11.5	30.5				
	11-14 years	4.6	0.0	11.5	16.7				
	15 or over	6.9	9.1	23.2	16.7				
2. What was there about ___ that made you/them think he/she might be retarded?	Slow development	48.8	30.4	19.2	14.7	<.005 [b]	<.001 [b]	NS [b]	NS [b]
	Physical symptoms	20.9	17.3	26.9	11.8				
	Behavioral problems	20.9	21.7	15.4	17.6				
	Couldn't learn in school	9.3	30.4	38.5	55.9				
3. Who was the most important person in getting you to place ___ in the ___ hospital?	Family	27.9	43.4	48.1	25.6	<.01 [b]	<.001 [b]	NS [b]	<.01 [b]
	Medical or psychological person	37.2	30.4	11.1	2.5				
	Police or welfare	13.9	17.3	18.5	64.1				
	Schools or other	20.9	8.6	22.2	7.6				

[a] The Kolmogornov-Smirnov Test of two independent samples was used.

[b] The Log-Likelihood Ratio Test was used. (Barnett, Wolf, The Log-Likelihood Ratio Test [The G-Test]: Methods and Tables for a Test of Heterogeneity in Contingency Tables," *Annals of Human Genetics*, 21:4 [June, 1957], 397-409).

such as police and welfare are primary forces in placement, the patient is more likely to return home.

We interpret these findings to mean that when the family—or persons whose advice is solicited by the family, i.e., medical persons—is "most important" in placing a person in a hospital for the retarded, the primary groups have themselves first defined the individual as a deviant and sought professional counsel. When their own suspicions are supported by official definitions, they are more likely to leave the patient in an institution.

Conversely, when a person is labeled retarded by an authoritative, governmental agency whose advice is not solicited and who, in the case of the police, may be perceived as a punishing agent, the family frequently rejects the official definition of the child as retarded and withdraws him from the institution at the first opportunity. This attitude was clearly exemplified by one mother who, when asked why the family had taken the child from the hospital, replied, "Why not? He had served his time."

The influence of the police as a factor in labeling the low-status person as retarded may actually be greater than than shown in Table 27.5. Fifty percent of the low-status retardates had some type of police record while only 23 percent of the high-status subnormals were known to the police, a difference significant beyond the .01 level.

CHARACTERISTICS OF PRIMARY SOCIAL SYSTEMS

We have seen that there is a significant difference between the images which high-status parents and low-status parents have of their children. Although the children in both groups are equivalent, from a clinical perspective, in the amount of retardation, the high-status parent is more convinced that his child is retarded, has classified him as retarded at a younger age, is more likely to believe that nothing will change his condition, and sees him as likely to have a future in which he will be dependent either in an institution or at home. On the other hand, the low-status parent lived with his child for a longer time before anyone labeled him as retarded and is less willing to say, unequivocally, that the child is retarded. He is more likely to believe the condition is amenable to change and is more prone to believe the patient will be able to assume adult occupational and marital roles. These differences were revealed in their most striking form when the two modal categories were compared.

From the social system perspective, it is our interpretation that these differences exist mainly because the style of life and normative expectations of the low-status family are widely discrepant from those of the high-status family. In ascertaining whether or not the differences in the style of life of various social levels which were found in other studies apply to this sample, we compiled Table 27.6 showing some of the characteristics of the primary social systems from which these patients came.

Persons with low intelligence scores are noticeably limited in their ability

Table 27.6. Characteristics of primary social systems

Characteristic	Response Categories	High Status resident (43) %	High Status released (23) %	Low Status resident (27) %	Low Status released (39) %	Significance Levels high status / low status	resident high released low	resident high released high	resident low released low
1. Education of the mother	Some college	26.8	14.2	3.8	0.0				
	High school graduate	39.0	19.0	7.6	10.5				
	Partial high school	17.0	23.8	7.6	13.1	<.001[a]	<.001[a]	<.01[a]	NS[a]
	Junior high or less	17.0	42.8	80.7	76.3				
2. Education of oldest siblings who have completed schooling	Some college	46.0	57.8	10.5	5.5				
	High school graduate	23.0	21.0	36.8	41.6	<.005[a]	<.01[a]	NS[a]	NS[a]
	Less than high school	30.6	21.0	52.6	52.7				
3. Number of siblings labeled retarded	None	97.6	91.3	85.1	66.6				
	One or more	2.3	9.5	14.8	33.3	<.02[b]	<.001[b]	NS[b]	NS[b]
4. Dependence status of family at admission	Financially independent	95.2	86.9	54.2	65.8				
	Supported by relatives or agencies	4.7	13.1	45.8	34.2	<.001[b]	<.001[b]	NS[b]	NS[b]
5. Ethnic status	Caucasian	79.0	74.0	37.0	46.1				
	Mexican or Negro	20.9	26.0	62.9	53.8	<.001[c]	<.01[c]	NS[c]	NS[c]

[a] The Kolmogornov-Smirnov Test of two independent samples was used.

[b] The Log-Likelihood Ratio Rest was used. (Barnett, Wolf. The Log-Likelihood Ratio Test [The G-Test]: Methods and Tables for a Test of Heterogeneity in Contingency Tables," *Annals of Human Genetics*, 21:4 [June, 1957], 397-409.)

[c] The Chi Square Test was used.

to acquire basic educational skills even in the most elementary academic disciplines. Inspection of the educational level of the mothers of low-status retardates reveals that many of them are not significantly more proficient than the patient. Over 75 percent of the mothers of low-status patients had completed junior high school or less and none of the low-status, modal mothers had gone to college. It should be noted that even within the high-status group, the mothers of released patients have significantly less education than the mothers of resident patients.

Although parents may be limited in the amount of education they themselves achieve, they may still have high expectations for their children. The education of the oldest sibling who had completed his education was used as an index of the education which a "normal" child in the family is expected to achieve. Over half of such siblings of low-status patients had dropped out of school before completing high school and less-than 10 percent had any college training. In contrast, only about a fourth of the high-status siblings had dropped out of school and approximately half had had some college training. Clearly, the minimal educational attainment of the patient would not appear so deviant to a low-status family in which other family members also had limited educations as it would to a high-status family in which many family members of the retardate's generation have had college training.

Looking at the other end of the scale, 33.3 percent of the modal, low-status retardates had one or more siblings who had also been labeled retarded. Only 2.3 percent of the resident high-status patients had such siblings.

The adult with low mental ability tends to be a person who must be dependent on other people for support. He is often able to function in the community only if he can establish a dependency relationship with some other adult, usually a parent or normal spouse, or if he is able to lean on a public or private agency for support. When the records of the families were studied to determine family dependency at the time of admission to the hospital, 37 percent of the low-status families was found to have been dependent upon public agencies or relatives while only 8 percent of the high-status families had depended upon outside assistance. With such a high rate of dependency in low-status families, an adult who depends upon Aid to the Totally Disabled or other sources of support would not be greatly different from others in his group. In fact, he is frequently regarded as an asset, since his welfare payments provide additional family income.

There was further evidence that the low-status families occupied a more peripheral relationship to the core social structure than the high-status families. Although ethnic group was controlled in the original matching of resident and released groups, when the sample was subdivided by social status, the Mexican and Negro groups, not surprisingly, were concentrated in the lower social levels. These ethnic minorities have been marginal to the mainstream of American life and are least likely to share the achievement orientations of the core groups.

When a retardate lives in an environment in which dependency is a common way of life, minimal education the rule rather than exception, and occupational achievement limited, his own dependent, educationally deficient, occupationally restricted mode of life does not deviate markedly from that of his family and associates. Under these circumstances, his intellectual deficit is less obvious and his role performance more acceptable to his group than in an environment in which his parents and siblings are highly educated, adult persons are self-supporting, and upward mobility is commonplace.

Discussions and Conclusions

The life space of the individual may be viewed as a vast network of interlocking social systems through which the person moves during the course of his lifetime. Those systems which exist close to one another in the social structure tend, because of overlapping memberships and frequent communication, to evolve similar patterns of norms. Most individuals are born and live out their lives in a relatively limited segment of this social network and tend to contact mainly social systems which share common norms. When an individual's contracts are restricted to a circumscribed segment of the structure, this gives some stability to the evaluations which are made of his behavior and to the labels which are attached to him.

However, when the person's life career takes him into segments of the social network which are located at a distance from his point of origin, as when a Mexican-American child enters the public school or a Negro child gets picked up by the police, he is then judged by a new and different set of norms. Behavior which was perfectly acceptable in his primary social systems may now be judged as evidence of "mental retardation." At this point, he is caught up in the web of official definitions. However, because he has primary social systems which may not agree with these official labels, he may be able to return to that segment of the social structure which does not label him as deviant after he has fulfilled the minimal requirements of the official system. That is, he can drop out of school or he can "serve his time" in the state hospital and then go home. By changing his location in social space, he can change his label from "retarded" to "not much different from the rest of us." For example, the mother of a Mexican-American, male, adult patient who had been released from the hospital after being committed following an incident in which he allegedly made sexual advances to a young girl, told the author, "There is nothing wrong with Benny. He just can't read or write." Since the mother spoke only broken English, had no formal schooling, and could not read or write, Benny did not appear deviant to her. From her perspective, he didn't have anything wrong with him.

The child from a high-status family has no such recourse. His primary social systems lie structurally close to the official social systems and tend to concur on what is acceptable. Definitions of his subnormality appear early in his life and are more universal in all his social groups. He cannot escape the retarded label because all his associates agree that he is a deviant.[21]

It is interesting to consider the role which a public institution for the retarded may play in making it possible for high-status persons to find a new location in social space. Observation of release histories of some persons discharged following work placement programs seems to reveal that an institution for the retarded may serve as a social leveler, an escalator which carries the high-status person away from high-status primary social systems and downward in the social structure. After a period of institutionalization, he may be released to occupy a position as a domestic servant, common laborer, or other of the less demanding roles found at the bottom of the social structure. Downward social mobility may well be a latent function of the public institution for the retarded which is seldom recognized. To a lesser extent this same process seems to operate when higher-status patients are placed in foster homes following a period of institutionalization. These homes are frequently found in less affluent neighborhoods and are run by persons of lower social status, often members of ethnic minorities.

In conclusion, tentative answers may be given to the three questions raised earlier in this discussion. "Who sees whom as retarded?" Within the social system perspective, it becomes clear that persons who are clinically similar may be defined quite differently by their primary social systems. The person from lower-status social systems is less likely to be perceived as mentally subnormal.

"What impact does this differential definition have on the life career of the person?" Apparently, these differential definitions do make a difference because the group which diverges most widely from official definitions is the group in which the most individuals are released from the institution to their families.

Finally, "What are the characteristics of the social systems which diverge most widely from official definitions?" These social systems seem to be characterized by low educational achievement, high levels of dependency, and high concentrations of ethnic minorities.

A social system perspective adds a useful dimension to the label "mental retardation" by its focus on the varied definitions which may be applied to behavior by different groups in society. For those interested in the care and treatment of persons officially labeled as mentally subnormal, it may be

21. Lewis Anthony Dexter, "On the Politics and Sociology of Stupidity in our Society" in *The Other Side: Perspectives on Deviance*, Howard S. Becker, ed. (Glencoe, Ill.: The Free Press, 1964), pp. 37-49.

beneficial in some cases to seek systematically to relocate such individuals in the social structure in groups which will not define them as deviant. Rather than insisting that a family adopt official definitions of abnormality, we may frequently find it advisable to permit them to continue to view the patient within their own frame of reference and thus make it easier for them to accept him.

28

DAVID MECHANIC

Some Implications of Illness Behavior for Medical Sampling

An adequate and representative sample is an important prerequisite for competent studies of etiologic processes in disease. Most medical studies, however, depend largely on populations of sick persons who come to clinics, hospitals, and other medical facilities for diagnosis and treatment. Such populations are accessible and convenient, and research based on them is relatively economical. Moreover, the assumption is often made that sampling problems are less acute when basic human processes are being studied. However, to the extent that known clinic and hospital populations are not representative of those having a particular disorder, and to the extent that selection of these persons as patients occurs on some *systematic basis*, biases that may lead to incorrect and unwarranted conclusions are introduced into studies.

The basic research problem to be posed, then, concerns the variables that affect the arrival of ill persons to medical settings for diagnosis and treatment. To the extent that there are systematic influences in referral practices, these must be taken into account in sampling patients for medical studies.

It is these considerations that make necessary studies of *illness behavior*. This term refers to the ways in which different symptoms may be variously perceived, evaluated, or acted (or not acted) upon by different kinds of persons. Whether by reason of earlier experiences with illness, differential training in recognition of symptoms, or whatever, some persons will make light of symptoms, shrug them off and avoid seeking medical care; others will respond to the slightest twinges of pain or discomfort by quickly seeking

Reprinted from the *New England Journal of Medicine*, 269 (1963), pp. 244-247, by permission of the author and publisher.

This paper is a modified version of a lecture presented at the University of Washington School of Medicine in February, 1963. The data presented were gathered with the assistance of a research grant (MF-8516) from the National Institute of Mental Health, National Institutes of Health, United States Public Health Service.

446

such medical care as is available. Variables affecting illness behavior come into play before medical scrutiny and even determine whether diagnosis and treatment will begin at all. Differential patterns of illness behavior may thus be responsible for making "hospital" and "clinic" cases of particular diagnostic categories inadequate populations for the study of particular disease processes.

Examples are two kinds of studies in which such considerations may be important. In one study[1] long-term patterns of health and illness were examined among 2934 employees of a large organization that had maintained excellent medical records for its personnel. The investigators found that, over long periods, the frequency of known illness (including the more common ones and regardless of the body system involved) was closely associated with various occupational and social conditions that frustrated the needs and aspirations of the employees studied or placed heavy or conflicting demands upon them, or both. As a consequence, the authors regarded social and interpersonal stresses as important etiologic factors in "all forms of illness," and they concluded, "In the population in general, those who are attempting to adapt to such difficult life situations are those who exhibit a major proportion of the illnesses occurring in the adult population."[2] It is important to note, however, that if stress and conflicting demands are important factors influencing the initiation of a medical visit, one would expect to find that known patients—regardless of illness—tend to be under stress. The etiologic significance of stress, therefore, is still subject to question.

A second type of study to which these comments are relevant concerns the incidence of somatic disease in psychiatric patients. Examination of clinic records show correlations between status as a psychiatric patient and a high incidence of somatic disease, but etiologic significance cannot be established from such data. Although investigators who work in this area prefer a "psychosomatic" explanation, no study available adequately rules out the more simple hypothesis: that persons who are likely to bring mood and behavior complaints to a psychiatric clinic are also likely to be sensitive to physical symptomatology.

The most recent and probably the most adequate study in this area[3] attempted to provide a control group "whose medical records were the next like-sex in the medical clinic files." Since there were cards in the file

1. L. E. Hinkle, Jr., and H. G. Wolff, "Health and Social Environment: "Experimental Investigations," in *Explorations in Social Psychiatry*, A. H. Leighton, J. A. Clausen, and R. W. Wilson, eds. (New York: Basic Books, 1957), pp. 105-132.

2. *Ibid.* p. 132.

3. Interdisciplinary Research Conference, University of Wisconsin, 1961. *Physiological Correlates of Psychological Disorder: Proceedings Sponsored by the Wisconsin Psychiatric Institute and the Department of Psychiatry of the University of Wisconsin Medical Center*, R. Roessler and N. S. Greenfield, eds. (Madison: University of Wisconsin Press, 1962), pp. 257-267.

for the entire possible population using that medical clinic (a university student-health service), this was presumably an adequate control. The control group, however, is inadequate in two ways: information is lacking about whether persons in the control population actually used other medical facilities available to them rather than those of the clinic;[4] and no information is provided to demonstrate that the propensity to use medical services is similar among patient and control populations.

It is important to recognize the deficiencies in the control group, since on superficial examination the design of the study appears adequate. Persons in the patient group are known users of the medical facility being studied. No information is provided for the "controls." A void record, therefore, may mean either that the student did not report illness to any medical facility *or that he used some other medical facility*. Since the clinic studied is not used by the entire student population (with a significant number of students using other facilites), and since there are systematic differences in those who choose private physicians as opposed to the clinic, the control group is not a *true control*. Similarly, since persons in the patient group are "known" users of the available facilities, it is probably correct to assume that, as a group, they have a higher propensity to use medical facilities than the "controls."

The importance of sampling is of great relevance to all areas of medical inquiry, and some of the biases inherent in clinic populations were therefore examined through an investigation of 614 male students at a large university. The subjects were approximately the same age, and lived and ate their meals in the same university dormitory. Because of school requirements, the academic demands made upon them were also substantially similar. Data were obtained by means of both a questionnaire and an investigation of their medical records.[5] With the use of a series of hypothetical questions concerning whether these students would seek advice from a physician if they had various degrees of fever students with varied inclinations to seek medical attention could be distinguished. The concern of the investigators became threefold: to determine the relation between the inclination to seek medical attention and the actual use of medical facilities

4. In a study of 781 respondents carried out at the same university it was found that 48 percent of the students had never used the student health service, and that approximately 25 percent used local private physicians not associated with the university. Each of the students was asked the following question: "If you became sick and felt you needed medical care, how likely would you be to visit the University Health Service?" The replies were as follows: 43 percent, "very likely"; 23 percent, "fairly likely"; 18 percent, "not very likely"; and 16 percent, "not at all likely."

5. Since data in this study were obtained from both medical records and students, it was possible to determine who used physicians other than those provided by the medical clinic. Since this particular university was somewhat separated from the nearest community, approximately 90 percent of the students reported that they utilized the student health facilities. When students reported using other physicians this information was taken into account in the analysis.

as measured by the students' health records; to ascertain the social and personal factors associated with the expressed inclination to seek medical advice; and to find the diagnostic categories most affected by differential inclinations to seek medical advice. Since the findings have been reviewed in other papers,[6] the present discussion is exclusively concerned with the findings most relevant to the sampling problem.

One of the main concerns of the research was the effects of "stress" on illness and illness behavior. The concept of stress has not been adequately or precisely defined in behavioral studies. In general, it seems to signify a state of affairs characterized by anxiety, discomfort, emotional tension, and difficulty in adjustment; it may be temporary and situational, or protracted and recurrent. In the present study stress was operationally defined as the subject's report of the frequency with which he was bothered by "loneliness" and "nervousness." To evaluate the adequacy of this stress index, the responses were analyzed for such other responses as might be regarded as indicators of stress: reports of worry; difficulty in college; general dissatisfaction; perception of the college environment as stressful; and trouble with headaches, indigestion, and inability to sleep. In each case the stress index was significantly related to these measures at better than the 0.001 level. Despite its obvious defects the stress index does discriminate between various levels of reported stress on the part of respondents.[7]

Both "perceived stress" and the measure of inclination to use medical facilities (hypothetical questions), taken individually, were found to be significantly related to the frequency of medical visits. Table 28.1 shows the relation between "perceived stress" and frequency of visits to the student health service, as a control of the inclination to utilize medical facilities. An examination of this table reveals that, for the high-inclination group, stress is significantly related to medical visits, and that although there is an observable tendency in the same direction among low-inclination persons, the effect is a smaller one, and not statistically significant. This suggests that among those who are already inclined to use medical facilities, stress plays an important part in the initiation of a medical visit. Of those persons with a high inclination to use medical facilities and under high stress, 73 percent were in the high-visit group; only 30 percent of the low-inclination persons

6. D. Mechanic, "Concept of Illness Behavior," *Journal of Chronic Diseases* 15 (1962), 189-194; D. Mechanic and E. H. Volkart, "Stress, Illness Behavior and the Sick Role," *American Sociological Review*, 26 (1961), 51-58; D. Mechanic and E. H. Volkhart, "Illness Behavior and Medical Diagnoses," *Journal of Health and Human Behavior*, 1 (Summer, 1960), 86-94.

7. Since data were collected from respondents on only one occasion, test-retest reliability for the independent measures could not be obtained. However, lack of reliability on these measures would tend to contribute to random effects and therefore would probably lower the predicted relations. The results, however, should be viewed with some caution since statistical correlation does not exclude the hypothesis that medical experience may influence responses on the independent variables.

under low stress were in the high-visit group. Reorganization of the data in Table 28.1 shows that, when level of stress is controlled, inclination to use medical facilities is a significant factor affecting medical visits in all stress groups. Frequency of medical visits is a function, then, of both inclination to use medical facilities and stress, but, in general, the inclination to use medical facilities is the more influential variable.

Table 28.1. Relation between level of stress and frequency of visits to student health center with expressed inclination to utilize medical facilities controlled

Frequency of Visits	Level of Stress			
	high	moderately high	moderately low	low
	%	%	%	%
High inclination to use medical facilities (N = 310):				
High (3 or more)	73	60	49	46
Low (0-2)	27	40	51	54
N	(30)	(70)	(154)	(56)
x^2 (3 df) = 8.46; p < 0.05.				
Low inclination to use medical facilities (N = 284):				
High (3 or more)	42	40	34	30
Low (0-2)	58	60	66	70
N	(19)	(67)	(125)	(73)
x^2 (3 df) = 2.12; p < 0.70.				

Although the investigation showed a relation between the inclination to use medical facilities (hypothetical questions) and actual use of such facilities it was also concerned with evaluating how various diagnostic categories were related to differential inclinations to use medical facilities. In the analysis of diagnostic data illnesses were classified on a matrix that permitted focus on illness "sites," irrespective of etiology (such as gastrointestinal tract and skin), on a given etiologic category, irrespective of site (for example, viral or traumatic), or on the possible combinations of etiologies and sites (such as viral respiratory or bacterial skin). Since the population studied was a comparatively healthy one, many of the diagnostic conditions more common in older populations did not comprise significant categories for analysis. Sixteen diagnostic categories were used in the analysis of the data. For the purposes of this paper it is not necessary to review all these data, but rather to show how illness behavior may influence the adequacy of samples drawn from clinic cases. Table 28.2 shows the relation between the measure of the inclination to use medical facilities and a viral respiratory diagnostic status. Similar patterns were observed for all respiratory, all viral, all bacterial and bacterial respiratory categories.

On examination of Table 28.2 it becomes apparent that if a sample of persons with viral respiratory conditions was taken from the particular clinic population studied, it would be overrepresented with persons of high and moderately high inclinations to use medical facilities. Such persons are known to differ from those with lower inclination in systematic ways: social class; religious and cultural background; and extent of stress.[8] It is also likely that they differ in various other personality and behavior traits. Various incorrect conclusions are possible on the basis of such biased samples—for example, since stress is a factor that helps produce a medical visit and medical diagnosis, it is common to find that patients with various pathologic conditions are under stress. The investigator must be particularly careful, however, to refrain from arguing that stress is an important etiologic factor in these illnesses on the basis of such data. The hypothesis may have some merit, but such data on the basis of analysis of clinic cases are not adequate for investigating the hypothesis.

Table 28.2. Viral respiratory conditions among various inclination groups

Level of Expressed Inclination	Viral Respiratory Conditions			
	none	1	2 or more	total
	%	%	%	%
High (N = 89)	45	37	18	100
Moderately high (N = 225)	54	32	15	101
Moderately low (N = 87)	67	25	8	100
Low (N = 202)	73	21	5	99

x^2 (6 df) = 31.16; p < 0.001.

In the analysis of other diagnostic categories considerable bias was found, the magnitude tending to be related to the extent to which the various diagnostic categories were routine. Categories of illness that occurred frequently among the population, that were relatively familiar and relatively predictable, and that did not threaten serious danger were those showing the most extreme bias. Illness behavior seemed to play a more important part in medical visits for symptoms usually regarded as not very serious. With more extreme and serious illness it is likely that the role of illness behavior is somewhat less important, although it may be closely related to delay in treatment. In any event, the data clearly show the importance of considering the role of illness behavior in relation to the adequacy of samples drawn from clinic and hospital populations.

In short, the intent of this paper is not to dispute the validity of particular theoretical positions regarding the etiology of disease; the intent is to emphasize the necessity of adequate and reliable data for substantiating

---

8. Mechanic, *op. cit.*, and Mechanic and Volkart (1960.1961), *op. cit.*

such views. Often, the conclusions based on studies derive more from the investigator's theoretical positions than from the data themselves. It is particularly important that studies be designed precisely enough to rule out obvious alternative explanations.

The core of the argument is that clinic and hospital cases used for the study of some illnesses, especially the more "routine" ones, may represent highly select and biased cases from which generalization to the larger group of persons in the general population having that illness may not be possible. The observation, for example, that persons who are ill (with whatever diagnosis) are also under stress is inadequate for any assertion of causality. Those with similar medical conditions who are not under stress may not seek medical advice. For some illnesses, at least, appearance in medical statistics may be a result as much of patterns of illness behavior and situational events as of the symptoms experienced.

Finally, it is extremely important that certain kinds of hypotheses be tested with the use of "normal populations." The epidemiologic approach not only is valuable for exploration but also may be used fruitfully for investigating specific hypotheses involving expectation systems, social attitudes, and other characteristics of personality and group related to disease.

29

DEREK L. PHILLIPS

Data Collection as a Social Process: Its Implications for "True Prevalence" Studies of Mental Illness

As it has become more and more apparent that official records and statistics provide an unsatisfactory estimate as to the number of people who are mentally ill,[1] investigators have increasingly turned to the utilization of other techniques for determining the "true prevalence" of mental illness in American society.[2] Several studies have utilized field interviews of non-hospitalized populations, conducted by nonmedical personnel, as a means of obtaining data concerning the quantity and quality of psychiatric disorder. Probably the best known of these investigations are the "Midtown"[3] and "Stirling County"[4] studies. Among other investigations utilizing field interviews for estimating mental illness are those by Dohrenwend, Elinson, Gurin, et al.; Leighton et al.; Manis and his associates; Phillips; and researchers at the University of Puerto Rico.[5]

I wish to thank Eliot Freidson for his helpful comments on an earlier draft of this paper.

1. Data on treatment rates are unsatisfactory in that they are, among other things, dependent upon the availability of treatment facilities, and public attitudes toward those utilizing them.

2. For a discussion of several of these studies, see Bruce P. Dohrenwend and Barbara Snell Dohrenwend, "The Problem of Validity in Field Studies of Psychological Disorder," *Journal of Abnormal Psychology*, 70 (February, 1965), 52-69; and Bruce P. Dohrenwend, "Social Status and Psychiatric Disorder: An Issue of Substance and an Issue of Method," *American Sociological Review*, 31 (February, 1966), 14-34.

3. Thomas S. Langner and Stanley T. Michael, *Life Stress and Mental Health* (New York: The Free Press, 1963); Leo Srole, Thomas S. Langner, Stanley T. Michael, Marvin K. Opler, and Thomas A. C. Rennie, *Mental Health in the Metropolis: The Midtown Study* (New York: McGraw-Hill, 1962).

4. Alexander H. Leighton, *My Name Is Legion* (New York: Basic Books, 1959); Dorothea C. Leighton, J. S. Harding, D. B. Maklin, A. M. MacMillian, and A. H. Leighton, *The Character of Danger* (New York: Basic Books, 1963).

5. Bruce P. Dohrenwend, *op. cit.*; Jack Elinson, Elena Padilla, and Marvin E. Perkins, *Public Images of Mental Health Services* (New York: Mental Health Materials Center, 1967); Gerald Gurin, Joseph Veroff, and Shiela Feld, *Americans View Their Mental Health* (New York: Basic Books, 1960); Alexander H. Leighton, T. A. Lambo, C. C. Hughes, D. C. Leighton, J. M. Murphy, and D. B. Macklin, *Psychiatric*

Although the Midtown and Stirling County studies employed other measures as well, all of these true prevalence studies relied heavily on psychiatric inventories. All contain questions asking people: "Do you feel somewhat apart or alone even among friends?"; "Do you feel that nothing turns out for you the way you want it to?"; "Do you have personal worries that get you down physically?" In other words, psychiatric evaluations are made on the basis of responses to interviewers' inquiries regarding certain feelings, experiences, and behaviors that are considered by "experts" to be indicative of mental disorder or malfunctioning. This means, of course, that figures concerning the true prevalence "rates" of mental illness in general populations ultimately rest on people's *reporting* or *admitting to* the kinds of symptoms (feelings, experiences, etc.) contained in these inventories.

Is it correct to assume that people *will* report or reveal their troubles to a stranger in an interview situation? Or is there reason to believe that many persons may be less than completely open in their responses? In order to answer these questions, it is necessary to consider first what happens when people come together in "everyday" situations. I will then review briefly some of the available evidence pertaining to what occurs in the collection of much social science data.

When an individual is in the presence of other people, he will tend to organize his behavior in light of what he feels the "others" expect is appropriate for someone like him in that kind of situation. The individual considers the meaning his behavior will have for others; he assesses his proposed behavior in light of the responses it will evoke in them; and then acts (or changes his action) so as to achieve the anticipated responses that he wants. Other actors in the situation do the same. In short, people take account of one another in most social situations and act according to their definitions of the situation.

The above is now almost a banality in the sociological literature. For we all know that an individual's attitudes, opinions, and behavior are influenced by his perceptions and evaluations of the situations in which he finds himself. Despite the fact that we all "know" this, many sociologists seem unwilling to view the administration of an interview in a field survey or the filling out of a questionnaire as forms of social interaction—either real or symbolic.

Although social investigators are sensitive to the importance of   ascer-

---

Disorder Among the Yoruba (Ithaca, N.Y.: Cornell University Press, 1963); J. G Manis, M. J. Brawer, C. L. Hunt, and L. C. Kercher, "Estimating the Prevalence of Mental Illness," *American Sociological Review,* 29 (February, 1964), 84-89; Derek L. Phillips, "The 'True Prevalence' of Mental Illness in a New England State," *Community Mental Health Journal,* 2 (Spring, 1966), 35-40; University of Puerto Rico School of Medicine and Department of Health and Welfare, "A Continuing Master Sample Survey for Puerto Rico as a Community Health Service Project," reported in Elinson et al., *op. cit.*

taining both objective and subjective kinds of data—or, if you like, the "facts" and the respondents' perceptions of the facts—they are frequently insensitive to the possibility (or probability) that the respondents' replies to their questions will be influenced by people's perceptions of what the interviewers want, or what is right, or best, or most desirable, as *they* *define* "right" or "best" or "desirable," and as they perceive these are defined by the interviewer, by significant others, or by people into whose hands the results may fall. While Goode and Hatt state that "interviewing is a process of social interaction,"[6] and Hyman et al., note that the data obtained in the interview are "derived in an interpersonal situation,"[7] sociologists generally fail to recognize the extent to which these "miniature social situations"[8] are characterized by the *same* social processes that are found in other everyday activities. As Riecken has noted: "The process of collecting data about human behavior is itself a social process and shares features in common with other situations and events of human interaction."[9]

Webb and his associates have estimated that about 90 percent of social science research is based upon interviews and questionnaires.[10] This means that most of our scientific conclusions are based upon materials secured by asking an individual to reveal—either in his own words or through acceptance or rejection of standardized items—his feelings, beliefs, attitudes, or experiences regarding some issue, idea, behavior, or other area of interest to the investigator. It seems especially important, therefore, that close scrutiny be given to possible sources of bias and invalidity in interview and questionnaire studies.

Whenever one engages in social research, there will always be nonrelevant factors which may influence the respondents' reports. Cicourel puts it this way:

> The respondent's and interviewer's stock of knowledge and their definition of the situation will determine their mutual reaction to the question posed. The relevances not related to the substance of the interview *per se* will also determine the amount of extra-interview bias or error which exists. This is a necessary consequence of not treating each other only as objects for rational consideration; their attractiveness or unattractiveness to one another, their bodily presence, the social, physical, and role distance, all produce bias and

6. William J. Goode and Paul K. Hatt, *Methods in Social Research* (New York: McGraw-Hill, 1952), p. 186.

7. Herbert Hyman, W. J. Cobb, J. J. Feldman, C. W. Hart, and C. H. Stember, *Interviewing in Social Research* (Chicago: University of Chicago Press, 1954), p. 20.

8. Herbert Hyman, "Inconsistencies in Attitude Measurement," *Journal of Social Issues*, 5 (1949).

9. Henry W. Riecken, "A Program for Research on Experiments in Social Psychology," in N. F. Washburne, ed., *Decision, Values, and Groups*, vol. 2 (New York: Pergamon Press, 1962), p. 25.

10. Eugene J. Webb, Donald T. Campbell, Richard D. Schwartz, and Lee Sechrest, *Unobtrusive Measures: Nonreactive Research in the Social Sciences* (Chicago: Rand McNally, 1966), p. 1.

error *naturally* because these are basic to the structure of everyday conduct.[11]

These biases and errors which Cicourel mentions may, consequently, affect the validity of social science measuring instruments. Speaking of this problem as it pertains to the measurement of attitudes, Cook and Selltiz state that: "Ideally, the goal would be to develop one or more measures from which the effects of all possible determinants other than the attitude toward the relevant object would be removed."[12] While an attempt to remove these response determinants (or unwanted influences) is obviously a commendable goal, it is first necessary that they be *identified*. By and large, they are not clearly identified in the sociological literature. Although most books on social science methodology discuss various procedures for minimizing or avoiding the influence of factors other than those being considered in the research, these factors remain largely unspecified. In survey research, special attention is paid to the importance of assuring anonymity, emphasizing that our studies are "scientific," stressing the need for "honest" answers, creating rapport so that the respondents know that the interviwer will not "disapprove" of any response, assuring people that they are just a "number" and that their answers will be kept confidential, and selecting samples in the proper manner. But the student is hard-pressed to locate empirical evidence for the effects of undesired response determinants. Perhaps this should not be surprising in that the books and manuals are written by "true believers" who are not apt to raise serious doubts about the very techniques which they are discussing, and frequently advocating.

However, if the student were encouraged to look around, he would find that there is evidence which indicates that in the interview situation factors other than those being measured do affect people's responses. For instance, there are several studies pertaining to the influence of various interviewer characteristics: race,[13] age,[14] religion,[15] social class,[16] and the interactions of age and sex.[17] Several reports in the psychological literature pertain to laboratory experiments and have strong implications for survey research. These

11.   Aaron V. Cicourel, *Method and Measurement in Sociology* (New York: The Free Press, 1964), pp. 79-80.

12.   Stuart W. Cook and Claire Selltiz, "A Multiple-Indicator Approach to Attitude Measurement," *Psychological Bulletin,* 62 (July, 1964), 37.

13.   K. R. Athey, J. E. Coleman, A. P. Reitman, and J. Tang, "Two Experiments Showing the Effect of the Interviewer's Racial Background on Responses to Questionnaires Concerning Racial Issues," *Journal of Applied Psychology*, 44 (1960), 244-246.

14.   David Riesman and J. Ehrlich, "Age and Authority in the Interview." *Public Opinion Quarterly*, 25 (1961), 39-56.

15.   Hyman et al., *op. cit.*

16.   Gerhard E. Lenski and John C. Leggett, "Caste, Class, and Deference in the Research Interview," *American Journal of Sociology*, 65 (1960), 463-467; David Riesman, "Orbits of Tolerance, Interviewers and Elites," *Public Opinion Quarterly*, 20 (1956), 49-73.

17.   Mark Benney, David Riesman, and Shirley Star, "Age and Sex in the Interview," *American Journal of Sociology*, 63 (1956), 143-152.

studies show that the subject's behavior is influenced by the sex of the experimenter,[18] his race,[19] his personality,[20] and whether he is perceived as friendly or hostile.[21] Other response determinants in laboratory experiments are experimenter bias (the unintended communication of his hypothesis), which has been studied by several investigators,[22] evaluation apprehension,[23] and the subject's desire to "put his best foot forward."[24]

In addition to the effects of certain attributes or characteristics of the interviewer and experimenter, there is also the influence of the "social distance" between the interviewer and respondent,[25] of response set,[26] and of social desirability.[27] "Response set" refers to the tendency of some persons to agree (or disagree) with items regardless of their content, while "social desirability" refers to people's tendency to endorse (or reject) items that appear socially desirable or undesirable.

18. A. Binder, D. McConnell, and Nancy A. Sjoholm, "Verbal Conditioning as a Function of Experimenter Characteristics," *Journal of Abnormal and Social Psychology*, 55 (1957), 309-314.

19. I. Katz, J. M. Robinson, E. G. Epps, and P. Waly, "The Influence of the Experimenter and Instructions Upon the Expression of Hostility by Negro Boys," *Journal of Social Issues*, 20 (1964), 54-59.

20. A. Sapolsky, "Effect of Interpersonal Relationships Upon Verbal Conditioning," *Journal of Abnormal and Social Psychology*, 60 ((1960), 241-246.

21. I. G. Sarason and J. Minard, "Interrelationships Among Subject, Experimenter, and Situational Variables," *Journal of Abnormal and Social Psychology*, 67 (1963), 87-91.

22. Neil Friedman, *The Social Nature of Psychological Research* (New York: Basic Books, 1967); Martin T. Orne, "The Nature of Hypnosis," *Journal of Abnormal and Social Psychology*, 58 (1959), 277-299; Martin T. Orne, "On the Social Psychological Experiment: With Particular Reference to Demand Characteristics and Their Implications," *American Psychologist*, 17 (1962), 776-783; Robert Rosenthal, "The Effect of the Experimenter on the Results of Psychological Research," in Bruce A. Maher, ed., *Progress in Experimental Personality Research* (New York: Academic Press, 1964); Robert Rosenthal, *Experimenter Effects in Behavioral Research* (New York: Appleton-Century-Crofts, 1966); Robert Rosenthal and K. Fode, "Psychology of the Scientist: V. Three Experiments in Experimenter Bias," *Psychological Reports*, 12 (April, 1963), 491-511.

23. Milton J. Rosenberg, "When Dissonance Fails: On Eliminating Evaluation Apprehension from Attitude Measurement," *Journal of Personality and Social Psychology*, 1 (January, 1965), 28-42; Milton J. Rosenberg, "The Conditions and Consequences of Evaluation Apprehension," in Robert Rosenthal and R. Rostow, eds., *Sources of Artifact in Social Research* (New York: Academic Press, 1969).

24. Riecken, *op.cit.*

25. Barbara Snell Dohrenwend, John Colombotos, and Bruce P. Dohrenwend, "Social Distance and Interviewer Effects," *Public Opinion Quarterly*, 32 (Fall, 1968), 410-422.

26. Arthur Couch and Kenneth Keniston, "Agreeing Response Set and Social Desirability," *Journal of Abnormal and Social Psychology*, 62 (January, 1961), 175-179; Arthur Couch and Kenneth Keniston, "Yeasayers and Naysayers: Agreeing Response Set as a Personality Variable," *Journal of Abnormal and Social Psychology*, 60 (March, 1960), 151-174; Lee J. Cronbach, "Further Evidence on Response Sets and Test Design," *Educational and Psychological Measurement*, (1950), 3-31.

27. E. L. Edwards, "Social Desirability and Personality Test Construction," in B. M. Bass and I. A. Berg, eds., *Objective Approaches to Psychology* (New York: Van Nostrand, 1959), pp. 101-116.

The above studies all represent investigations which attempted to ascertain the manner in which certain factors existing in the interview or laboratory situation affect people's responses. Certainly the list of factors is sufficiently long so as to give pause to anyone ready to accept the validity of all social science research. But there is another source of evidence which must also be considered in assessing the extent of error in our research. I am referring to those investigations showing sharp discrepancies between what people say and what they do.[28] If we assume that there should be fairly strong relationships between attitudes and behavior (and, after all, we are usually most interested in overt behavior—although we seldom study it), we might anticipate that so many instances of a lack of relationship would have generated numerous investigations to discover why this should be the case. For the most part, such investigations are rather scarce in the literature of sociology.

The studies mentioned seem to suggest that many of our findings may be due to factors other than those of concern to the investigator: for example, characteristics of the interviewer (age, sex, social class, etc.), situational factors (social distance between the interviewer and respondent, for instance), and respondent bias (response set and assessments of social desirability). Furthermore, the meaning of the responses may be other than sociologists frequently assume, in that attitudes and behavior are often not strongly related to one another. While the factors cited as error and bias may occur as a "natural" consequence of individuals interpreting one another as social objects, the evidence cited should make us quite skeptical about the accuracy and meaningfulness of much sociological research.

Studies of Deviant Behavior

If there is reason to question the accuracy of much social science research, it would seem that this should especially be the case with studies of "deviant" behavior. For as Maccoby and Maccoby note:

> when people are being interviewed (or are filling out questionnaires) directly concerning behavior about which there is a strong expectation of social approval or

28. R. Bastide and P. Van den Berghe, "Stereotypes, Norms, and Interracial Behavior in Sao Paulo, Brazil," *American Sociological Review*, 22 (December, 1957), 689-694; Wilbur B. Brookover and John B. Holland, "An Inquiry into the Meaning of Minority Group Attitude Expressions," *American Sociological Review*, 17 (April, 1952), 196-202; Irwin Deutscher, "Words and Deeds: Social Science and Social Policy," *Social Problems*, 13 (Winter, 1966), 235-254; Howard J. Ehrlich and James W. Rinehart, "A Brief Report on the Methodology of Sterotype Research," *Social Forces*, 43 (May, 1965), 564-575; Linton C. Freeman and Turkoz Ataov, "Invalidity of Indirect and Direct Measures Toward Cheating," *Journal of Personality*, 28 (December, 1960), 443-447; Edward Hassinger and Robert L. McNamara, "Stated Opinion and Actual Practice in Health Behavior in a Rural Area," *The Midwest Sociologist*, (May, 1957), 93-97; Richard T. LaPiere, "Attitudes vs. Actions," *Social Forces*, 13 (March, 1934), 230-237; Lawrence S. Linn, "Verbal Attitudes and

disapproval, and in which there is considerable ego involvement, they then tend to err in the direction of idealizing their behavior.[29]

There have been very few attempts to examine this tendency toward idealization in sociological studies of deviant or disapproved behavior. Hence, it seems important to consider at some length a recent study which had this task as its goal. This study by Clark and Tifft was concerned with validating a self-administered questionnaire pertaining to several types of deviant behavior; they wanted to know whether people who had "really" committed various acts would admit to them.[30] While any attempt to validate a social science measure always encounters problems, this study seems to be on relatively solid ground. They first asked people whether or not they had ever engaged in each of thirty-five different deviant behaviors. Then they asked these same people to submit to a polygraph ("lie-detector") examination. Prior to their taking the examination, each person was interviewed and told that he could select his questionnaire and make whatever modifications (in private) were necessary to achieve 100 percent accuracy. In the words of the authors, Clark and Tifft:

> By the time the polygraph examinations were completed, all respondents had made corrections to their questionnaire responses. About 58 percent of the total number of changes between the initial questionnaire responses and the final responses were made at the time of the personal "interview" and 42 percent during the polygraph examination. Three-fourths of all changes increased the frequency of admitted deviance, the remainder were in the opposite direction.[31]

If we accept the use of the polygraph as an appropriate validation technique—and there is reason to believe that a properly administered polygraph has great accuracy[32] —we must conclude that many people do not tell the truth about certain deviant behaviors in self-administered questionnaires. For instance, of those whom the polygraph indicated "Had sex relations with a person of the same sex," only 14 percent revealed this fact on the original questionnaire.[33] Asked whether they had "falsi-

---

Overt Behavior: A Study of Racial Discrimination," *Social Forces*, 43 (March, 1965), 353-364; W. J. McGuire, "Attitudes and Opinions," *Annual Review of Psychology*, 17 (1966), 475-514; L. C. Robbins, "The Accuracy of Parental Recall on Aspects of Child Development and Child Rearing Practices," *Journal of Abnormal and Social Psychology*, 66 (1963), 261-270; Charles R. Tittle and Richard J. Hill, "Attitude Measurement and Prediction of Behavior: An Evaluation of Conditions and Measurement Techniques," *Sociometry*, 30 (June, 1967), 199-213; Michael Zunich, "A Study of the Relationship Between Child Rearing Attitudes and Maternal Behavior," *Journal of Experimental Education*, 30 (December, 1961), 231-241.

29. Eleanor Maccoby and Nathan Maccoby, "The Interview: A Tool of Social Science," in Gardner Lindzey, ed., *Handbook of Social Psychology*, vol. 1 (Reading, Mass.: Addison-Wesley, 1954), p. 482.

30. John P. Clark and Larry L. Tifft, "Polygraph and Interview Validation of Self-Reported Deviant Behavior," *American Sociological Review*, 31 (August, 1966), 516-523.

31. *Ibid.*, p. 520.

32. *Ibid.*, pp. 519-520.

33. This figure is based on my calculations from the data presented from item number 21 on page 518 in Clark and Tifft, *op. cit.*

fied information while filling out an application form or report," 43 percent of those whom the polygraph showed had done so denied it initially.[34] And of those whom the polygraph indicated had "masturbated," one-third initially failed to admit it.[35]

Clark and Tifft attempted to locate some of the factors involved in these "systematic errors," as they termed them. They assumed that deviant behavior might be in conflict with either personal or group norms to which individuals usually conform. Therefore, the respondents were questioned about their feelings as to the acceptability of the behaviors described in each of the items. In 66 percent of the instances in which the individuals did not initially admit an act but later did, they stated that the act was "never permissable" according to their own feelings. And in 36 percent of the instances in which respondents initially denied but later admitted an act, they stated that the act was "never permissible" according to the perceived standards of their reference group.[36] Clark and Tifft conclude from this that: "There is strong evidence that errors on questionnaires are directly associated with perceived discrepancies between individual acts and personal and group norms. The errors represent an attempt to make reported behavior compatible with perceived norms."[37]

I have dealt at length with this validation study of self-reported behavior because it demonstrates so forcefully the doubtful accuracy of responses to questions about deviant behaviors. Speaking of their attempt to validate items used in many delinquency estimates, Clark and Tifft conclude: "Those items most frequently used on delinquency scales were found to be rather inaccurate. These findings dictate the need for concern for the validity of indicators and the patterns of response bias to self-report data-gathering techniques."[38]

With so much inaccuracy in the case of a self-administered questionnaire where the individual can answer questions without having to face an interviewer, what should we expect of the situation where the respondent must consider the interviewer's presence? Let us consider, as an instance, survey studies of the "true prevalence" of homosexual behavior. In American society, when two adult males are seen kissing, holding hands, or engaged in sexual relations with one another, it is likely that they will be labeled homosexual[39] and probably treated as such by others who have witnessed, or heard about, their behavior. They may also come to define themselves as homosexual, which they might not have done were it not for the public definition. Now imagine a young man being interviewed in a field survey

34. Based on my calculations from the data for item number 25.
35. Calculated from data for item 29.
36. Clark and Tifft, *op. cit.*, p. 522.
37. *Ibid.*, p. 522.
38. *Ibid.*, p. 523.
39. See, for example, John I. Kitsuse, "Societal Reaction to Deviant Behavior: Problems of Theory and Method," in Howard S. Becker, ed., *The Other Side* (New York: The Free Press, 1963), pp. 87-102.

—typically by a young graduate student or by a middle-class housewife. For purposes of argument, let us say that the young man *has* had sexual relations with another male but has never been witnessed or found out by others (that is, he is not a "deviant"). The interviewer asks him if he has ever engaged in sexual relations with another male. Assuming that he is aware of the societal definition of sexual relations with another male as evidence of homosexuality, he may very well answer no. If he does answer "no" (that is, lies), he might feel somewhat ashamed for not having told the truth, and his sense of integrity may perhaps suffer. On the other hand, if he were to answer "yes," he might feel virtuous for having told the truth. But by answering affirmatively, he would also have placed himself in a position where he could be labeled homosexual and where he would risk the interviewer's disapproval, and where he would, by admitting it to himself in the presence of another, *define himself* as homosexual.

The above example illustrates the fact that in the interview situation, as in other social situations, the individual (in this case, the respondent) must make an assessment as to the rewards, costs, and profits he may realize by responding in a given manner.[40] He then strives to perform in such a way as to maximize the profits to be earned in his exchange with the interviewer. The interviewer and the situation itself are, therefore, appraised in terms of potential profit to the respondent (in terms of the ratio of costs and rewards).

But what are the rewards that respondents seek from their interaction with an interviewer in a field survey? One clear reward is a positive evaluation from the interviewer. The respondent, like all other people, wants to be evaluated in socially desirable terms. In short, he seeks *social approval*. And, as Blau notes: "A basic reward people seek in their associations is social approval. . . .[41] This means that the sheer fact of being interviewed is likely to arouse the respondent's needs and anticipations related to social evaluation.

While all people seek social approval, they obviously differ in the strength of their need to be thought well of by others. The implications of this are clearly stated by Crowne and Marlowe:

> for those whose need is high, we could assume a generalized expectancy that approval satisfactions are attained by engaging in behaviors which are culturally sanctioned and approved. . . .[I]t is simply not considered desirable in the contemporary social milieu to indicate on a test that one is anxious, frustrated, unhappy, and beset by all sorts of strange thoughts and impulses. It is not consistent behavior if one is dependent upon the acceptance, recognition, and approval of others.[42]

40. George C. Homans, "Bringing Man Back In," *American Sociological Review*, 29 (December, 1964), 809-818.

41. Peter Blau, *Exchange and Power* (New York: John Wiley, 1964), p. 17.

42. D. P. Crowne and D. Marlowe, *The Approval Motive* (New York: John Wiley, 1964), p. 7.

Thus we should anticipate that individuals will bend their responses to serve their need for social approval. Crowne and Marlowe have shown that persons with a high need for social approval are more sensitive than others to perceived situational demands and are more likely to respond affirmatively to social influences; they tend to terminate psychotherapy more quickly than people with less need for social approval; and they produce less revealing projective-test protocols.[43] It appears, then, that individuals who are high in the need for social approval are more conforming and cautious, and their responses are more normatively anchored, than is the case with persons less in need of social approval.

In addition to the influence of the need for approval (and other individual needs or goals) in determining behavior, there are the effects of people's *expectancies* and the *meaning of the situation* for them.[44] By expectancies, I mean people's assessments as to how their behavior or interview responses will be evaluated. The situation itself, of course, serves to influence an individual's expectancies in that his "definition of the situation" determines his assessment of the rewards and costs ensuing from various behaviors or responses. People's expectations with regard to obtaining social approval in the interview are obviously dependent partially on whether they define the interview situation as an examination of their knowledge, opinions, attitudes, moral worth, health, or emotional stability.

Although in the past few pages I have given some attention to the effects of differences in the need for social approval on people's responses, in the remainder of the paper I will no longer be concerned with these differences. Rather, I will assume that *all* people seek the approval of others and that this need is randomly distributed in the population. My assumption about the universal need for social approval is, I think, reasonable. As to my confidence in the assumption regarding the random distribution of this need, there appears to be little conclusive evidence regarding the antecedents and determinants of the strength of the approval need. Therefore, it seems safe to make the assumption of a random distribution—especially since it allows for an emphasis in the following discussion on other influences on people's responses, with need for approval assumed to be *held constant*.

Let us turn, then, to a further consideration of the ways in which people's responses may be affected by their definition of the situation and their, consequent, expectations regarding the profits ensuing from different responses. A question of prime importance here is whether or not people differ in their perceptions as to the *purpose* and *implications* of the interview. It seems reasonable to argue that if people do correctly perceive

43. *Ibid.*

44. J. B. Rotter, "Some Implications of a Social Learning Theory for the Prediction of Goal Directed Behavior From Testing Procedures," *Psychological Review*, 67 (1960), 301-316.

the purpose and implications of certain kinds of questions, they may, because of a need for approval, distort or repress certain kinds of behaviors or responses.

Studies of Mental Illness

My concern here is with whether or not people's location in the social structure (their sex, ethnicity, or social class position) may influence their definition of the interview situation and their expectancies in such a way that these, in turn, affect their responses. That is, I am concerned with some possible sources of "error" in psychiatric interviews in survey research. There are obviously other sources of errors in these interviews, but my focus is on some which have not received much attention in field studies of mental illness. My interest here is in "constant" rather than "random" errors. While validity is affected by both types of error, random (or variable) errors are less troublesome than constant or systematic ones. Probably because of this, most sociologists seem content to assume that errors are random unless proven otherwise.

First, let us ask to what extent people differ in their knowledge or awareness that these inventories contain questions pertaining to their mental health status. That is, are people's abilities to correctly define the situation as one in which they are being psychiatrically evaluated systematically related to their position in the social structure? This is a difficult question, and I have no ready answer. But it would certainly seem that there may be a systematic relationship between people's socioeconomic status, for instance, and their ability to recognize the purpose of the questions contained in mental health inventories. Individuals occupying a high social class position are probably better able than others to correctly define the situation as one in which their mental health is being assessed. Because of their greater education, they are more likely than people with less schooling to have encountered similar instruments and measures as part of the content of their schooling (in sociology and psychology courses, for instance), as well as having experienced these as part of the application procedure for college and for jobs. Not only are they more likely than less-educated and lower-class persons to have experience with such instruments, but they are also more apt to have been apprised as to the purpose of such instruments. As Gurin and others have noted, those with more education are more psychologically sophisticated in general, and are also better able to recognize the signs and symptoms of mental illness.[45] It seems correct to suggest, then, that there are class-linked differences in people's ability to recognize that questions concerning "nervousness," "trouble

---

45. Gurin et al., *op. cit.*; Derek L. Phillips, "Education, Psychiatric Sophistication, and the Rejection of Mentally Ill Help-Seekers," *Sociological Quarterly*, (Winter, 1967), 122-132.

sleeping," and so forth are being used as a means for estimating their mental health status. While these differences may also be systematically related to other variables such as age, sex, and ethnicity, it certainly seems correct to argue that they are highly likely to be related to socioeconomic status.

Consider now the question as to the *implications* of their responses. Here, too, it seems apparent that there are class-linked differences. Individuals who are more psychologically sophisticated are undoubtedly better able to recognize that their responses to inventory questions may be put to a number of uses. In the case of a work situation, they may be aware that replies to similar questions are frequently used as one basis for hiring, promotion, demotion, and firing. Similar differences in knowledge probably exist when people respond to verbal questioning or fill out self-administered questionnaires when applying for medical or life insurance or for a license to drive an automobile or own a gun. That is, individuals of higher class standing are probably more apt to recognize that responding affirmatively to questions that may classify them as mentally ill may have negative consequences for them. High-status persons, therefore, are more likely than others to have learned that the "correct," "right," or "best" answers regarding questions pertaining to mental health are those that deny any troubles or problems.

An example of the possible distortions of certain kinds of inventories is seen in the advice offered by W. H. Whyte to men who must take certain "personality" tests:

> When an individual is commanded by an organization to reveal his innermost feelings, he has a duty to himself to give answers that serve his self-interest rather than that of the Organization. In a word, he should cheat. . . . When in doubt about the beneficial answer to any question, repeat to yourself: I love my father and my mother, but my father a little bit more. I like things pretty much the way they are. I never worry about anything.[46]

In other words, Whyte is counseling people to decide about any item which alternative would result in the most socially favorable self-description. This is, of course, the same strategy which people with a high need for social approval have evoked for themselves.

In determining what is the most favorable (or least unfavorable) self-description, an individual must, in a sense, make an evaluation as to what is "appropriate" or "inappropriate" for someone occupying his status(es). Thus, he must ask himself: "What is expected of someone like me in a situation like this?" It seems clear that his perceptions as to what others expect of him is dependent on his sexual status, his ethnicity, and his social class position. Let us, then, consider three different studies that

46. William H. Whyte, Jr., *The Organization Man* (New York: Doubleday Anchor, 1956), p. 179, pp. 196-197.

are suggestive as to the influence of people's perceptions regarding "appropriate" behavior upon responses in an interview concerned with mental illness.

The first of these studies was concerned with the relationship between sexual status and psychiatric symptoms. In this investigation, Bernard Segal and I hypothesized that women would report more psychiatric symptoms than would men with the same number of physical illnesses.[47] We used the number of physical illnesses which people had as a rough indicator of "stress," for we wanted to compare the responses of men and women under approximately equal stress conditions. We reasoned that women would be more likely than men to *report* certain acts, behaviors, and so forth that lead to their being categorized as mentally ill. Our argument was simply that it is more culturally appropriate and acceptable in American society for women to be expressive about their difficulties.[48] As Barker and others have noted, it seems more appropriate for women in our society to have problems, especially problems of illness.[49] Women are granted more indulgence. The other side of our argument was that men are subject to different expectations. It is less permissible for them to be sick, emotionally disturbed, or upset, because they are expected to exert more self-control, and, if difficulties do occur, they are expected to bear them with greater equanimity.[50]

Data collected from two interviews (one year apart) with 278 adult respondents of a small New England town provided strong support for our hypothesis. We used as our measure of mental health status the 22-Item Mental Health Index developed by Langner[51] as part of the Midtown Studies and since used by other investigators.[52] On the mental health index, we found that a considerably greater percentage of women than men reported a high number of psychiatric symptoms. This was true for the data collected in each of the two interviews. These results were consistent with

47. Derek L. Phillips and Bernard E. Segal, "Sexual Status and Psychiatric Symptoms," *American Sociological Review*, 34 (February, 1969), 58-72.

48. See Kitsuse, *op. cit.*; Erwin L. Linn, "Agents, Timing, and Events Leading to Mental Hospitalizations," *Human Organization*, 20 (Summer, 1961), 90-99.

49. Roger Barker, *Adjustment to Physical Handicap and Illness* (New York: Social Science Research Council, 1953).

50. See, for instance, Richard R. Korn and Lloyd W. McKorkle, *Criminology and Penology* (New York: Holt, Rinehart and Winston, 1962); David Krech and Richard S. Crutchfield, *Individual in Society* (New York: McGraw-Hill, 1962); Talcott Parsons and Robert F. Bales, *Family, Socialization, and Interaction Process* (Glencoe, Ill.: The Free Press, 1955); Alice S. Rossi, "Equality Between the Sexes; An Immodest Proposal," *Daedalus*, 93 (Spring, 1964), 607-652; Morris Zelditch, Jr., "Role Differentiation in the Nuclear Family: A Comparative Study," in Norman W. Bell and Ezra Vogel, eds., *The Family* (Glencoe, Ill.: The Free Press, 1960).

51. Thomas S. Langner, "A Twenty-Two Item Screening Score of Psychiatric Symptoms Indicating Impairment," *Journal of Health and Human Behavior*, 3 (Winter, 1962), 269-276.

52. Dohrenwend, *op.cit.*; Elinson et al., *op.cit.*; Manis et al., *op.cit.*; Phillips, 1966, *op.cit.*

those of other "true prevalence" studies of mental illness, showing women with a higher rate of psychiatric disturbance than was the case with men.[53] We believe that these results may be due not to "true" sex differences in frequency of disturbance but rather to a greater *reluctance* on the part of men to admit to or report certain unpleasurable feelings and sensations, a reluctance based on a recognition and awareness of cultural expectations regarding expressive control.

While our findings and interpretations are supportive of the above conclusion, there are obvious gaps in the study. Of most importance with regard to our explanation is the fact that we employed no measure as to what men and women saw as appropriate or desirable behavior for someone of their sexual status. However, there is another study which does begin to deal with this problem. This investigation was conducted by Bruce Dohrenwend[54] and uses the same 22-item index of mental illness which we employed.

Dohrenwend's study was concerned mainly with the influence of social class position and ethnicity on people's mental health status. After finding that with social class held constant Puerto Ricans had a higher rate of mental illness than Jews, Irish, or Negroes in a sample of New York City residents, Dohrenwend asked whether these differences in rates might not reflect culturally patterned differences in the modes of *expressing* distress and/or culturally patterned *willingness* to express distress. He then asked a different group of respondents to rate the items in the psychiatric inventory as to their "social desirability." This rating revealed that on 17 of the 22 items the Puerto Ricans gave a *less* undesirable rating than did the other three groups.[55] Dohrenwend suggested, therefore, that because the Puerto Ricans regarded the characteristics in the screening instruments as less undesirable than did members of the other ethnic groups, they might also be more willing than the other groups to admit to such characteristics. If this were true, then they may actually have a very much lower rate of mental illness than their reported rate of symptoms would suggest.[56]

However, there is another possibility which Dohrenwend suggests. It may be that "the reason Puerto Ricans see these symptoms as strongly undesirable may both indicate the same thing—higher actual rates of disorder."[57] Unfortunately, Dohrenwend's data did not allow him to choose between these alternative hypotheses.

Although Dohrenwend's data did not allow for a choice between these competing hypotheses, a third study did consider these alternatives. Before

53. James A. Davis, *Stipends and Spouses* (Chicago: University of Chicago Press, 1962); Gurin et al., *op. cit.*; Langner and Michael, *op. cit.*; Leighton et al., *op. cit.*; Phillips, 1966, *op. cit.*
54. Dohrenwend, *op. cit.*
55. *Ibid.*
56. *Ibid.*
57. *Ibid.*, p. 24.

discussing this investigation, let us consider further Dohrenwend's two hypotheses regarding the relationship between people's assessments as to the social desirability of the 22 mental health items and their reports of such symptoms. Dohrenwend's first hypothesis suggested that the desirability of the items can vary independently of the prevalence of the symptoms among members of one's own group; that an individual's perceptions of what is or is not desirable can be determined by forces *external* to his traditional reference group of family, friends, or neighbors of similar socioeconomic and cultural background.

The second of Dohrenwend's hypotheses suggested that an individual comes to learn or perceive the desirability or undesirability of a given symptom by observing the *prevalence* of that symptom among people like himself, other people of his ethnic and/or socioeconomic background. He argues that if symptoms are common among one's own status group—in his case, family, friends, and neighbors—then the desirability of the items will be higher than if the symptoms are not common.

This latter interpretation suggests that the social environment of an individual determines his evaluations as to the desirability of given symptoms, and that the most important aspect of this "social environment" is the actual (or perhaps, more properly, the perceived) prevalence of these symptoms among a man's traditional reference group. This may or may not be the case, for this line of reasoning does not account for the efforts of some Negroes to "pass," the striving of the Irish, Negroes, Germans, Italians, Jews, and now, Puerto Ricans, to lose their native "accents," nor for other similar everyday instances where members of a given group seem to consider characteristics highly common within that group to be undesirable.

If we assume for the moment that Dohrenwend is correct and if we assume that both variables relate to an individual's score on a mental health inventory, then we would expect a desirability measure and some measure of the symptom prevalent among the respondent's traditional reference group to be highly correlated and thus to be redundant predictors of an individual's mental health score. Hence, a test of this hypothesis would be to undertake an analysis so as to determine whether people's evaluations as to the social desirability of the items and the prevalence of psychiatric symptoms are, in actual fact, independent or redundant predictors of mental health scores. If Dohrenwend's second hypothesis is supported, then we no longer need to concern ourselves with questions about the desirability bias in terms of the 22-Item Mental Health Inventory.

The third study to be considered here was one I conducted with Kevin Clancy[58] in an attempt to choose between the two hypotheses offered by

58. Kevin J. Clancy and Derek L. Phillips, "Some Sources of Artifact in Social Research: An Examination of the Literature and an Analysis of a Psychiatric Inventory," unpublished manuscript, 1968.

Dohrenwend. We predicted that: (1) people's scores on the 22-item inventory would be related to their assessment as to the desirability of the items; and (2) people's assessments of the desirability of the inventory items would reflect something other than the estimated prevalence of these symptoms within their traditional reference groups. Thus, we expected that people's assessment of the desirability of the items and their estimates as to the prevalence of such symptoms would be independent predictors of mental health scores.

To test these hypotheses, telephone interviews were completed with a sample of 115 adults residing in metropolitan areas of over 1 million population. In this study we were also interested in the extent to which the three variables discussed above—assessment of social desirability, estimated prevalence, and mental health scores—were related to people's social class position.

Our main concern was with trying to choose between Dohrenwend's two hypotheses. If people's assessment as to the desirability of the inventory items were determined solely by their estimates of the prevalence of these symptoms within their reference groups, then their social class positions should exercise no independent effects as to item desirability. If, on the other hand, people's assessments of item desirability were not determined by their estimates as to the prevalence of similar conditions among people they know but rather by their degree of psychiatric sophistication regarding the signs and symptoms of mental illness and the purpose of the inventory, then higher-status persons should view the items as more undesirable than do lower-class persons.

Before reporting the findings concerning the above question, we must note that our first hypothesis—regarding the relationship between people's views about the desirability of the inventory items and the number of symptoms which they report—was supported by the data. The less undesirably people saw the items, the more symptoms they reported. Turning now to our second hypothesis, we found that people's assessments regarding the desirability of the symptom items were independently related to *both* their social class position and their estimates of prevalence among people they know. The higher their social class position and the greater their estimates as to the prevalence of similar symptoms within their reference groups, the larger the number of symptoms reported. Furthermore, the independent effects of these two variables on assessments regarding social desirability were of about equal magnitude.

What this means, then, is that people's views about the desirability or undesirability of the inventory items are, as Dohrenwend suggested, determined partially by their looking around and making a judgment as to how many of their "significant others" show similar characteristics. But people's views with regard to desirability are also influenced by their location in the social class hierarchy. I suggested earlier that these social class differentials are due to a greater awareness on the part of higher-status persons as to both the purpose of psychiatric inventories and the implications of various responses.

Our data allowed us to make another important examination. This concerned the frequently demonstrated inverse relationship between social class position and mental illness. We wanted to determine whether this relationship might be partially accounted for by the above mentioned social class differentials in people's assessments as to the social desirability of the items constituting the 22-Item Mental Health Inventory. Examining the data we found that introducing social desirability into the analysis of the relations between social class and mental health status reduced considerably the magnitude of the relationship. In fact, when the independent effects of social class position and social desirability on people's scores on the mental health inventory were compared, it was found that their assessment of the desirability of the 22 mental health items had a *greater* influence upon their index scores than did their social class position.

Implications

The three studies discussed above raise questions as to the possibility of systematic errors in other investigations utilizing psychiatric interviews in survey research on mental illness. That is, if people's social class position, ethnicity, and sexual status all influence their assessments about the desirability of inventory items, and these assessments of desirability, in turn, affect people's reports about the presence or absence of the symptoms in themselves, then similar errors may operate in other studies concerned with the same variables. Taken together, the three investigations cited here raise questions as to whether women "really" have higher rates of mental illness than do men, whether social class and mental illness do "actually" bear an inverse relationship to one another, and whether Puerto Ricans "really" have higher rates of mental illness than other ethnic groups. My own suspicion is that if we were able, in a sense, to control for the effects of social desirability, the *direction* of the frequently demonstrated relationships concerning mental illness and the three variables of social classs, sex, and ethnicity would be maintained, but the *magnitude* of the relations would be reduced considerably.

The perspective of the above argument is, of course, consistent with the theory of deviance set forth by Becker and others.[59] In this view, deviance is to be seen not just as a quality of the acts a person commits, but rather

59. Howard S. Becker, *Outsiders* (New York: The Free Press, 1963); Kai T. Erikson, "Notes on the Sociology of Deviance," *Social Problems*, 9 (Spring, 1962), 307-314; Kitsuse, *op cit.*; Edwin M. Lemert, *Human Deviance, Social Problems, and Social Control* (Englewood Cliffs, N.J.: Prentice-Hall, 1967); Edwin M. Lemert, *Social Pathology* (New York: McGraw-Hill, 1951); Thomas J. Scheff, *Being Mentally Ill* (Chicago: Aldine, 1966).

as a consequence as well of the way that the public or certain designated "experts" respond to them. I consider that when actors and witnesses are aware of the cultural standards of appropriateness that obtain in and for different status categories, we can expect to find that people will generally be inclined to avoid, and will be capable of not carrying out, such acts as would lead others to respond to them negatively. What this means, as I have emphasized, is that differences in the prevalence of some types of acts defined as deviant, among people who occupy different statuses, reflect differences in the actor's willingness to engage in or make visible certain acts or behaviors.

Of greater concern than the problems of studying mental illness and other types of deviance are the implications of my presentation for social research in general. What I have been arguing is that in all research involving human beings there exist artifact variables. Thus, in social science investigations, variation in the dependent variable may be explained by reference to two sets of variables. One set involves the "independent" variables which our theory leads us to hypothesize as being related (in a certain direction or of a certain magnitude) to the dependent variable. The second set consists of "artifact" variables which are related to the dependent variables (and perhaps to the independent variables as well), and arise as part of normal interpersonal relations.

The most important question concerning these artifact variables is *how much* effect they have. Are these artifact variables only a source of minor annoyance or are they a major source of contamination in our research? This is, of course, an empirical question, and its answer undoubtedly differs from one research situation or activity to another. It seems, though, that most social researchers have tended to minimize the importance of these artifacts. This is perhaps understandable, though unfortunate. For I think that the burden of proof should be on showing that these artifacts *are not* seriously affecting our results and conclusions. This means, as I remarked earlier in the paper, that our first task should be to identify these undesired sources of influence. I have listed many of them throughout the paper, and there are undoubtedly others yet to be discovered.

Identifying these artifacts is only one task to be considered. But there is obviously another question to be posed. Is it possible to develop artifact-free measures? I think that the answer to this query is a clear and resounding *no.* As long as we gather our data through field-research methods (interviewing and participant observation), the presence of an investigator or interviewer will always influence the results to some extent. This is, of course, because the same social processes involved in other encounters are bound to occur in field research.[60] A discussion of these processes is provided by Goffman:

60. The problems cited with regard to the use of interviews in survey research concerned with mental illness exist also in the clinical situation. Psychiatrists' clinical

Underlying all social interaction there seems to be a fundamental dialectic. When one individual enters the presence of others, he will want to discover the facts of the situation. Were he to possess this information, he could know, and make allowances for, what will come to happen and he could give the others present as much of their due as is consistent with his enlightened self-interest . . . . Full information of this order is rarely available; in its absence, the individual tends to employ substitutes—cues, tests, hints, expressive gestures, status symbols, etc.—as predictive devices. In short, since the reality that the individual is concerned with is unpredictable at the moment, appearances must be relied upon in its stead.[61]

Schutz made a similar point when he stated: "we take the position that the social sciences have to deal with human conduct and its commonsense interpretation in the social reality, involving the analysis of the whole system of projects, and motives of relevances and constructs."[62] He then went on to say that "such an analysis refers by necessity to the subjective point of view, namely, to the interpretation of the action and its settings in terms of the actor."[63]

One thing we seem to need in sociological research, then, is a model of the actor. And this model must provide us with some principles of social interaction that will guide us in conducting our research. As Cicourel puts it: "If it is correct to assume that persons in everyday life order their environment, assign meanings or relevances to subjects, base their social actions on their common-sense rationalities, then one cannot engage in field research or use any other method of research in the social sciences without taking the principle of subjective interpretation into consideration."[64]

A model of the actor with some principles of subjective interpretation is a clear need in sociological research. Another need is further research in what might be termed "the social psychology of social research." For in-

---

judgments as to the presence or absence of symptoms, their views of the severity of such symptoms, and their placement of individuals in various diagnostic categories are all based largely on what people say (or admit to, or report) and on how they comport themselves. Here too, then, the individual frequently asks himself: "What is expected of someone like me in this situation?" His concern with the appropriate behavior for someone occupying his status continues, of course, throughout his "career" as a mental patient. See, for instance, Ernest Becker, "Socialization, Command of Performance, and Mental Illness," *American Journal of Sociology*, 67 (1962), 494-501; Erving Goffman, "The Moral Career of the Mental Patient," *Psychiatry*, 22 (1959), 125-131.

Thus, understanding what the field interview situation means to various types of people also has implications for what goes on in the clinician's office and on the wards of hospitals for the mentally ill. See Ken Kesey, *One Flew Over the Cuckoo's Nest* (New York: Signet Books, 1962).

61. Erving Goffman, *The Presentation of Self in Everyday Life* (New York: Doubleday Anchor, 1959), p. 249.

62. Alfred Schutz, "Common-Sense and Scientific Interpretations of Human Action," *Philosophy and Phenomenological Research*, 14 (1953), 27.

63. *Ibid.*

64. Cicourel, *op. cit.*, p. 61.

stance, we should have more investigations as to the meaning of the interview situation for the respondent. An example of regarding people's expectancies, or "evaluation apprehensions" as Rosenberg[65] calls them, concerns the meaning of an experimental situation. An extension would be research to determine the meaning of various research situations for different groups—social classes, ethnic groups, etc. The importance of such research was suggested almost 30 years ago by C. Wright Mills:

> Perhaps the central methodological problem in the social sciences springs from recognition that often there is a disparity between lingual and social-motor types of behavior. . . . [Systematic investigations] should enable the methodologist to build into his methods standard margins of error, different rates of discount for different *milieux*. They would show (for various cultural actions, types of subjects, and various modes of verbalization) how much and *in what direction* disparities between talk and action will probably go. In this way factual investigation should provide a basis for rules for the control and guidance of evidence and inference.[66]

It is about time that we considered Mills' suggestion seriously. For we cannot engage in meaningful research until we have a better understanding of what the research situation means to different kinds of people. Thus, in our research activities, as in other social situations which we study, we should be concerned with social action as defined by Max Weber as consisting of "all human behavior when and insofar as the acting individual attaches a subjective meaning to it. . . and takes account of the behaviors of others and is thereby oriented in its course."[67]

---

65. Rosenberg, *op. cit.*

66. C. Wright Mills, "Methodological Consequences of the Sociology of Knowledge," *American Sociological Review*, 64 (December, 1940), 320.

67. Max Weber, *The Theory of Social and Economic Organization*, A. M. Henderson and Talcott Parsons, trans. (New York: Oxford University Press, 1947), p. 88.

Name Index

473

Subject Index

Printed in the United States
205939BV00003B/1-51/P

9 780202 362083